A Practical Guide to Point of Care Ultrasound (POCUS)

Arunangshu Chakraborty
Balakrishnan Ashokka
Editors

A Practical Guide to Point of Care Ultrasound (POCUS)

Springer

Editors
Arunangshu Chakraborty
Department of Anaesthesia
Critical Care and Pain, Tata
Medical Center
Newtown, Kolkata, West Bengal, India

Balakrishnan Ashokka
Department of Anaesthesia
National University Hospital
Singapore, Singapore

ISBN 978-981-16-7686-4 ISBN 978-981-16-7687-1 (eBook)
https://doi.org/10.1007/978-981-16-7687-1

This Springer imprint is published by the registered company Springer Nature Singapore Pte Ltd.
The registered company address is: 152 Beach Road, #21-01/04 Gateway East, Singapore 189721, Singapore

I dedicate this work to my better half Ananya, for her unrelenting support and our children, Anwesh and Agniv for being my inspiration.

Arunangshu Chakraborty

I dedicate this academic journey to 'Tanvi Ashokka', my tween twinkle, for helping me 'Focus' on that matters beyond the 'POCUS'.

Balakrishnan Ashokka

Foreword

Although the concept of ultrasound is over 200 years old, the history of using ultrasound as a medical diagnostic tool began only about 70 years ago. Soon, the principle was also found to be an excellent tool for viewing the heart, and echocardiography was born. Strictly being in the radiologists' domain for the first 50 years, it caught the attention of the intensivists and the emergency physicians. They found ultrasound to be an excellent tool for inexpensive, non-invasive and bedside imaging. They started using it for even hitherto uncharted areas like lung ultrasonography. These physicians were not trained radiologists, but they needed this valuable imaging tool throughout the day. So, a term point-of-care ultrasonography was born. It was the use of the ultrasound machine to answer some specific questions and assist in some specific procedures, especially needed in critical care. We are already seeing the future when an ultrasound transducer attached to our smartphone will replace the stethoscope for the emergency and critical care physicians.

With this background my former colleague Dr. Arunangshu Chakraborty along with Dr Ashokka Balakrishnan has written this excellent book on point-of-care ultrasound. The book is meant for the critical care physician, the emergency physician and the anaesthesiologist. These physicians will find it to be comprehensive, yet handy. The book addresses all aspects of critical care ultrasonography and transthoracic echocardiography, including its use in the diagnostics and the common bedside procedures. The authors also provide excellent illustrations to explain the salient points. Each chapter ends with a set of self-assessment questions. It also comes with some high-quality videos as an additional feature. This book will teach the beginner and stay with the regular user of point-of-care ultrasonography as a quick reference. I foresee a wide acceptance of this book among the critical care physicians.

Department of Critical Care
AMRI Hospitals
Kolkata, West Bengal, India

Susruta Bandyopadhyay

Preface

Point-of-care ultrasound (POCUS) is defined as a goal-directed, bedside ultrasound examination performed by a healthcare provider to answer a specific diagnostic question or to guide the performance of an invasive procedure. The field of POCUS is vast and the scope is infinite, so much so that it is difficult to cover all of them in a single volume. What we wanted was to present a clear and concise description of the most common day-to-day uses of point-of-care ultrasound (POCUS) in a pocket-sized manual for the residents and trainees of the multifaceted disciplines of anaesthesia, intensive care and emergency medicine. This book is more focused on the practical applications than theoretical discussions. Although ultrasound-guided regional anaesthesia (USRA) has been included in some of the POCUS textbooks, we have not included it in this book as we believe that USRA is a larger topic and deserves its own textbook. There are many indeed, including our primer *Blockmate—A Practical Guide to Ultrasound Guided Regional Anaesthesia* by Springer Nature.

Currently, there is a shortage of textbooks in the field, and few cover all the necessary areas that are needed for the learners in the aforementioned disciplines. Each chapter in this book has been written by authors who are active practitioners of POCUS in their respective fields, and therefore tackles the practical issues comprehensively and they also host training sessions and workshops teaching these principles. The chapters contain multiple choice questions for the learners to hone their knowledge and prepare for the examinations.

A special feature of this book is the wonderfully curated video library, created by Dr. Amit Dikshit and Dr. Sudhakar Subramani. Readers of *A Practical Guide to Point of Care Ultrasound* will have access to these videos through the book. These step-by-step approaches demonstrated in the videos will enable the reader, who may be even a novice to the field, to be able to start practising POCUS on his own.

POCUS is going to be one of the most sought-after areas in medicine in the coming decades. This book will be useful for the learners in anaesthesia, critical care, emergency medicine and trauma as well as the clinical specialists who did not have POCUS in their curriculum but want to pick up foundations in knowledge, contemporaneous technical skills, to keep abreast with the modern-day nuances of medical practice.

Kolkata, West Bengal, India — Arunangshu Chakraborty
Singapore, Singapore — Balakrishnan Ashokka

Contents

Basics of Point-of-Care Ultrasound

1

Arunangshu Chakraborty
and Balakrishnan Ashokka

1.1 Basics of Ultrasound: Physics and Physiology

Sound waves are waves of compression and rarefaction in a medium such as air. For propagation of sound, the most important factors are its frequency, wavelength, and the qualities of the medium it travels through.

Only a part of the sound waves present in nature is audible to human ears, which is known as the **hearing range**. Human hearing range is between 20 and20,000 Hz, although individual capabilities may vary. Any sound which has a frequency lower than 20 Hz is not audible to most humans and known as infrasound. On the other hand, sound of frequency greater than 20,000 Hz is also inaudible to human ears and known as **ultrasound**. In the animal kingdom, animals such as elephants can generate and hear the infrasound that allows them to communicate over a long distance, whereas bats and dolphins can generate and receive ultrasound which endows them survival edge in navigation and spatial orientation.

Ultrasound has steadily gained importance and popularity in medical imaging since its introduction in the early 1960s [1]. It has evolved rapidly through scientific discoveries and advancement in computing. When ultrasound was used for the first time in regional anesthesia in the 1990s, the ultrasound output was a chart of dots. Now it provides a real-time image which is easily relatable to the anatomy. Ultrasound is safer compared to ionizing radiation and it is portable. The side effects of clinical ultrasound are negligible. The use of ultrasound by anesthesiologists for the purpose of interventions such as vascular cannulations and regional anesthesia has made those techniques safer and more reliable compared to landmark-based techniques [2, 3].

1.1.1 Mechanism of Action

Ultrasound is created by the piezoelectric effect (PE) converting electrical energy into mechanical vibrations (Fig. 1.1). The word piezo is derived from the Greek word "piezein," meaning "to press." It was discovered by Pierre Curie in 1880 in quartz crystals.

When a varying voltage is applied, the PE material starts to vibrate, with the frequency of the voltage determining the frequency of the sound waves produced. When placed in contact with skin via an "acoustic coupling" jelly, the "transducer" (commonly called "probe") transmits and receives the ultrasound beam.

A. Chakraborty (✉)
Department of Anaesthesia, Critical Care and Pain, Tata Medical Center, Newtown, Kolkata, West Bengal, India

B. Ashokka
Centre for Medical Education (CenMED), National University Health System, Singapore, Singapore

A. Chakraborty, B. Ashokka (eds.), *A Practical Guide to Point of Care Ultrasound (POCUS)*,
https://doi.org/10.1007/978-981-16-7687-1_1

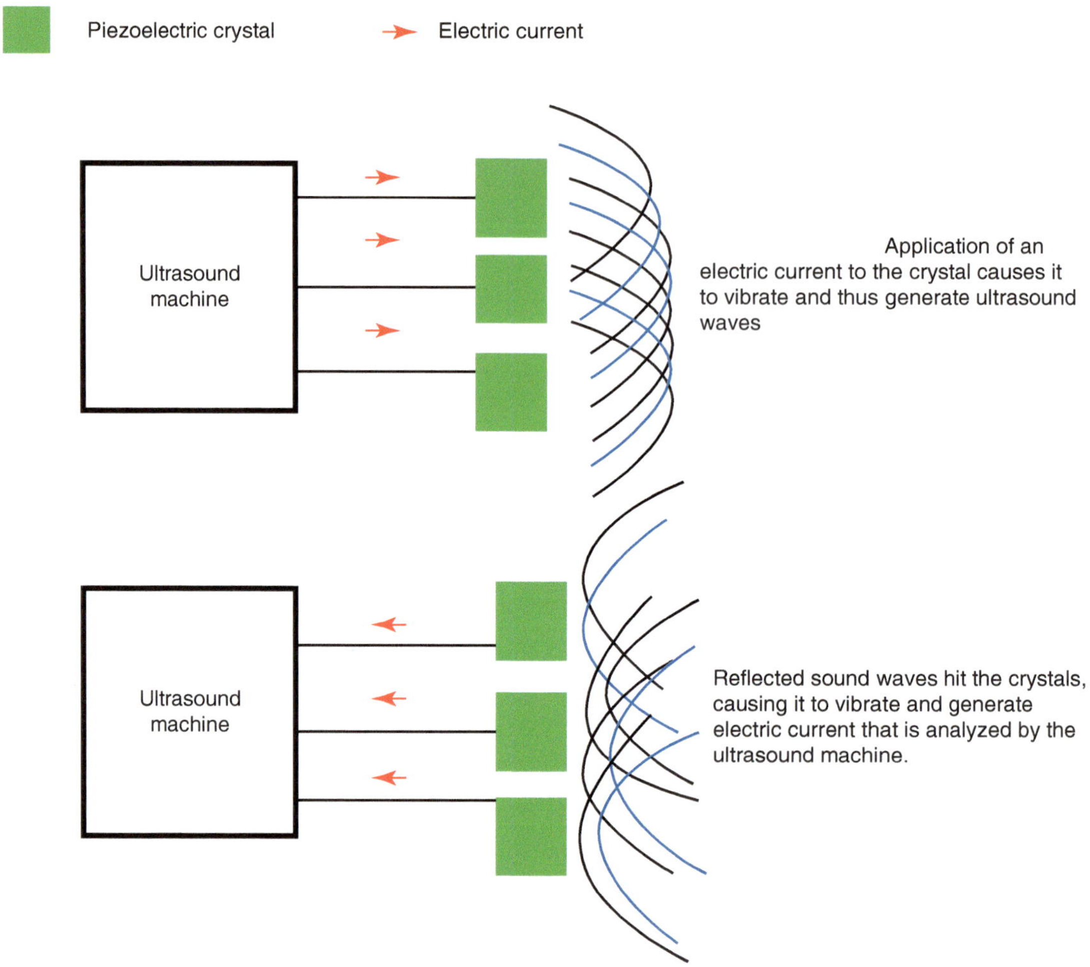

Fig. 1.1 Ultrasound created by piezoelectric effect converting electrical energy into mechanical vibrations

The pulse wave that is generated at the transducer is transmitted into the body of the subject, reflected off the tissue interface, and returned to the transducer again. These returning ultrasound waves cause the PE elements to vibrate within the transducer which causes a voltage to be generated. Thus, the same crystals are used to send and receive ultrasound waves. An image is created out of the returning signal.

With advancements in digital signal processing and software tools, the ultrasound image has evolved from a grayscale chart to a 3D image over the last four decades.

Key Concepts [4–6]

1. **Acoustic velocity (c)** is the speed at which sound waves travel through a medium. It is directly proportional to the density and stiffness of the medium
   - The velocity is fastest in solids and slowest in air.

   The average speed of propagation of ultrasound in body tissue is about 1540 m/s.

2. **Acoustic Impedance** is the product of the sound velocity and tissue density. The difference in acoustic impedance between two tissues influences the amplitude of the returning echo.
3. **Resolution** is the ability to distinguish between two structures that are positioned close to each other.

   Resolution depends on the frequency of ultrasound. Wavelength of the ultrasound beam is inversely proportional to the frequency. Smaller the wavelength, the better is the resolution. Thus, higher frequency gives better resolution.

   Resolution can be classified as spatial and temporal.

Spatial Resolution: It is the ability of ultrasound to distinguish between two objects lying side by side. It can be of two types, axial and lateral.

- *Axial Resolution:* This is the ability to separately discern two structures lying along the ultrasound beam axis as separate and distinct. Affected by the frequency of the beam (Fig. 1.2). For example, when an abdominal wall is imaged, the ultrasound beam traverses the skin, subcutaneous tissue, and the abdominal wall muscles with their fasciae, peritoneum, and abdominal contents depending on the depth setting. A good resolution allows us to distinguish between each of these structures separately.
- *Lateral Resolution:* It is the ability to distinguish between structures lying perpendicular to beam axis, i.e., structures lying side by side. It is affected by the beam width. For example, when the ultrasound scan is done for an axillary block, the ultrasound beam has to clearly distinguish between the axillary artery, axillary veins, the median, radial, and ulnar nerves as well as the muscle layer and fasciae (Fig. 1.3).

Temporal Resolution: The word temporal is derived from the Latin root "tempus" which means time. Temporal resolution is the ability to precisely locate moving structures at given time instants. This has an important role in cardiological imaging. It depends on the processing speed and refresh rate of the ultrasound machine.

1.1.1.1 Interactions of Ultrasound with Tissue

The ultrasound wave is subjected to a number of interactions as it travels through a medium. They are (Fig. 1.4)

- Reflection.
- Transmission.
- Attenuation.
- Scattering.

1.1.2 Reflection

Reflection is the phenomenon in which a part of the energy is sent back to the medium from which the energy originates (Fig. 1.5).

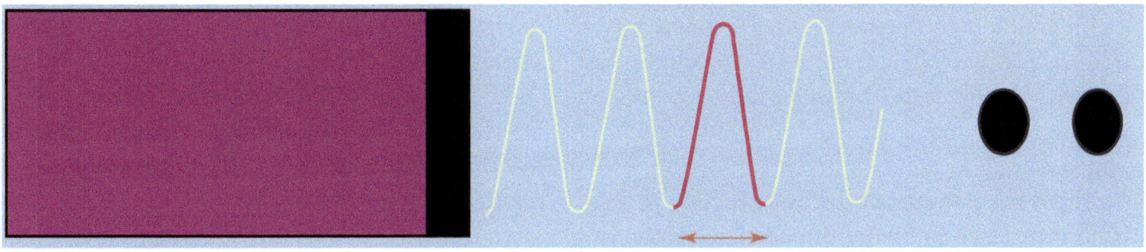

Fig. 1.2 Axial resolution

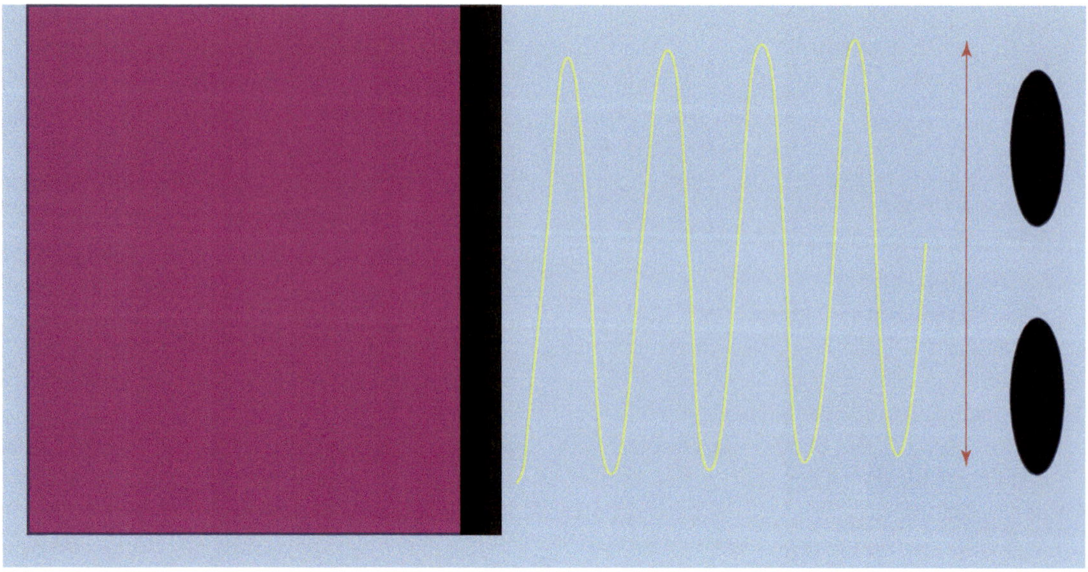

Fig. 1.3 Lateral resolution

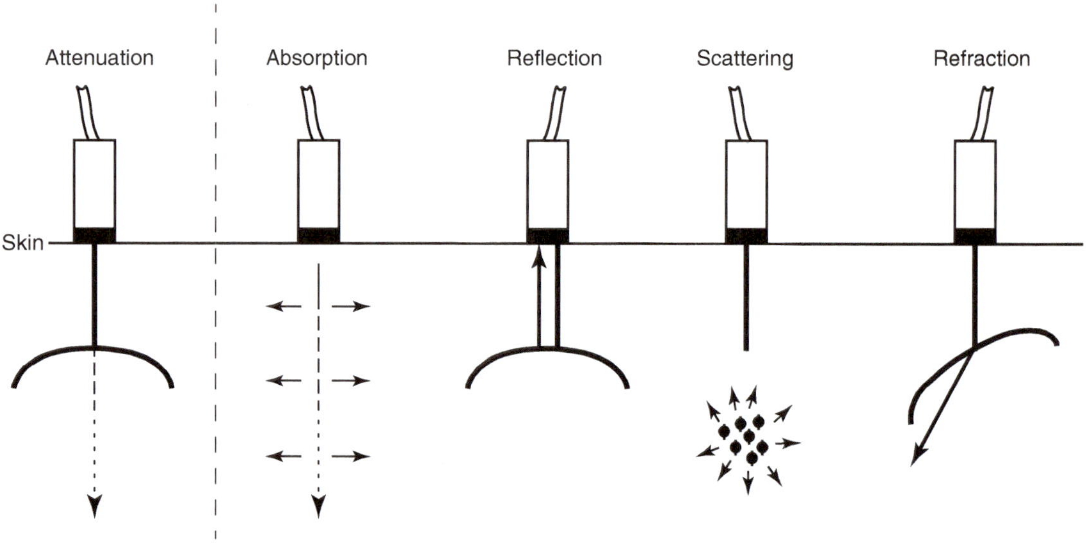

Fig. 1.4 Interaction of ultrasound with tissue

Like all electromagnetic waves, sound waves also exhibit the phenomenon of reflection. The amount of reflection from a surface depends on the angle of incidence and the difference in impedances between two media.

There is an absence of echo/reflection if there is no difference in media impedances. However, in an interface between lung or bone and soft tissues, there is a significant difference between the media impedances which results in creation of strong echoes.

Ultrasound is almost totally reflected at the interface between tissue/liquid and air, producing the brightest echo. E.g., the echo produced by pleura in a normal lung.

Refraction is the change of direction of sound while crossing the interface between two media. The radiological significance of this phenomenon

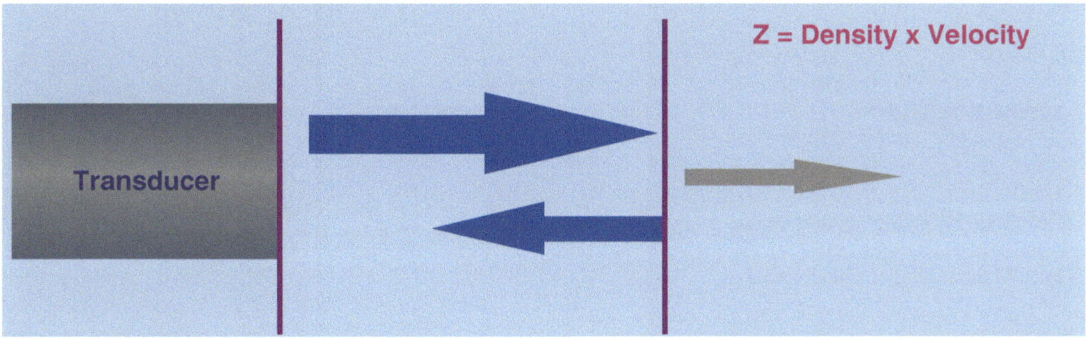

Fig. 1.5 Reflection

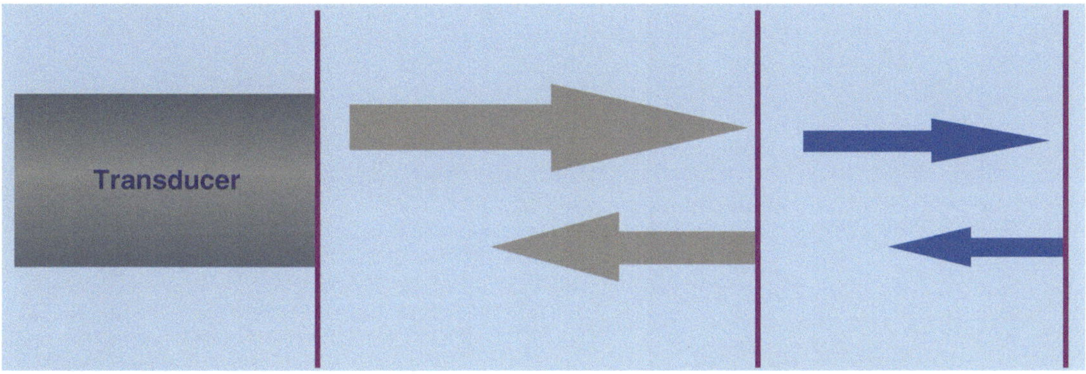

Fig. 1.6 Transmission of waves

is the creation of artifacts such as those seen under larger vessels on USG.

1.1.3 Transmission

Not all waves are reflected when passing through dissimilar media, some are transmitted (Fig. 1.6). The transmitted waves generally produce weaker echo therefore with increasing depth the amplitude and resolution of ultrasound weaken.

1.1.4 Attenuation

The amplitude of the sound waves decreases with increasing depth of penetration in the body. This is known as attenuation. It happens due to loss of the sound energy. Lost energy is absorbed by the medium producing heat. The loss of energy, and thus attenuation is directly related to the frequency of the ultrasound beam.

Thus, greater the frequency, more the attenuation, and lesser is the penetration of the ultrasound wave.

Attenuation coefficient is a measure of attenuation caused by each tissue as a function of the ultrasound wave frequency. The practical aspect of this, for example, is that tissues such as bones have a high attenuation coefficient which greatly limits the transmission of the ultrasound beam. Also, this means penetration shall decrease with increasing frequency.

Scattering: This is the redirection of sound waves in different directions caused due to interaction with a rough surface or small reflector (Fig. 1.7).

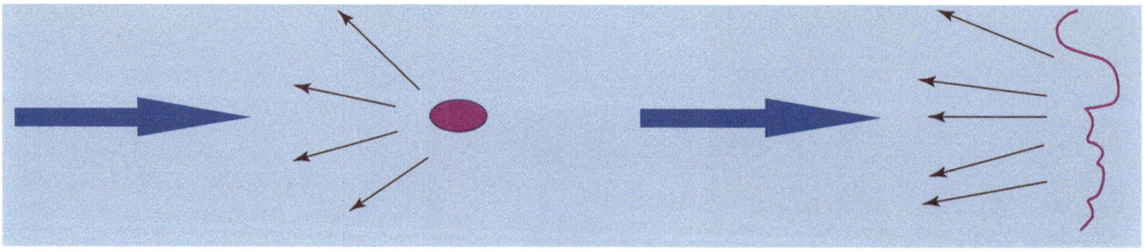

Fig. 1.7 Scattering of sound waves

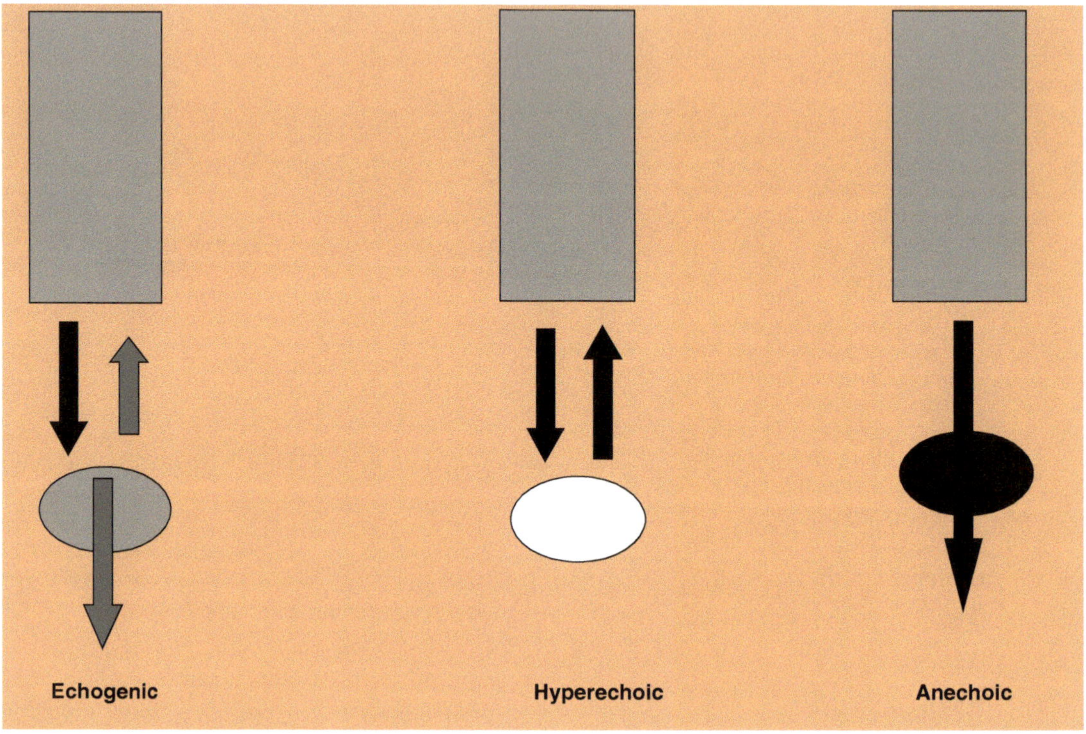

Fig. 1.8 Basis of echogenicity

1.1.5 Echogenicity

The ultrasound waves reflected by tissues return to the transducer to produce image. This phenomenon is similar to echoes that we hear in an empty hall. The property of tissues to generate echo is called echogenicity (Figs. 1.8 and 1.9).

The tissue which produces a similar echo to its surrounding tissue is called isoechoic, the tissue that causes lesser echo hypoechoic, e.g., muscles; the tissue that causes more echo is called hyperechoic, e.g., fascia, bones, pleura; the tissue that produces minimal or no echo is called anechoic, e.g., liquid filled cavity such as blood vessels and pleural effusion.

1.1.5.1 Modes of Imaging

Although medical ultrasound began with A-mode, gradually more and more complex modes have been added. The mode most commonly used in regional anesthesia practice is B-mode, which is also known as 2D ultrasound. Table 1.1 summarizes different modes of ultrasound in medical imaging.

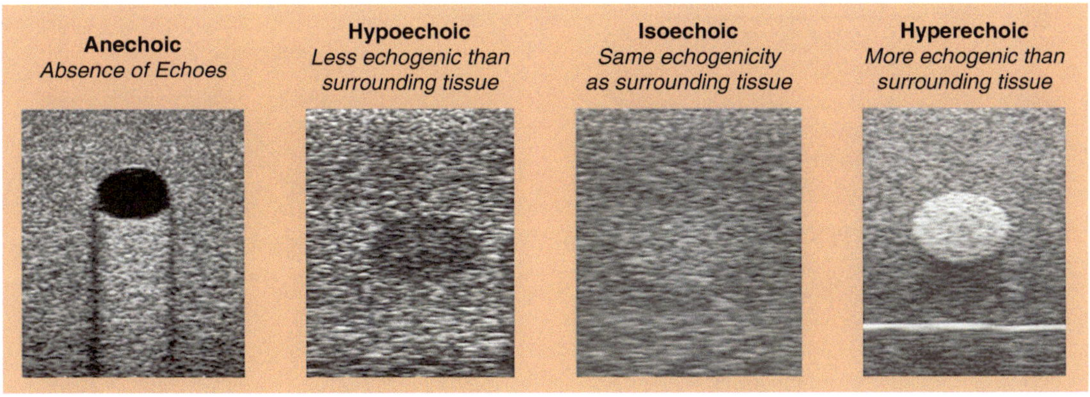

Fig. 1.9 Basis of echogenicity—anechoic, hypoechoic, isoechoic, and hyperechoic tissues

Table 1.1 Modes of imaging

A-Mode	This is the most basic mode and works by displaying the reflected sound pulses on a time axis from a single line scan. This mode is not of much use in clinical anesthesia
B-Mode	This is a 2D version of the A-mode and the most popularly used mode in anesthesia. On passing through a slice of tissue, the reflected ultrasound beam is displayed which depicts the anatomical cross section
M-Mode	This mode can detect the movement of reflecting media along a single line scan. Often used along with the B-mode, this mode is popularly used in cardiological imaging to visualize heart valve movement
Doppler Mode	This mode is based on the doppler effect which is described by a change in the frequency of sound due to the relative motion between the source and receiver of sound. In this mode, the reflected sound waves, when ultrasonic waves are beamed along an artery or vein, have a doppler change in frequency due to the motion of blood
Colour Doppler	This provides a color coded image of doppler shifts. The direction of blood flow depends on the direction of motion towards or away from the transducer. By convention, red and blue colors are selected for the identification of direction and velocity of blood
Power Doppler	Nearly five times more sensitive than color doppler and is used to scan smaller vessels more accurately. This mode however does not provide any information on the speed and direction of flow

1.1.5.2 Transducers

The ultrasound transducer, commonly called "probe" is the part held by the operator's hand that comes in contact with the patient. It is a vital part of the machine as it contains the PE crystals that emit and receive ultrasound. Transducers come in various sizes and shapes. The shape of a probe governs the field of vision while the frequency of sound waves emitted governs the image resolution and depth of penetration (Fig. 1.10).

The linear probe emits a linear array of ultrasound and produces a rectangular image. It is usually of high frequency and low penetration. The higher frequency gives the linear probe better image resolution and is favored for superficial interventions where high accuracy is required.

The curvilinear probe emits a curved array of ultrasound beams and produces a curved image. It has a lower frequency but a wider area of imaging and greater depth. Due to low frequency, the image resolution is grainy and inferior compared to a linear probe. However, for deeper blocks, imaging and interventions it is the transducer of choice.

1.1.5.3 Time Gain Compensation

This is an operator-controlled amplification technique to make up for the sound attenuation as ultrasound waves travel through tissue. It must be manually adjusted for each tissue type to be scanned and manipulated for best image optimization.

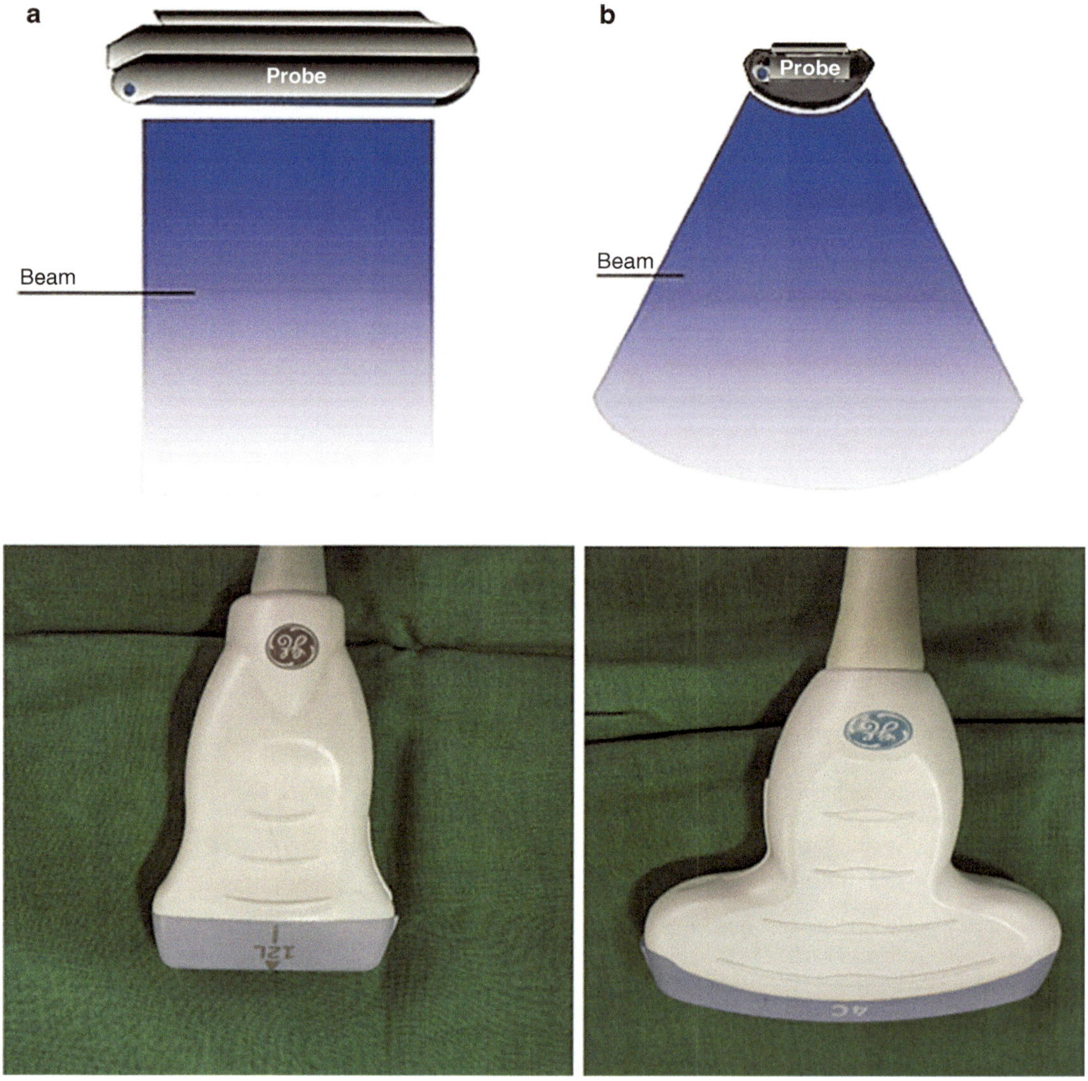

Fig. 1.10 (**a**) Linear and (**b**) Curvilinear transducers and their ultrasound beam pattern

The TGC control layout differs from one machine to another. The presence of slider knobs is a popular design; each knob in the slider set controls the gain for a specific depth, which gives a well-balanced image (Fig. 1.11). Accordingly, the sliders are called near field TGC and far field TGC.

1.1.5.4 Practical Aspects

The ultimate objective of learning the basics of ultrasound imaging is to be able to obtain an optimal image. For image optimization, the following points should be kept in mind [7–9]:

- Frequency of the transducer.
- Depth adjustment.
- Gain.
- Focus.
- Compound imaging use (Fig. 1.12).

Frequency: Higher frequency is usually selected for superficial interventions that require greater resolution. With decreasing frequency, tissues at greater depth can be imaged, at the cost of resolution (Fig. 1.13).

Depth: Depth of the image has to be adjusted to the depth of the object to be blocked or the depth of the intervention endpoint. The depth selected should be at least a few centimeters more than the

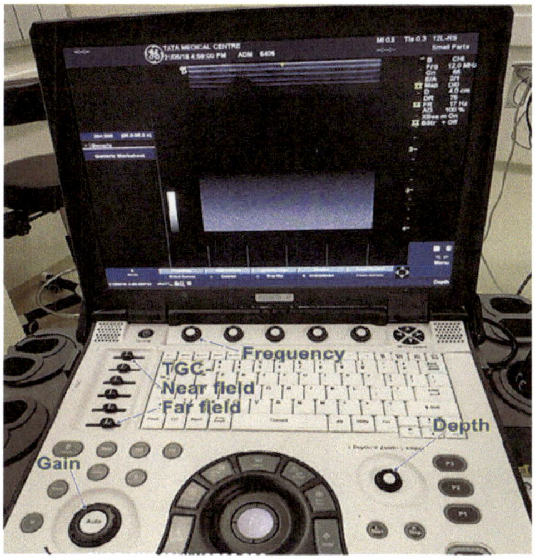

Fig. 1.11 The TGC layout in a standard USG machine

depth of the target. That way, if the needle overshoots the target it can be seen. Also, the nearby anatomical structures would remain visible.

Decreasing the depth increases magnification and vice versa. For superficial blocks, by decreasing the depth setting, greater details can be appreciated.

Gain: The gain function is used to increase overall screen brightness. An optimum gain should be used to obtain the best possible contrast between the muscles and the connective tissue (fascia) for a nerve block because usually the nerves produce echo that is similar to the connective tissue. While TGC controls are used to modify the gain at different depths, overall gain can be adjusted using the gain button (Fig. 1.14).

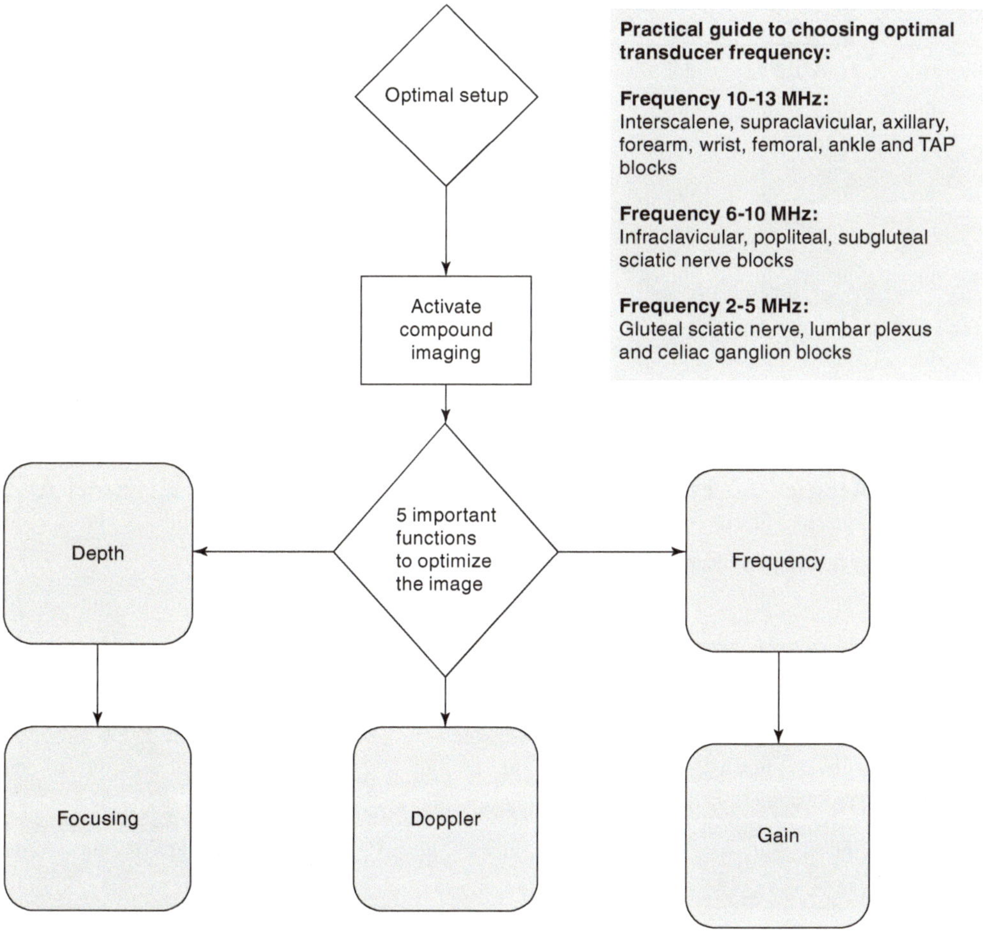
Optimal setup
Activate compound imaging
5 important functions to optimize the image
Depth
Focusing
Doppler
Frequency
Gain
Practical guide to choosing optimal transducer frequency:
Frequency 10-13 MHz:
Interscalene, supraclavicular, axillary, forearm, wrist, femoral, ankle and TAP blocks
Frequency 6-10 MHz:
Infraclavicular, popliteal, subgluteal sciatic nerve blocks
Frequency 2-5 MHz:
Gluteal sciatic nerve, lumbar plexus and celiac ganglion blocks

Fig. 1.12 Algorithm for optimum imaging with ultrasound

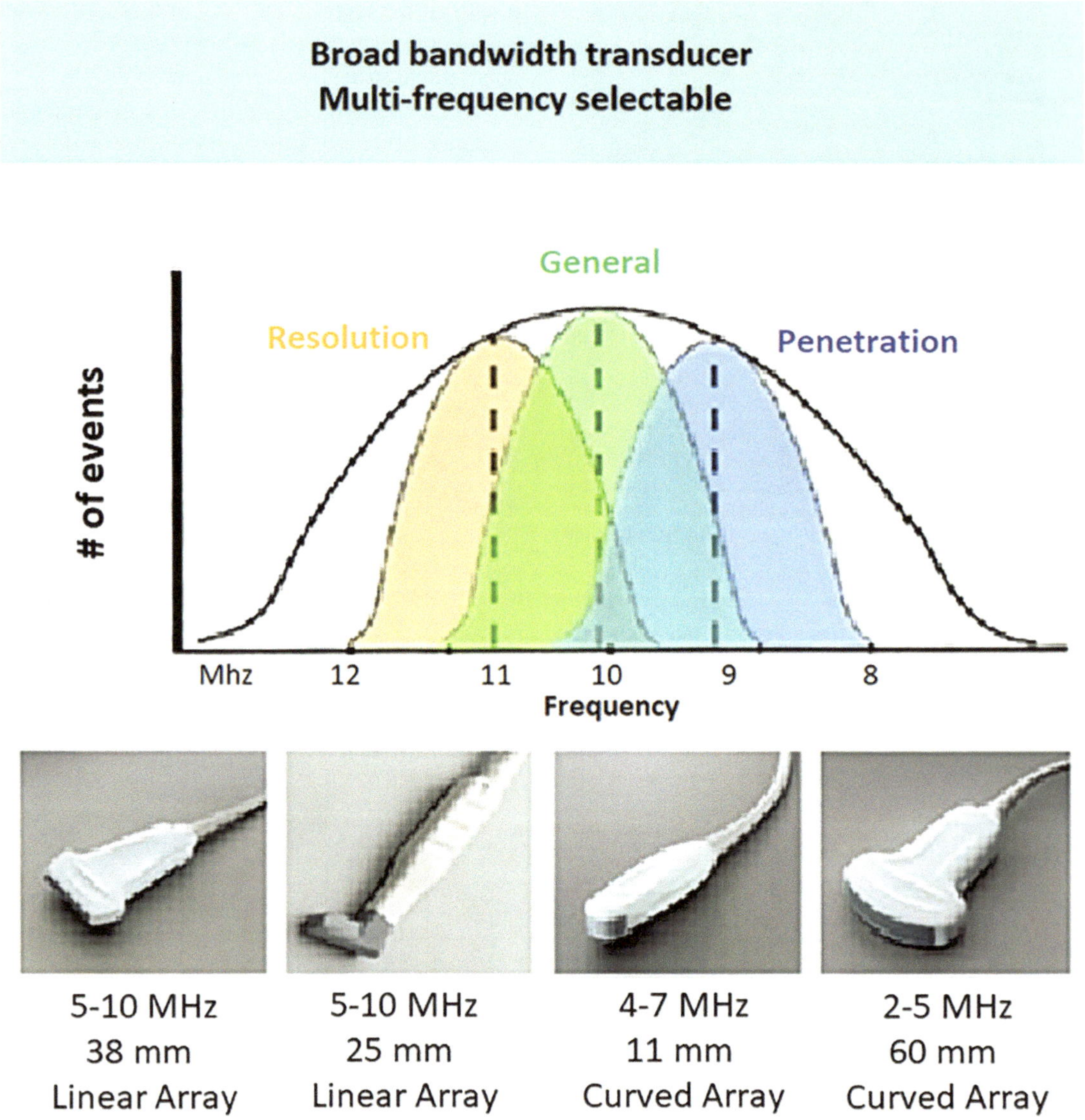

Fig. 1.13 Frequency and transducers

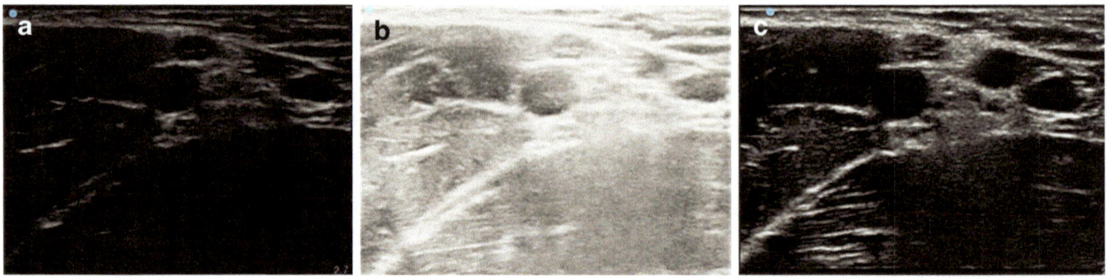

Fig. 1.14 Gain adjustment: Ultrasound scan of the axillary area with gain adjustment: (**a**) low gain, (**b**) high gain, (**c**) optimal gain

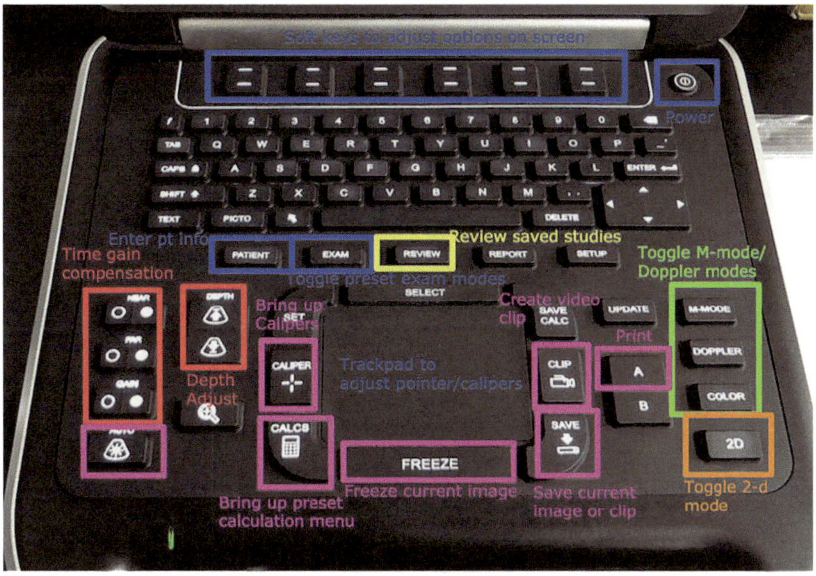

Fig. 1.15 US console showing frequently used functions

Focus: Focus of the ultrasound image is the narrowest point of the ultrasound beam. It is the point where the image resolution is best. Modern ultrasound machines have electronic focus adjustment capacity. It is best to place the focus just at the level of or slightly below the object to be viewed for optimum image quality.

The ultrasound machine **console** (Fig. 1.15) contains the buttons and sliders for modifying all the above factors such as frequency, depth, and focus. One must be well versed with the console to obtain the best image and to be able to store and retrieve images.

Compound Imaging

It is the technology that combines multiple coplanar images (spatial compounding) with images obtained from multiple frequency spectra (frequency compounding) to form a single image. This decreases artifacts and speckles and improves resolution [10] (Fig. 1.16).

Maneuvering the US Probe: PART

Even after optimizing the image setting, an optimal image may not be obtained. For that, the ultrasound probe needs to be held and maneuvered (Fig. 1.17).

Pressure: By putting mild pressure with the probe, subcutaneous fat can be displaced and a better image can be obtained.

Alignment: Proper alignment of the probe in the recommended plane is required to obtain a clinically useful image. E.g., The US probe is held transversely for a TAP block, but sagittally for a SAP block.

Rotation: The probe may need to be slightly rotated to align it perfectly with the underlying tissue and the block needle. E.g., For the supraclavicular brachial plexus block, the probe needs to be slightly externally rotated.

Tilt: Slight cephalad, caudal, lateral, medial, or oblique tilt may be necessary for the optimal image. Because of the direction of the nerve fibers, some nerves seem different at different angles and a little tilt is required to obtain the perpendicular cross section and hence the best image. This property of tissues is called ***anisotropy***. E.g., Caudal tilt is required for imaging the supraclavicular brachial plexus.

Needling Techniques

The Ultrasound beam travels in a straight line, like a thin sheet, perpendicular to the probe. How the intervening needle is visualized depends on how much of its length is in alignment with the ultrasound beam [11, 12].

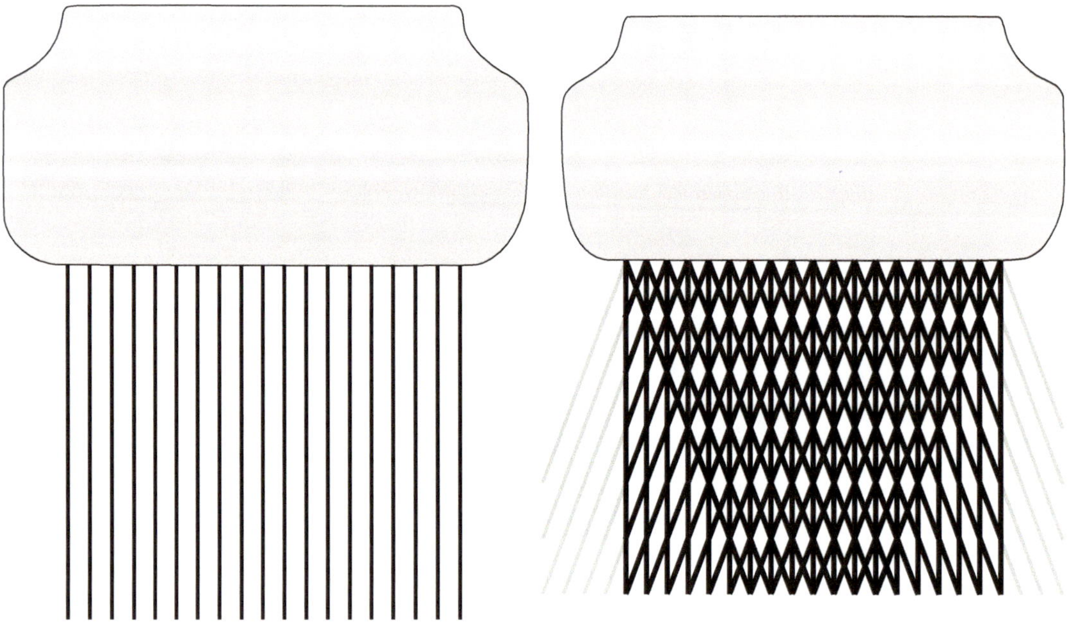

Fig. 1.16 Compound image combines multiple coplanar images with images obtained from multiple frequency spectra to form a single image

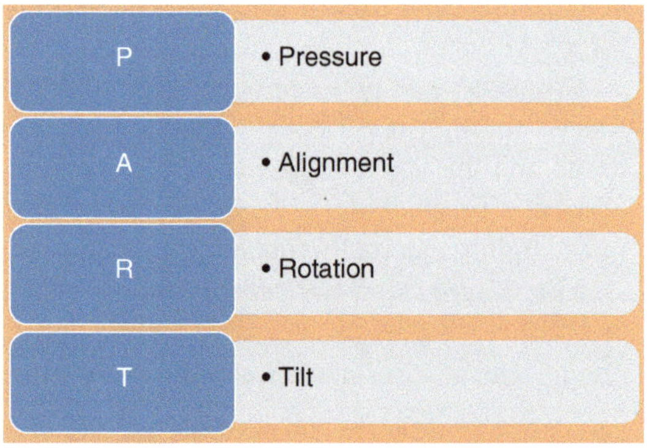

Fig. 1.17 PART maneuver to obtain optimal image

In-Plane

The needle is placed parallel to the transducer. The needle shaft and tip are both visible (Figs. 1.18 and 1.19).

Example: axillary block.

This approach is safe and easy to learn but is difficult to practice in deeper blocks. The quality

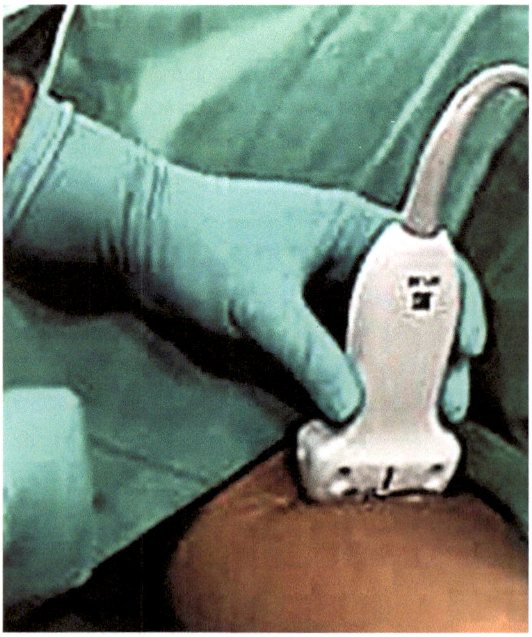

Fig. 1.18 In-plane needling technique

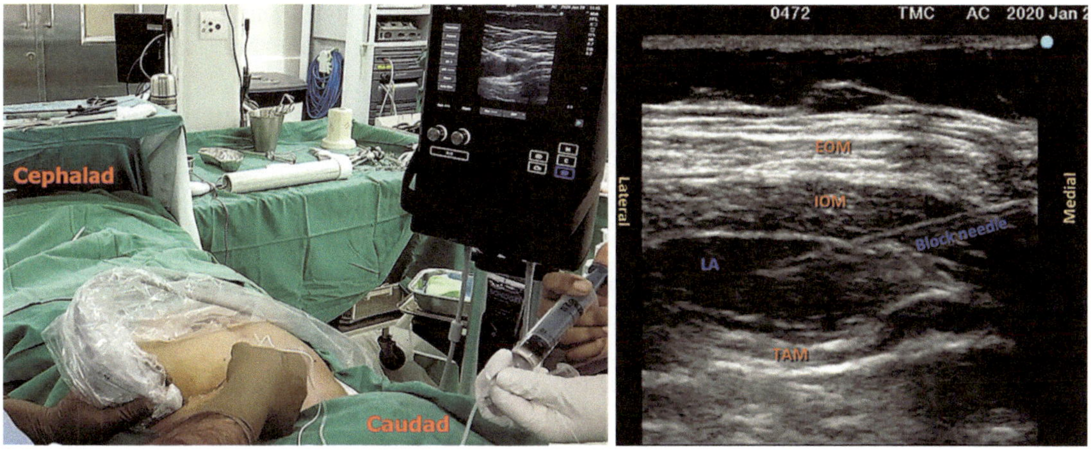

Fig. 1.19 In-plane needling technique. Note that the entire length of the needle and its tip is imaged in real time

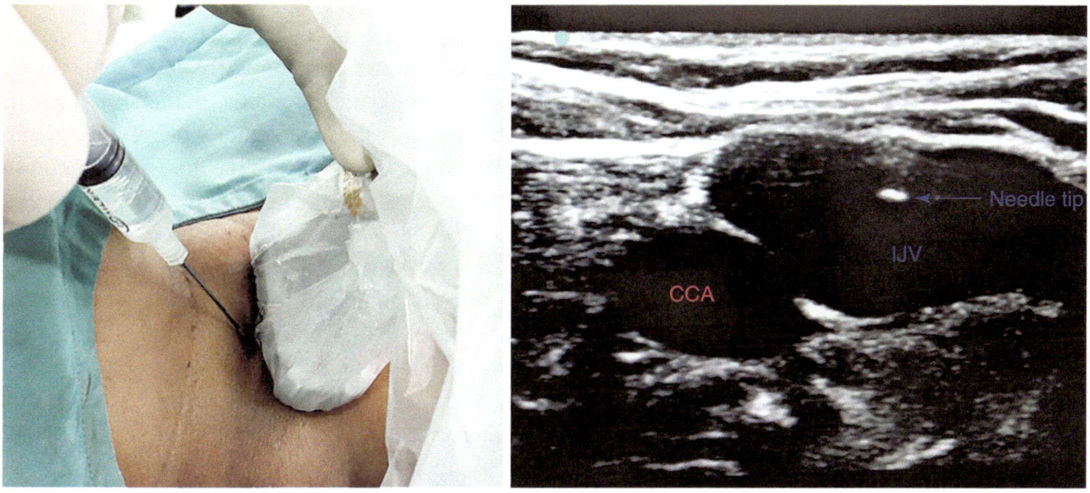

Fig. 1.20 Out of plane cannulation of internal jugular vein (IJV): Left panel shows the probe holding and needle entering out of plane at a right angle to the probe. The ultrasound image on the right shows the sonoanatomy and the tip of the needle being seen as a bright hyperechoic spot. *CCA* common carotid artery lies medial to the IJV

of needle visualization depends on the angle of entry of the needle. ***The flatter the angle (acute angle), the better is the image.*** To reach deeper objects, a more perpendicular angle is required, which makes needle visualization in this technique difficult.

1.1.5.5 Out of Plane

The needle is placed perpendicular to the transducer probe. The tip of the needle may be difficult to locate accurately in this approach and use of echogenic tip needles is advised. ***It is important to observe tissue displacement by the advancing needle tip as often the needle tip may not be seen.***

For superficial procedures such as internal jugular vein cannulation, it is a good strategy to estimate the depth of the target and calculate the entry point of the needle, angle of inclination, and angle of the ultrasound probe accordingly. For deeper structures, hydrodissection with 1–2 ml saline can be used to confirm the location of the needle tip.

Example: Vascular cannulations (Fig. 1.20).

1.1.5.6 Bioeffect and Safety

Ultrasound application produces biologic effects by thermal and nonthermal mechanisms. Heat is generated through absorption of ultrasound by tissues and is directly proportional to ultrasound intensity, frequency, and duration.

Two standard indices are displayed by an ultrasound machine (Fig. 1.21).

Thermal index (TI): It is the transducer acoustic power divided by the estimated power needed to increase tissue temperature by 1°.

Mechanical index (MI): It is the peak rarefactional pressure divided by the square root of the center frequency of the pulse bandwidth. The relative likelihood of thermal and mechanical hazard is indicated by TI and MI, respectively. TI or MI >1.0 is dangerous.

Different tissue and examination settings are saved and categorized in modern ultrasound machines to aid in imaging as well as reducing these bioeffects. For example, the ophthalmic mode is a low power setting that allows examination of the eyes without causing any tissue injury to the sensitive ophthalmic tissues such as the retina.

Artifacts: Artifacts are false images produced due to highly reflective tissue interfaces. There are various types of artifacts, such as comet tail artifacts and mirror image artifacts.

Some of the artifacts are misleading, whereas some are useful. Lung ultrasound artifacts such as A lines and B lines are pathognomonic and useful for the detection of clinical conditions.

These artifacts are described in detail in textbooks of point-of-care ultrasound.

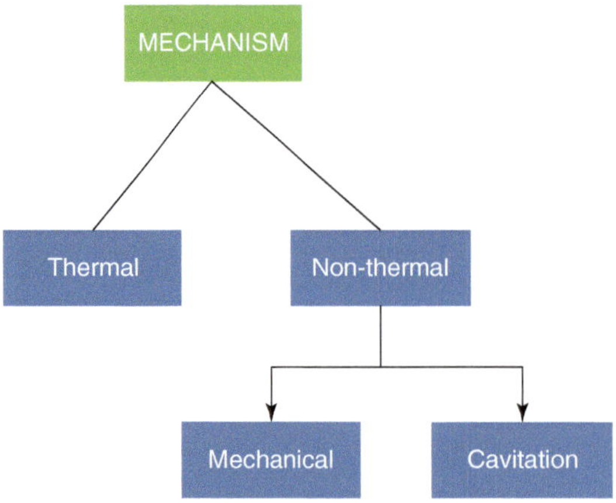

Fig. 1.21 Bioeffect and safety

1.2 Point-of-Care Ultrasound: Concept and Limitations

Like the five elements of nature, the human body is also composed of solid tissue (earth), liquid tissue (water), and gas-filled spaces (air). While imaging with ultrasound, we refer to tissue in terms of "echogenicity" or "echo signature." Water offers least resistance to the passage of ultrasound thereby providing the least echogenicity which is called anechoic. Of all parts in the body, water containing tissues such as blood, pleural fluid, and amniotic fluid have the least echogenicity, the echogenicity being directly proportional to the density of the fluid and it increases if there are suspended particles. Thereby, an exudative pleural fluid will have more echogenicity than a serous fluid. The sludge in the gallbladder can be distinguished from normal bile because of the suspended particles, which reflect ultrasound and produce a higher echogenicity.

Solid tissues reflect ultrasound based on their water content. Thereby, muscles are less echogenic than the adipose tissue and the fibrous septae that separate them. The nerves being solid, with lesser water content than muscle can be identified too, but their echogenicity changes from their origin to the end. Nerves at their origin as nerve roots tend to be less echogenic and appear as hollow circles or "bubbles" in the short axis (SAX) view, but as the roots unite to form divisions and the divisions unite to form nerves, they gather more and more fatty layers of perineural tissue and the nerves appear as "honeycomb" in the SAX view.

Bones are the most dense tissue in the body and they do not allow ultrasound to pass. Therefore, the bones appear hyperechoic due to the reflection of ultrasound by the shiny bony surface and we see an "acoustic shadow" beneath them, like the shadow cast by a solid object under the sun.

Air also does not allow the passage of ultrasound, but the tissue-air interface reflects the ultrasound almost completely, producing the highest hyperechoic image that appears shiny and glistening.

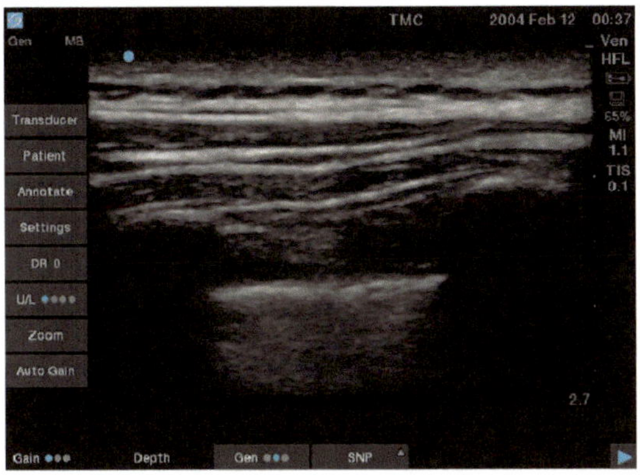

View of ribs and pleura: Note the acoustic shadow cast by the ribs, which are hyperechoic

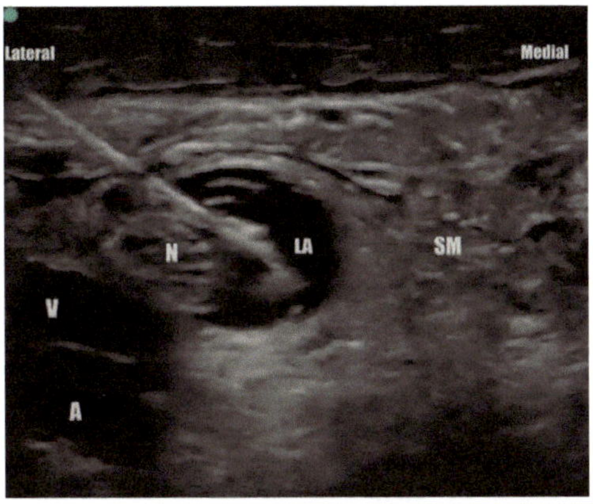

Honeycomb appearance of peripheral nerves, note the anechoic nature of the blood vessels and the injected local anesthetic (LA) in contrast to the nerve and the surrounding tissue

The purpose of Point-of-care ultrasound (POCUS) is not to train the anesthetist, the intensivist, or the emergency physician as a radiologist. POCUS is defined as a goal-directed, bedside ultrasound examination performed by a health care provider to answer a specific diagnostic question or to guide the performance of an invasive procedure. With the specific question in mind, the examination becomes brief and it does not have to bear the level of precision expected from a radiologist. With the training on POCUS, the physician should be able to identify the different tissues and carry out the specific objectives.

Key Concepts

- Knowledge of ultrasound physics is needed for image optimization. The key understandings are
  - Appropriate transducer selection.
  - Gain settings.
  - Depth settings.
  - Tissue echo characteristics.
  - Ultrasound artifacts.
- For optimal imaging, it is important to adjust the *pressure, alignment, rotation, and tilt* (PART) of the probe.
- The best needle image is obtained when the needle forms an acute angle with the ultrasound probe as more US waves reflect off the needle. The steeper the angle, the lesser the needle visibility. The best image is produced by a needle that is parallel to the ultrasound probe, i.e., perpendicular to the ultrasound beam.
- For deeper tissues, it is useful to enter the needle 2–3 cm away from the edge of the ultrasound probe so that a reasonably acute angle can be formed.

Self Assessment Questions

1. In-plane approach uses
   A. Long axis view
   B. Short axis view
   C. Both views can be used
   D. None of the above
2. Echogenicity of blood is known as
   A. Hypoechoic
   B. Hyperechoic
   C. Anechoic
   D. Both A and C
3. Which ultrasound transducer provides better resolution?
   A. High-frequency linear array
   B. Low-frequency curved array
   C. Phased array doppler
   D. All of the above
4. Which of the following tissues appear brightest in an ultrasound image?
   A. Tip of the bones such as spinous process of vertebrae
   B. Bony surface such as pelvic bones
   C. Pleura with an inflated lung underneath
   D. Peripheral nerves
5. Gain is increased to
   A. Increase contrast of the image
   B. Increase resolution of the image
   C. Freeze the image
   D. Increase overall brightness of the image
6. Time gain control (TGC) allows to
   A. Increase or reduce the speed of ultrasound scanning
   B. Increase or reduce the brightness of a particular depth of the scanning area
   C. Increase contrast of the image
   D. Increase gain of the overall image
7. Focus of the ultrasound beam should be set at
   A. At the middle of the image
   B. At the bottom of the image
   C. At or just below the target tissue
   D. Anywhere, it does not matter
8. Which of the following is true?
   A. Lower frequency transducers produce better resolution
   B. Higher frequency transducers have lesser depth of penetration
   C. Frequency and depth of penetration are directly proportional
   D. Image quality does not change with increasing depth of the tissue
9. Which of the following statements is NOT correct?
   A. Axial Resolution is the ability to separately discern two structures lying along the ultrasound beam axis as separate and distinct
   B. Lateral Resolution is the ability to distinguish between structures lying perpendicular to the ultrasound beam axis
   C. Temporal resolution is the ability to precisely locate moving structures at given time instants
   D. Resolution is inversely proportional to the frequency of ultrasound
10. Artifacts are created due to
    A. Reflection
    B. Refraction
    C. Transmission
    D. Attenuation

References

1. Marhofer P, Chan VW. Ultrasound-guided regional anesthesia: current concepts and future trends. Anesth Analg. 2007;104:1265–9.
2. Neal JM, Brull R, Chan VW, Grant SA, Horn JL, Liu SS, et al. The ASRA evidence-based medicine assessment of ultrasound-guided regional anesthesia and pain medicine. Executive summary. Reg Anesth Pain Med. 2010;35:S1–9.
3. Cory PC. Concerns regarding ultrasound-guided regional anesthesia. Anesthesiology. 2009;111:1167–8.
4. Brull R, Macfarlane AJ, Tse CC. Practical knobology for ultrasound-guided regional anesthesia. Reg Anesth Pain Med. 2010;35:S68–73.
5. Merritt CR. Physics of ultrasound. In: Rumack CM, Wilson SR, Charboneau JA, editors. Diagnostic ultrasound. 3rd ed. St. Louis, MO: Elsevier Mosby; 2005.
6. Sites BD, Brull R, Chan VW, Spence BC, Gallagher J, Beach ML, et al. Artifacts and pitfall errors associated with ultrasound-guided regional anesthesia. Part II: a pictorial approach to understanding and avoidance. Reg Anesth Pain Med. 2007;32:419–33.
7. Bigeleisen PE, editor. Ultrasound-guided regional anesthesia and pain medicine. London: Lippincott Williams and Wilkins; 2010.

8. Pollard BA, Chan VW. Introductory curriculum for ultrasound-guided regional anesthesia. Toronto, ON: University of Toronto Press Inc.; 2009.
9. Tsui BC. Atlas of ultrasound and nerve stimulation-guided regional anesthesia. New York: Springer; 2007.
10. Brian DS, Macfarlane AJ, Sites VR, Chan VW, Brull R, et al. Clinical sonopathology for the regional anesthesiologist. Reg Anesth Pain Med. 2010;35:272–89.
11. Maecken T, Zenz M, Grau T. Ultrasound characteristics of needles for regional anesthesia. Reg Anesth Pain Med. 2007;32:440–7.
12. Pollard BA. New model for learning ultrasound-guided needle to target localization. Reg Anesth Pain Med. 2008;33:360–2.

2 Ultrasound-Guided Vascular Cannulation

Arunangshu Chakraborty, Rakhi Khemka, Sudhakar Subramani, and Li Jia Fan

2.1 Introduction

Central venous cannulation was one of the earliest clinical applications of point-of-care ultrasound. It has been widely accepted [1] that using ultrasound for central venous cannulation reduces the number of attempts to cannulate and increases safety by reducing complications such as common carotid artery puncture, trauma to pleura, and the brachial plexus. Meta-analyses of RCTs comparing real-time ultrasound-guided venipuncture of the internal jugular with an anatomical landmark approach report higher first insertion attempt success rates [1–14], higher overall success rates [1–25], lower rates of arterial puncture [2–15, 18, 20], and fewer insertion attempts *(Category A1-B evidence)* [1–25]. RCTs also indicate reduced access time or times to cannulation with ultrasound compared with a landmark approach *(Category A2-B evidence)*. It is considered the Gold standard now to cannulate the internal jugular vein with ultrasound guidance.

A. Chakraborty (✉)
Department of Anaesthesia, Critical Care and Pain, Tata Medical Center, Newtown, Kolkata, West Bengal, India

R. Khemka
Tata Medical Center, Kolkata, West Bengal, India

S. Subramani
Department of Anesthesia, University of Iowa, Iowa City, IA, USA

L. J. Fan
Division of Critical Care, Department of Paediatrics, Khoo Teck Puat—National University Children's Medical Institute, National University Hospital, Singapore, Singapore

2.2 Principle of Vascular Cannulation

2.2.1 Identification of the Blood Vessel

The blood vessels are clearly distinguishable from the surrounding tissue due to their hyperechoic wall and hypoechoic content (blood). The posterior wall of the blood vessel and the tissue directly underneath often display a typical enhancement artifact. The smaller blood vessels such as the radial artery when thrombosed may sometimes look similar to a tendon or a nerve under ultrasound. It is useful to scan both up and downstream to identify the blood vessel by identification of the continuity of the image pattern.

The hallmark of a vein is its collapsibility under pressure of the ultrasound transducer (UST). While it is useful in identifying the veins, it must be kept in mind that-

A sufficient pressure will obliterate even the arteries.

While performing the cannulation the pressure from the UST must be carefully kept to the minimum to facilitate the procedure.

A. Chakraborty, B. Ashokka (eds.), *A Practical Guide to Point of Care Ultrasound (POCUS)*,
https://doi.org/10.1007/978-981-16-7687-1_2

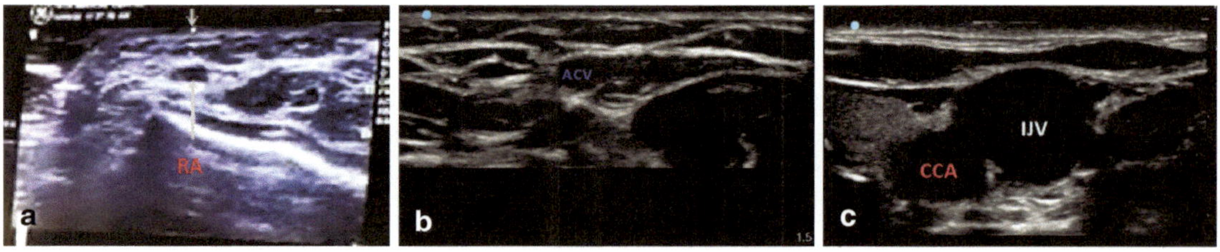

Fig. 2.1 Blood vessels: (**a**) Radial artery, (**b**) Cubital vein, (**c**) Internal jugular vein and common carotid artery

One should also remember some practical but commonly overlooked aspects such as position of the blood pressure (BP) cuff and its state of inflation at the time of an arterial access. Often after induction of anesthesia when the BP is low, or in general in a hypotensive patient, arterial cannulation is a challenge. In such patients, it is important to remember to lighten the pressure of the UST while cannulating the artery (Fig. 2.1).

2.2.2 Depth, Distance, and Angle

Unlike nerve blocks and other ultrasound-guided procedures, vascular cannulations are mostly performed using an out-of-plane technique. The choice of whether to use an in-plane or an out-of-plane technique depends on the diameter of the vessel and its depth. While a larger and superficial vessel can be cannulated in an in-plane technique, a smaller or deeper target generally necessitates the use of an out-of-plane technique.

For an out-of-plane approach to a blood vessel it is to be remembered that the needle tip is visible only where it crosses the plane of the ultrasound beam, making the window for error quite small. It is useful to mentally construct a right-angled triangle, with the plane of the ultrasound beam forming the perpendicular, distance from the midline of the probe to the point of entry to the base and the needle trajectory of the hypotenuse while holding the ultrasound transducer (UST) vertically and in a transverse orientation to the target vessel. For deeper and bigger targets the ideal angle of entry should be between 45 and 60° (Fig. 2.2). The distance of the point of entry from the UST must be measured accordingly to derive the angle of entry. For deeper and larger vessels such as the femoral vein, a steep needle angle is usually required to retain the direc-

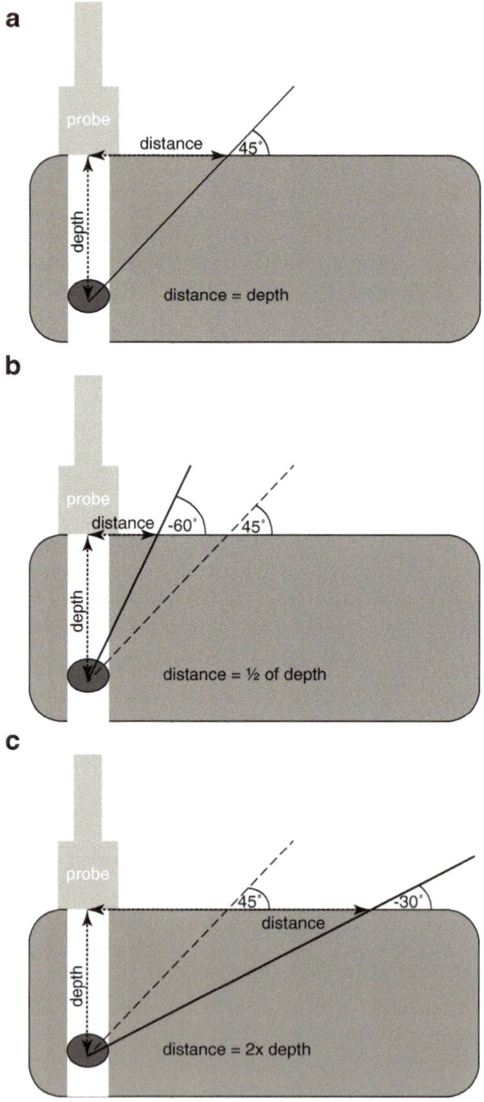

Fig. 2.2 Relationship between the depth of the target, distance of the point of entry from the transducer footprint, and the angle of the needle: (**a**) when the depth and the distance are equal, the angle is exactly 45°. (**b**) The angle increases when the distance reduces and (**c**) the angle decreases as the distance increases

tion. Even superficial but larger targets can be cannulated with a needle angle of 45° or more. For superficial and smaller targets a shallower approach is usually required for cannulation as a steeper angle may lead the needle to go through the posterior wall easily causing difficulty in cannulation, hematoma, and requiring multiple attempts. Superficial vessels such as radial artery cannulation usually require an angle of 30° or less. The distance of the point of entry of the needle needs to be calculated accordingly. Moving the probe up and down and tilting the probe would help visualizing the needle.

2.2.3 Selecting the Transducer and Mode

While imaging for vascular cannulations, it is important to rationalize the appropriate transducer and mode.

2.2.3.1 Transducer

A high-frequency (10–20 mHz) linear transducer is usually selected for cannulation of vessels up to the depth of 5 cm. Cannulation of deeper vessels such as the femoral vessels in an obese individual may require the curvilinear UST which has a lower frequency (7–10 mHz) but a greater depth of penetration. A transducer with a smaller footprint such as the hockey stick transducer is useful for cannulation in children or adults with small body parts.

2.2.3.2 Mode

2D mode is generally used for cannulation. A color Doppler mode can be selected to identify arteries from veins. Arteries have a pulsatile flow and the flow towards the transducer is usually colored in red and flow away blue in most of the ultrasound machines. Color mode is particularly useful for distinguishing between deeper and closely lying vessels such as the femoral artery and vein.

2.2.4 Preparation

2.2.4.1 Preprocedural Evaluation

- Review indications for cannulation.
- Decide the technique—Seldinger/catheter-over-needle.
- Decide the type and bore of cannula/catheter.
- Review relevant past medical history.

2.2.4.2 Positioning/Room Set Up/ Ergonomics

Patient

- Comfortably lying or sitting.
- Supine position with Trendelenburg for central venous cannulation of upper extremity.
- Arm well supported; arm board (if available) with the limb abducted and externally rotated.
- Adequate exposure to clean field.

Operator

- Ergonomically positioned: Sitting or standing.
- Align ultrasound monitor, patient and patient's access point within the operator's line of sight.
- Equipment close, reachable, and in order to be used.

Equipment

- Ultrasound machine.
  - Linear transducer (7.5–10 MHz): Superficial structures.
  - Curvilinear transducer (2–5 MHz): Deeper structures.
- Probe cover.
- Sterile gel.
- Tourniquet for peripheral venous cannulation.
- Gloves.
- Syringe of normal saline (flush).
- Skin preparation—alcohol/antiseptic wipes.
- Cannula.
  - Check the required flow rate to determine the gauge required.
  - Standard vs longer cannula dependent on the depth of vein being accessed.
- Adhesive transparent dressing (e.g., Tegaderm).
- ± blood vials for pathology (as required).

2.3 Central Venous Cannulation

Although the placement of a central venous catheter (CVC) is a routine procedure in intensive care medicine and in perioperative care, acute severe complications such as inadvertent arterial puncture or cannulation, hematoma, hemothorax, or pneumothorax occur in a relevant proportion of patients [26]. Traditionally, IJV central cannulation placement is performed using landmark techniques based on the knowledge of anatomic structures and palpation of arteries next to the veins. Unfortunately, these landmark techniques have their own limitations in detecting anatomic variations at the CVC insertion site as well as venous thrombosis that is especially common in oncologic and critically ill patients can make CVC placement impossible or dangerous for the patient [27]. The use of ultrasound has been proposed to increase the safety and quality of CVC placement by reducing CVC-related complications [28]. The meta-analysis of over 5000 patients from 35 trials demonstrated a reduced total rate of complications by using US compared with conventional landmark techniques (4.0% vs 13.5%, respectively). In addition, the overall success rate was higher in the US (97.6% vs 87.6%). The benefits of US-guided CVC placement with regard to the total complication rate, overall success rate, and number of attempts until success were consistent across experienced and inexperienced operators [29].

2.3.1 Internal Jugular Vein Cannulation

One of the earliest vascular cannulations that is performed using ultrasound guidance is the internal jugular vein (IJV) cannulation. The patient-awake or under anesthesia/sedation is placed supine, head turned to the other side and table/bed tilted to 10–15° Trendelenburg. The head down maneuver helps in engorging the vein and also prevents inadvertent venous air embolism (VAE). After antiseptic dressing and draping, the ultrasound probe, covered in a sterile plastic sheet is placed on the neck at the level of the cricoid cartilage and slided laterally to image the IJV and the common carotid artery (CCA). Small, linear array, high-frequency transducers (5–15 MHz) with scanning surface of 2–5 cm are best suited for IJV cannulation. An index mark corresponds with an orientation marker on one side of the US scan sector shown on the US device screen helps to obtain the correct probe orientation during US examination [30]. It is important to note here that the IJV and the CCA often have considerable overlapping, starting from 20% to even 100% at this level. When the CCA is directly below the IJV, even with the ultrasound guidance there is a considerable risk of inadvertent CCA puncture. Therefore, it is prudent to scan up and down the IJV to find out the position where the overlapping is minimum and choose that point for the puncture. Turning the head too much to the other side sometimes increases the overlap. These factors should be considered at the time of positioning. If the patient is awake, he/she can be advised to optimize the head turn to the optimal level.

The distance of the point of entry of the needle from the footprint of the UST should be kept in mind while inserting the needle and the angle adjusted accordingly.

Sometimes the needle would push the skin and subcutaneous tissue in a manner before actually piercing that it appears that the needle has gone past the vein. In such a situation the vein appears collapsed under the pressure of the needle. As soon as the needle enters the vein the pressure is relieved and the needle tip is seen as a bright echogenic point inside the hypoechoic lumen of the IJV.

While positioning the UST, the midpoint of the UST, which often has a mark, should be directly above the midpoint of the vein. Lateral and medial ends should be identified before entering the skin. In case of doubt, remember CCA lies medially and posterior (below) to the IJV.

US can be used in different ways to facilitate CVC placement. Using US prior to catheter placement only to visualize the IJV to determine patency and anatomical variants has been referred to as the US-assisted approach. However, the US-guided approach, which is real-time visualization of needle placement and advancement is generally recommended to prevent or minimize catheter-related complications [31]. US guidance during needle advancement can be performed using: a short-axis (SAX) probe orientation and an out-of-plane view of the needle; a long-axis (LAX) probe orientation and an in-plane view of the needle or occasionally an oblique orientation, a view that is halfway between the short-axis and the long-axis view with the US probe placed at approximately 45° with respect to the target vessel [32, 33]. In addition a new anteroposterior SAX but in-plane technique that combines the advantage of in-plane technique to track the needle tip and short-axis view of visualizing nearby anatomical structures by placing the probe on the side of the neck, oriented anteroposteriorly, perpendicular to the long axis of the neck have been described. This view visualizes IJV and its relationship to the carotid artery in the short axis [34].

With limited available data unable to predict superiority of one technique over another one. However, SAX out-of-plane approach is easier to learn for physicians not familiar with ultrasound [35]. The advantage of the SAX approach allows better visualization of the vein in relation to the artery might more sufficiently help to avoid accidental arterial puncture, but the needle is only visualized as an echogenic point which is not necessarily the tip of the needle [36]. The entire needle can be visualized in its complete course with LAX in-plane approach and the depth of the needle tip is also visualized simultaneously thereby reducing the risk of penetration of the posterior vessel wall [37] (Figs. 2.3, 2.4, 2.5, and 2.6).

2.3.2 Subclavian Vein Cannulation

2.3.2.1 Anatomy of Subclavian Vessels

The subclavian vein is the continuation of the axillary vein as it courses beneath the clavicle. At

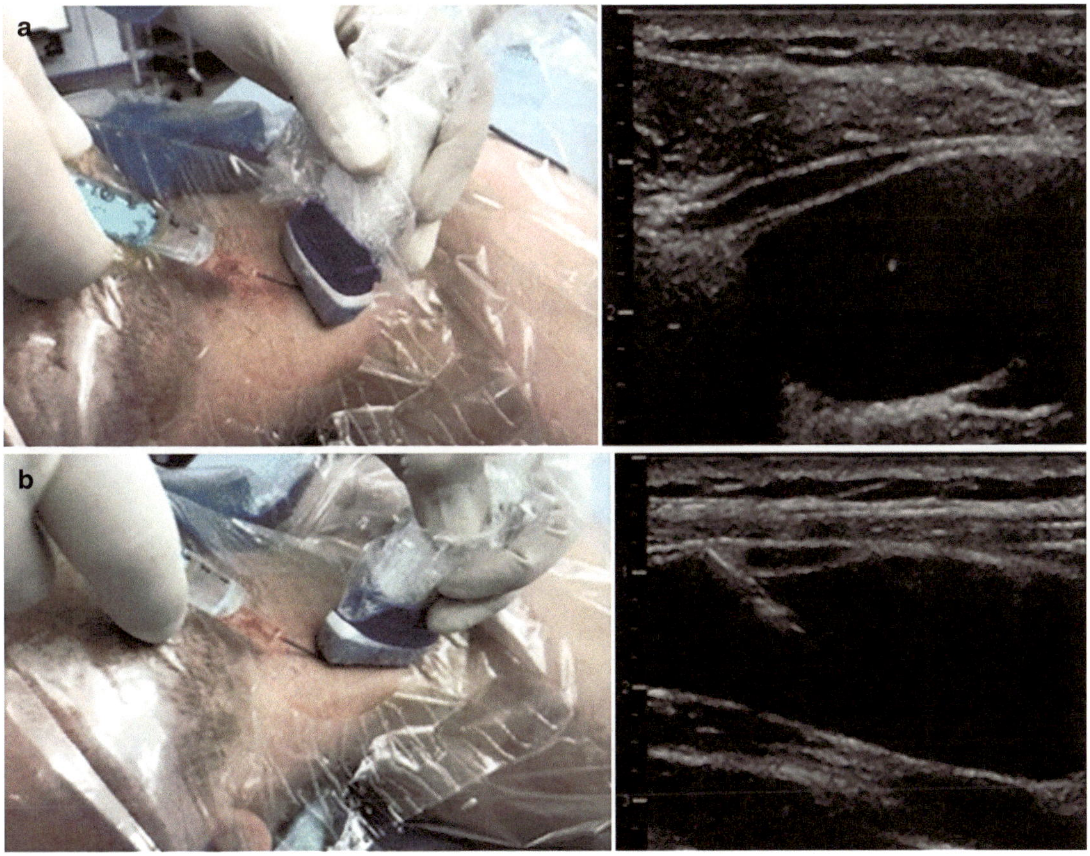

Fig. 2.3 US image of internal jugular vein in (**a**) short (out-of-plane view) and (**b**) long axis(in-plane view)

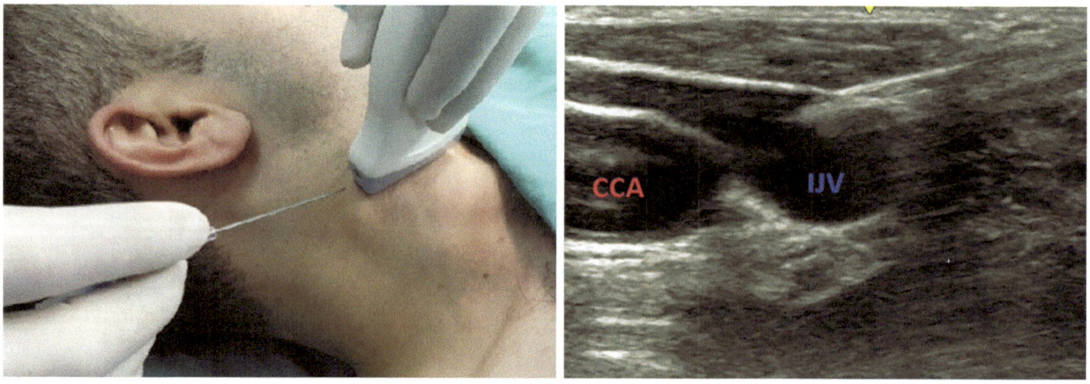

Fig. 2.4 Oblique approach for IJV cannulation

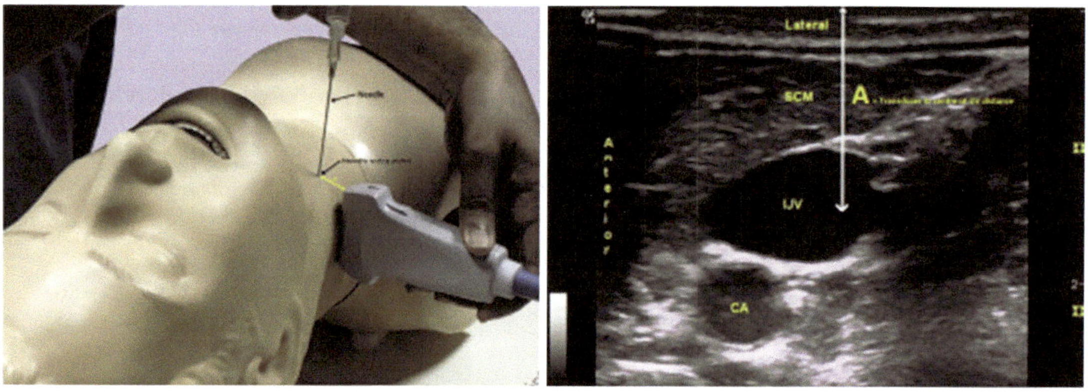

Fig. 2.5 Alternative in-plane technique for IJV cannulation

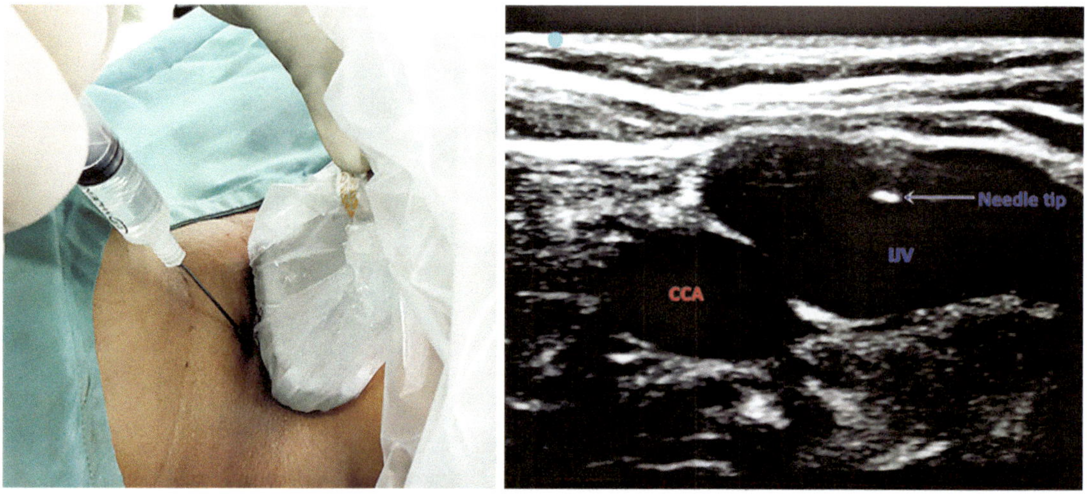

Fig. 2.6 Cannulation of the internal jugular vein (IJV): Left: Note the high-frequency linear UST being held in a transverse orientation and the needle entering at an angle of about 60°. Note that the distance from the UST footprint to the point of entry of the needle is shorter than the depth of the target vessel. Right: the needle tip is seen as a bright echogenic object inside the lumen of the IJV. Note the overlap of CCA and IJV to more than 30%

the lateral border of the first rib, it travels superiorly then under the clavicle travels medially until it joins the internal jugular vein to form the innominate vein. The subclavian artery runs posterior and superior to the subclavian vein. The brachial plexus courses superiorly and deep to the medial portion of the subclavian artery. On the left side, the thoracic duct lies close to the subclavian vessels. Most importantly, the lung and pleural cavity lie inferior and deeper to the subclavian vein and are particularly vulnerable to accidental puncture more often on the left chest where the apex of the lung can extend just above the first rib. Familiarity with anatomical variants of subclavian vessels are essential prior to any interventional procedures or cannulation of both vein and artery.

2.3.2.2 Ultrasound Assessment of Subclavian Vessels

Similar to IJV, 2D and color Doppler US are utilized to assess the morphology, patency, anatomical variants, and certain pathological conditions such as aneurysm, stenosis, or thrombosis of the vessels. Compared to US-guided cannulation of IJV there are limited data on the utilization of US for SV cannulation. Meta-analysis of over 2000 patients from nine studies showed that the use of US resulted in a reduced rate of accidental arterial puncture (0.8% vs 5.9%); and hematoma formation (1.2% vs 6.6%). However, there was no statistically significant difference between the use of US and the conventional landmark technique with regard to the total complication rate, the overall success rate, the number of attempts until success, the time to successful cannulation, and the success rate with the first attempt [38, 39]. Currently there is no strong evidence of using the US for SV cannulation from different societies (Fig. 2.7).

2.3.2.3 Ultrasound-Guided Subclavian Vein Cannulation Technique

While IJV cannulation with ultrasound is one of the basic techniques of POCUS, the subclavian vein (SCV) cannulation is a more advanced tech-

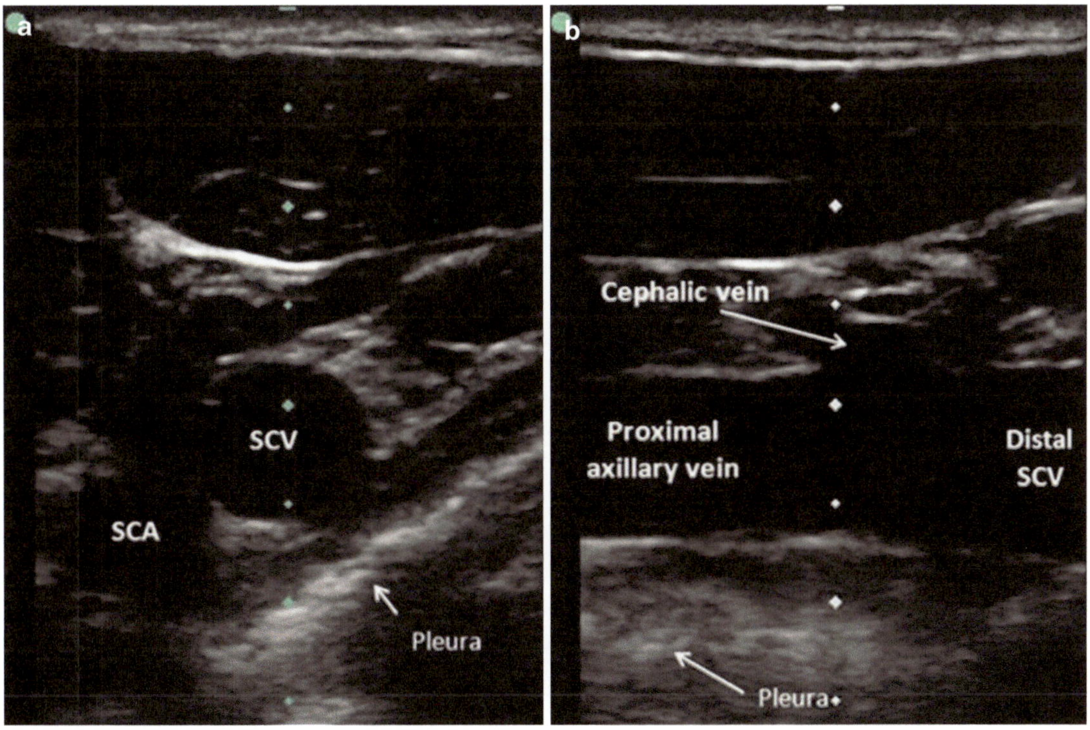

Fig. 2.7 US image of subclavian vessels. (**a**) Short axis image with probe in parasagittal orientation, (**b**) Long axis image, with the probe in coronal/transverse orientation

nique. The clavicle, which lies directly above the SCV, precludes ultrasound imaging. SCV being a deeper vein and the subclavian artery lying in close proximity makes the cannulation even more challenging. Subclavian vein (SV) can be visualized from infraclavicular (most common) or supraclavicular approach. High-frequency linear probes are commonly used to visualize subclavian vessels and for morbidly obese individuals, curvilinear probe with better penetration features is recommended. The UST is positioned perpendicular to the midline, i.e., in a coronal/transverse orientation, medial end of the UST lying on the midpoint of the clavicle. A little cephalad tilt of the UST allows imaging of the SCV and SCA. The artery would be imaged lying posterior to the vein. Before puncture, one should be sure that both the artery and the vein can be imaged separately. Vein can also be identified by its collapsibility under pressure and that it expands upon valsalva maneuver and by a Trendelenberg position. In case of difficulty of visualization, a more lateral site may be chosen.

An infraclavicular approach is a more traditional approach, although a supraclavicular approach has been described.

Infraclavicular Approach

For infraclavicular approach, either SAX out-of-plane or long-axis in-plane techniques have been implemented with limitations of each approach like in IJV cannulation. Compared to the landmark method, cannulation occurs more laterally.

The UST is held transversely at an angle of 90° to the midline just below the clavicle in a way that the medial side of the ultrasound image shows the clavicle and the shadow cast by it and the lateral side shows the subclavian vein on a little cephalad tilt of the transducer. The image is adjusted for depth, which is typically at 6 cm for thin individuals. As the transducer is slided laterally and tilted further cephalad, both subclavian vein and artery can be imaged. The angle of insonation is important to observe because the needle for an in-plane cannulation would travel in the same plane.

After instilling local anesthetic (LA) along the path of the needle entry, the central venous cannulation needle, fixed with an empty 2 cc (or 5 cc) syringe is inserted in-plane from lateral to medial. (Once the needle tip can be imaged inside the SCV, dark venous blood can be aspirated in the syringe attached to the needle. The syringe is then disconnected and the guidewire is introduced. The guidewire should be visualized in the superior vena cava and not in the SCA or the IJV by placing the UST on the neck and tilting the probe caudally. If the guidewire is found in the neck it is to be pulled back and negotiated in again. Only after confirmation of the guidewire location in the superior vena cava, the needle is withdrawn.

Proceduralist can stand either at head end or on the ipsilateral side for right subclavian vein cannulation. Ergonomics need to be ensured as it is a demanding procedure.

A short-axis view can be also obtained at this location by rotating the UST by 90° and an out-of-plane approach for cannulation can be performed.

In either approach, it is mandatory to identify and image the subclavian artery before beginning the process of cannulation. Currently no evidence of showing one method's superiority over other methods however a US-guided infraclavicular approach is feasible to visualize SCV in most of the clinical settings (Figs. 2.8 and 2.9).

Supraclavicular Approach

Ultrasound Assessment of SCV in the Fossa Above the Clavicle

The SCV runs from lateral to medial under the clavicle, just anterior to the subclavian artery (SCA). As it approaches the heart, the SCV is joined by the IJV, forming the brachiocephalic (innominate) vein. The supraclavicular approach attempts to cannulate the portion of the SCV just lateral to the clavicular head of the sternocleidomastoid muscle. The right SCV is preferred to the left since it forms a straighter angle with the IJV, offering a shorter distance for wire passage into

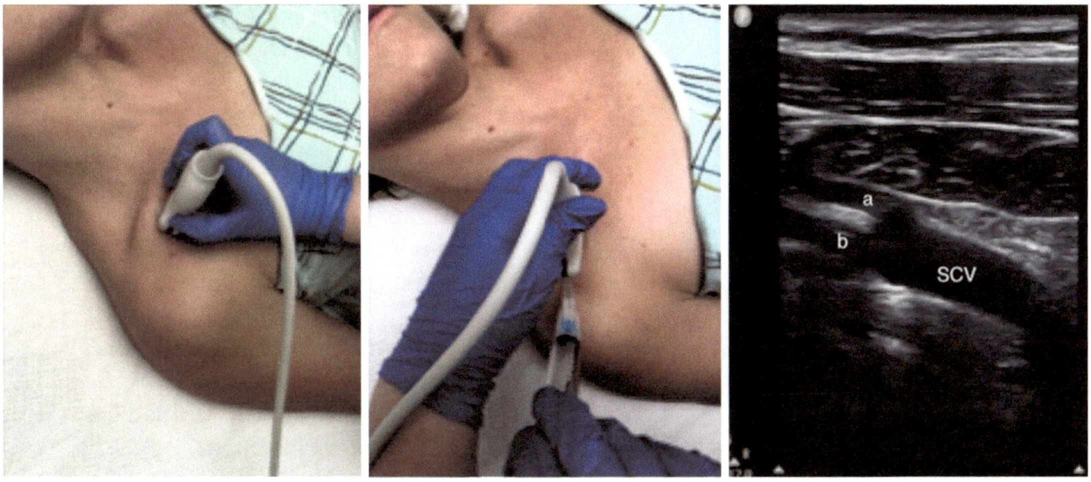

Fig. 2.8 Infraclavicular approach long axis

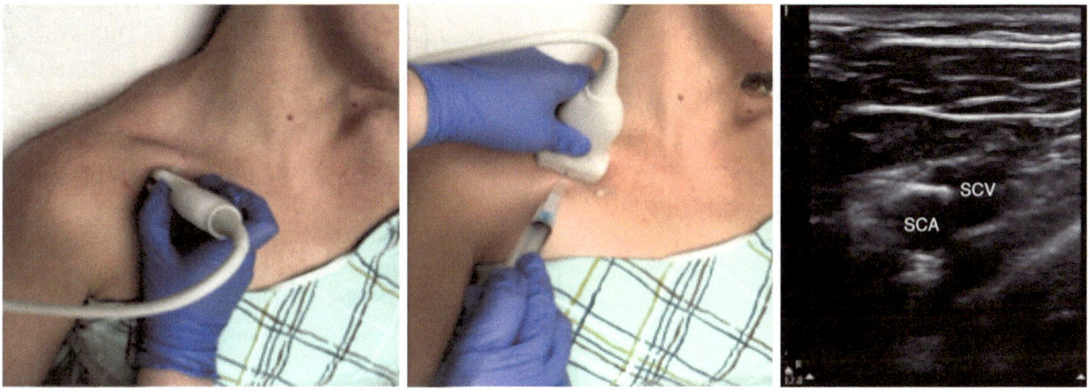

Fig. 2.9 Infraclavicular approach short axis

the superior vena cava, avoiding proximity to the thoracic duct, which drains into the left SCV. Place a high-frequency linear transducer (6–13 MHz) on the lateral neck just above the clavicle to locate the IJV and carotid artery. Slowly trace the IJV by moving the probe caudally into the supraclavicular fossa until the probe abuts the clavicle. While visualizing the most caudal aspect of the IJV, angle the probe anteriorly to visualize the confluence of the IJV and SCV (Fig. 2.11). At this proximal location, the SCV lies anterior to the SCA, and the operator should dynamically fan the probe from a posterior to anterior position to identify both vessels.

Ultrasound-Guided SCV Cannulation

Once visualize the SCV, turn the probe in the longitudinal plane prior to needle puncture. Enter the SCV from the lateral aspect using in-plane technique. Probe needs to be tilted more anteriorly (caudally) and stabilized against the clavicle. This approach has an advantage of placing SCV even during CPR. This approach has several advantages over landmark technique. SCV can also be accessed by short axis out-of-plane technique (Fig. 2.11). However, long-axis approach is preferred to avoid pleural puncture. Ultimately familiarity of SCV anatomy at this location and the operator skill determines the successful cannulation.

2.3.3 Femoral Vein Cannulation

The femoral vein (FV) cannulation is employed for central venous access where the superior extremity central venous access is otherwise ruled out and for temporary intravenous pacing. A high-frequency linear array UST is selected. The patient lies supine and the proceduralist stands on the ipsilateral side. The UST is placed transversely, just inferior to the inguinal crease. The superficial femoral artery can be easily identified as an anechoic pulsatile structure with the FV lying medial and inferior to it. The FV appears as an oval-shaped anechoic object which is compressible by the UST. After adjusting the UST, so that the FV lies in the center of the image, the block needle is inserted out of the plane. The UST is slided up and down to follow the needle trajectory till the tip of the needle appears at the upper surface of the vein as a bright dot, appears to indent on the vein wall and then pierces it. Dark venous blood can be aspirated with the syringe attached. Guidewire is passed down.

The entire procedure should be performed under direct ultrasound imaging. The needle is to be advanced only when visualized without any doubt.

The same process can be applied for a femoral artery cannulation.

2.3.3.1 Systematic Approach for USG Central Venous Catheter Placement

Irrespective of cannulation site, for clinical practice, the authors recommend a systematic approach using six steps:

1. To identify the anatomy of the insertion site and localization of the vein, it is recommended to perform a baseline scan prior to sterile preparation. It also helps to know anatomical variants.
2. To confirm patency of the vein by using various US features such as color Doppler, compression US or even spectral Doppler in rare occasions.
3. Use real-time US guidance for puncture of the vein, one should be familiar with the depth and angular orientation prior to placing the needle.
4. Confirm needle position in the vein, recommended to use LAX to complete the track of the needle inside the vessel and to avoid posterior wall puncture.
5. Confirm wire position in the vein and track all the way to IJ and SV junction if wire is placed in IJV to ensure wire enters the innominate vein prior to dilation over the guidewire.
6. Confirm catheter position in the vein.

2.3.3.2 Femoral Vein Cannulation

Limitations of Ultrasound-Guided Central Venous Catheter Placement

Although US is noninvasive and thus does not bear a risk to directly harm the patient, some limitations and disadvantages of US during central venous access are worth considering. One might argue that the risk of catheter-related bloodstream infections might be higher if US is used for CVC placement without applying a strict aseptic approach. US might give a false sense of security and mislead him/her to neglect traditionally taught principles with regard to needle direction especially for inexperienced users. To overcome these problems formal education and training including simulation with a structured certification of US skills for vascular access and the development of a consensus standard for these training programs have been suggested. Sometimes insertion site-related specific issues when using US. For example, shorter necks in morbid obese individuals might make LAX a challenge to visualize the IJV and might need curved-array probes even for IJ placement. For subclavian access, because the angle of cannulation is usually steeper when using US, it is especially important to align and constantly visualize the needle to avoid pleural injury.

2.3.4 Confirmation of the Correct Position of the Central Venous Catheter Tip

Prevention of central venous catheter tip malposition is of paramount importance, as it has been associated with significant complications, including central venous or superior vena cava thrombosis, arrhythmias, cardiac tamponade, and hemodynamic monitoring inaccuracy. Moreover, with malposition, appropriate treatment may be delayed with subsequent further related complications. In this regard, the intracavitary electrocardiographic (IC-ECG) method is currently recommended in international guidelines as accurate, well-tolerated, and cost-effective for assessing the proper location of the central venous catheter tip. However, this method is commonly considered to be applicable only when there is a well-defined and identifiable P wave in the ECG trace. Although a few studies have recently suggested that IC-ECG might also be used in patients with atrial fibrillation after some appropriate modifications of the basic technique, in patients with a pacemaker or with other arrhythmias, IC-ECG is still considered to be not applicable. As bedside chest radiograph has been shown to be inaccurate in identifying the catheter tip location due to the inaccuracy of the radiological landmark for the cavo-atrial junction, ultrasound imaging has been proposed as an alternative technique to IC-ECG and chest radiograph for tip location. Indeed, the application of ultrasound to vascular access should not be limited to venepuncture but should be extended to assist in all steps of the procedure. Specifically, in regard to the prevention of primary malposition, ultrasound may play two roles as a "tip location" and a "tip navigation" technique. Ultrasound-based tip navigation techniques can be used to confirm that the catheter or the guidewire is threading towards the cavo-atrial junction by sonographic visualization throughout the ipsilateral brachiocephalic vein, ruling out catheter misdirection into the ipsilateral IJV or other superior vena cava tributary veins (e.g., the contralateral brachiocephalic vein). Sonographic tip navigation may be performed with the same linear probe used for the puncture. As a tip location technique, ultrasound allows direct or indirect visualization of the catheter tip or the J-guidewire at the cavo-atrial junction, upper right atrium, or in the lower superior vena cava by means of transthoracic echocardiography. Different approaches and different protocols have been described in the literature on this topic. Four different echocardiographic views have been tested: the apical four-chamber view, the subcostal four chambers view, the subcostal bi-caval view and the suprasternal/supraclavicular view. Both of the four chambers views allow only evaluation of the right atrium without visualization of the superior vena cava or inferior vena cava. On the contrary, the subcostal bi-caval view, the most studied approach, allows visualization of the superior vena cava, cavo-atrial junction, right atrium, and inferior vena cava. Four groups of researchers have studied the suprasternal/supraclavicular view, which allows the identification of the confluence between the two brachiocephalic veins, the superior vena cava, the right branch of the pulmonary, artery and the aortic arch. These structures enable indirect identification of the cavo-atrial junction. Ultrasound-based tip navigation may be used during the procedure to help the operator in directing the guidewire.

2.3.4.1 The European Society of Anesthesiologists Recommends [40]

1. When an intracardiac electrocardiogram is not applicable, using real-time ultrasound to detect and prevent central venous catheter malposition, as it has been shown to be well-tolerated, feasible, quickly performed, and interpreted at bedside, and more accurate and faster than a chest radiograph (1C).
2. Combining vascular ultrasound for guidewire and central venous line tip navigation with transthoracic echocardiography for tip location (1C).
3. Performing pleural and lung ultrasound (PLUS) to rule out potential pleural-pulmonary complications (mainly pneumothorax) soon after the procedure in any difficult puncture of the subclavian or axillary vein and, particularly, if the patient complains of shortness of breath or discomfort that worsens after catheter placement (1B).
4. Using PLUS to monitor the development of a confirmed pleural-pulmonary complication or for follow-up of treatment (1B).
5. Ultrasound for diagnosis and follow-up of catheter-related thrombosis (1C).

2.4 Peripheral Venous Cannulation

Ultrasound-guidance is often useful for peripheral venous cannulation in patients in whom peripheral venous cannulation without guidance is difficult, e.g., burn patients, patients of cancer chemotherapy, patients with peripheral edema where the veins cannot be seen otherwise. Obese patients also benefit from ultrasound guidance in peripheral venous cannulation by reducing the number of attempts and increasing first pass and overall success rate [41–48]. The technique can be real-time ultrasound-guided or US-assisted—where the proceduralist may mark the location of the veins with the ultrasound and then proceed with cannulation with usual technique. The usual targets are the antecubital vein and the saphenous vein.

2.4.1 Indications

- Difficulty in locating veins via visualization or palpation due to.
  - Body habitus.
  - Edematous skin.
- Multiple unsuccessful blind insertion attempts.
- Severe dehydration.
- Multiple previous cannulations (e.g., intravenous drug use, chemotherapy).

2.4.2 Procedure

2.4.2.1 Initial Scout

Using the ultrasound transducer survey potential vessels for cannulation should be scanned. Start in the antecubital fossa with a transverse probe orientation. Targets in the upper limb are basilic, brachial, and/or cephalic veins. The basilic vein, while variably present, lacks flanking arteries and nerves, and is usually the more superficial target. In contrast, the deep brachial vein is near ubiquitously present, but has nerves and arteries in close proximity, and is found at a greater depth.

2.4.3 Confirm Vein

The blood vessel located should be confirmed as a vein using the following principles-

(a) Patent peripheral veins easily and completely collapse with gentle compression with the probe.
(b) Nonpulsatile.
(c) Color Doppler can be used.
(d) Pulsed wave Doppler also can be used to demonstrate the pulsatile flow pattern in adjacent arteries and the nonpulsatile, phasic flow in veins.

2.4.3.1 Identify the Appropriate Vein

The appropriate vein should be identified by applying the following principles

(a) Diameter, depth, path: The vein should be of an adequately large diameter, at an achievable depth, in a straight path.
  - Using a standard 48 mm angiocatheter, success rate drops to 0% when vessel depth is more than 1.6 cm.
  - No significant difference between more superficial veins at different depths,
  - The success rate increases with increasing venous diameter.
    - 56% when less than or equal to 0.3 cm
    - 92% when greater than or equal to 0.6 cm.

Desirable targets are therefore found between 0.3 cm and 1.5 cm from the surface, with an internal diameter of at least 0.4 cm

(b) Note and avoid venous valves.

2.4.3.2 Preparation

- Clean probe after initial scout.
- Place a cover directly on the clean probe.
- Apply a tourniquet to the upper aspect of the patient's arm.
- Prepare the skin over the previously identified venous target with alcohol/antiseptic wipe.

2.4.3.3 Needle Insertion

- Don sterile gloves.
- US probe is held in the nondominant hand with a stable grip.
- Apply sterile gel.
- Check probe orientation: Touch one end of the probe and watch for reaction on the monitor.
- Align for use on the patient so that the medial of the screen is medial of the patient and lateral is lateral.
- Locate the target, adjust depth.
- Transducer orientations-.
  - Transverse:
    Advantages: Improved ability to center needle to the midline of vessel.
    Disadvantages: Loss of direct needle tip visualization each time the probe or the needle is moved.
  - Longitudinal:
    Advantages: Entire needle visualized throughout the procedure with a better perception of depth within the vessel.
    Disadvantages: Inability to identify if the needle is off the midline of the vessel. For narrower vessels, it is difficult to keep the transducer centered on the vessel lumen in long axis.
  - Optional confirmation of position prior to insertion of needle by placing needle between transducer and skin to illicit shadow artifact.
  - Note the depth of the artery to approximate final insertion depth.
- Insert needle through skin at a 45° or lesser approach angle.
  - Concentrate on monitor after initial insertion,
  - Find needle tip through fanning or small movements of ultrasound prior to further movement. Tilting the probe towards the approaching needle in the short axis (transverse orientation) is helpful to locate the advancing tip without moving the probe from its position.
- Progressive targeted movement of needle towards vessel.
  - Incremental movements of 1 mm at a time directed towards vessel.
  - Process of moving ultrasound probe forward off the needle tip, stabilizing and then moving the needle further forward into the ultrasound's view.

2.4.3.4 Confirmation of Cannulation

1. Visualization of cannula and needle within the lumen of the vessel.
   (a) On transverse orientation: Bull's eye sign,
   (b) On longitudinal orientation: needle seen entering and lying within the lumen,
2. A positive "saline flush test."
   (a) Identify cannula in long axis and push 5–10 mL of saline,
   (b) Positive test is direct visualization of bubbles within the lumen,
   (c) May be aided by color Doppler 4,
3. Flashback of blood through the cannula.

The ultrasound probe can be put down at this point so that both hands can be used to advance the catheter, remove the needle, attach the bung, flush the cannula, clean the surrounding skin, and secure it in place with a transparent dressing.

2.4.3.5 Complications

In comparison to blinded techniques, complications associated with peripheral IV insertion under ultrasound guidance are typically minor but include:

- Nerve injury: Median or median cutaneous nerve.
- Arterial cannulation: Highlights the importance of confirming venous characteristics on ultrasound prior to cannulation.

2.5 Arterial Cannulations

2.5.1 Scout Scan

After proper positioning, an initial scan is important to locate the artery, confirm using color Doppler and or power Doppler. Note the depth and diameter of the artery.

2.5.1.1 Preparation

- Clean probe after initial scout.
- Place a sterile cover on the clean probe.
- Confirm position of the limb.
- Prepare the skin over the previously identified target with alcohol/antiseptic wipe.
- A window drape may be placed.
- Select the cannula/catheter.

2.5.1.2 Needle Insertion

- Don sterile gloves.
- The US probe is held in the nondominant hand with a stable grip.
- Apply sterile gel.
- Check probe orientation: Touch one end of the probe and watch for reaction on the monitor.
- Align for use on the patient so that the medial of the screen is medial of the patient and lateral is lateral.
- Locate the target, adjust depth.
- Transducer orientations-.
  - Transverse:

    Advantages: Improved ability to center needle to the midline of vessel.

    Disadvantages: Loss of direct needle tip visualization each time the probe or the needle is moved.
  - Longitudinal:

    Advantages: Entire needle visualized throughout the procedure with a better perception of depth within the vessel.

    Disadvantages: Inability to identify if needle is off the midline of the vessel. For narrower vessels, it is difficult to keep the transducer centered on the vessel lumen in long axis.
  - Optional confirmation of position prior to insertion of needle by placing needle between transducer and skin to illicit shadow artifact.
  - Note the depth of the artery to approximate final insertion depth.
- Insert needle through skin at a 45° or lesser approach angle.
  - Concentrate on monitor after initial insertion,
  - Find needle tip through fanning or small movements of ultrasound prior to further movement. Tilting the probe towards the approaching needle in the short axis (transverse orientation) is helpful to locate the advancing tip without moving the probe from its position.
- Progressive targeted movement of needle towards vessel.
  - Incremental movements of 1 mm at a time directed towards vessel.
  - Process of moving ultrasound probe forward off the needle tip, stabilizing and then moving the needle further forward into the ultrasound's view.

2.5.1.3 Confirmation of Cannulation

1. Visualization of cannula and needle within the lumen of the vessel.
   (a) On transverse orientation: Bull's eye sign,
   (b) On longitudinal orientation: Needle is seen entering and lying within lumen,
2. A positive "saline flush test."
   (c) Identify cannula in long axis and push 5–10 mL of saline,
   (d) Positive test is direct visualization of bubbles within lumen,
   (e) May be aided by color Doppler 4.
3. Flashback of blood through cannula.

The ultrasound probe can be put down at this point so that both hands can be used to advance the catheter, remove the needle, attach the pressure monitoring line, flush the cannula, clean the surrounding skin, and secure it in place with a transparent dressing or suture as deemed necessary.

2.5.1.4 Complications

In comparison to blinded techniques, complications associated with arterial cannulation under ultrasound guidance are negligible.

2.5.2 Radial Artery Cannulation

Radial artery cannulation is usually done without ultrasound guidance but ultrasound-guided technique is an important skill that each trainee must learn to be able to complete the task of radial artery cannulation even after a few missed attempts.

Radial artery is superficial and the diameter of the lumen is about 3–4 mm. Being a small and superficial target, it is easy to miss. Out-of-plane approach is generally preferred, in-plane approach is possible too! When performing the cannulation out-of-plane, slide the probe up and down and tilt towards the advancing needle to locate the tip. Once blood appears in the hub of the cannula, an attempt should be made to take a long-axis view and insert the cannula a few mm more inside the lumen. Then the catheter is slided in, keeping the stylet fixed with the other hand.

In the catheter-over-needle technique, as is most commonly performed, often it happens that blood appears at the hub indicating that the cannula has entered the artery, but upon advancement of the catheter it gets kinked and it has to be taken out and reinserted. The angle of the cannula should be kept acute, less than 30° so that after entering the artery, a few mm more can be inserted to avoid kinking of the catheter.

2.5.3 Femoral Artery Cannulation

Femoral artery is cannulated for percutaneous coronary intervention (PCI) and other intra-arterial interventions such as thrombectomy and recanalisation. It is sometimes used in cardiac anesthesia and cardiothoracic intensive care units for arterial pressure monitoring and intra-arterial balloon pump (IABP).

The process of cannulation is similar to the femoral vein cannulation. An out-of-plane approach and a Seldinger technique is used, i.e., a needle is inserted in the artery, upon obtaining pulsatile blood flow a guidewire is inserted, the needle is taken out followed by insertion of the catheter over the guidewire. For safety precaution against accidental dislodgement of the catheter thus inserted, many centers practice suturing the catheter hub with skin before taking the guidewire out.

2.5.4 Arteria Dorsalis Pedis Cannulation

Arteria dorsalis pedis (ADP) cannulation is useful for head and neck surgery with plastic reconstruction that would need a radial free flap. It is a small and superficial target, easy to miss. A short-axis view is to be obtained first to identify the artery. In contrast with most arteries, ADP is a superficial artery which is easily collapsible by the pressure of the UST. Therefore, after identification, use of color Doppler is warranted to confirm the artery. Once confirmed, the UST should be rotated by 90° while keeping it centered on the artery to obtain the long-axis view (LAX). Careful alignment of the UST is needed to get the complete LAX view. Colour Doppler is used again to confirm (Fig. 2.10). In-plane approach can be taken to cannulate the artery if a good LAX view can be obtained. Alternatively, an out-of-plane approach can be performed. When going out of plane, slide the probe up and down and tilt towards the advancing needle to locate the tip.

2.5.5 Posterior Tibial Artery Cannulation

The posterior tibial artery (PTA) cannulation can be useful for head and neck surgeries and particularly in children, in whom the radial or the ADP may be too small to cannulate. It is an important skill to learn.

Has been used in small children as an alternative to the radial artery as the lumen (ID>1.1 mm) can generally accommodate a 20 G arterial cannula [49].

2.5.5.1 Technique

Site: Midpoint between the medial malleolus and the Achilles tendon.

Position: Ankle dorsiflexion and eversion significantly increase the proximity to the skin surface. An assistant may be asked to hold the foot in position for cannulation.

Posterior tibial vessels lie in close proximity to the tibial nerve in a neurovascular bundle

Fig. 2.10 Cannulation of the subclavian vein (SCV)—stepwise approach. The needle (Arrowheads) enter lateral to medial. Subclavian artery (SCA) lies below the SCV

1. Subclavian vein (SCV) and artery (SCA) are identified in the long axis view

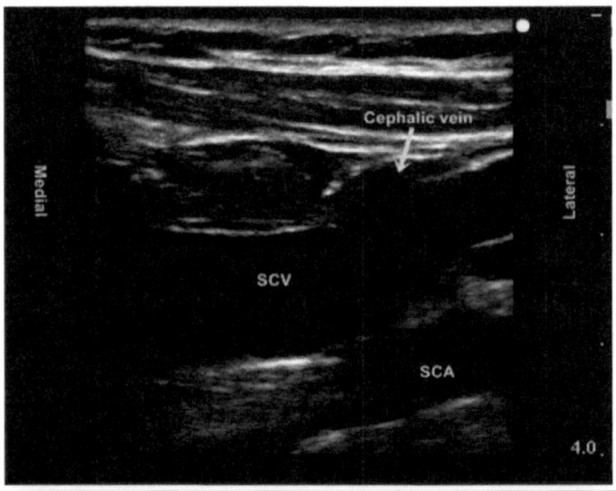

2. In-plane cannulation is performed. Note the needle tip (arrows) in the center of the vein

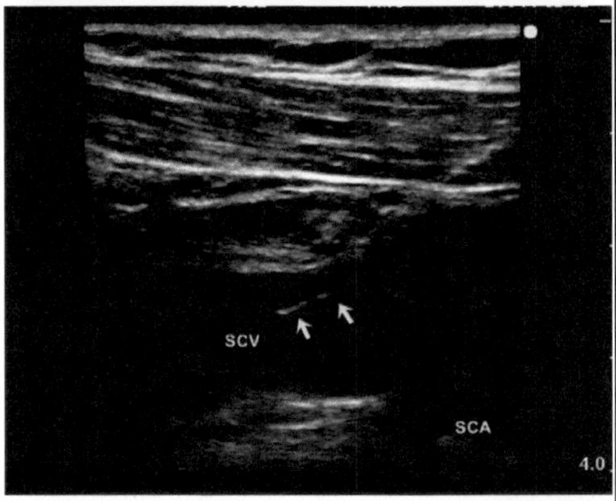

3. Guidewire (arrows) is inserted and imaged with ultrasound

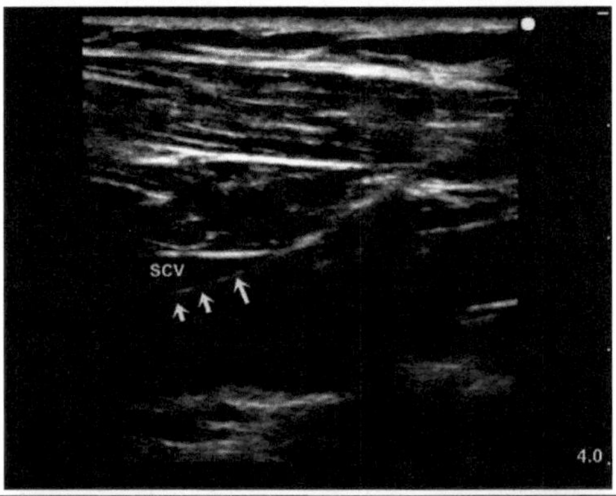

4. Ultrasound transducer is placed above the clavicle and tilted caudally to observe the guidewire (arrows) entering the Superior vena cava (SVC). The guidewire appears as a shiny line moving with each heartbeat.

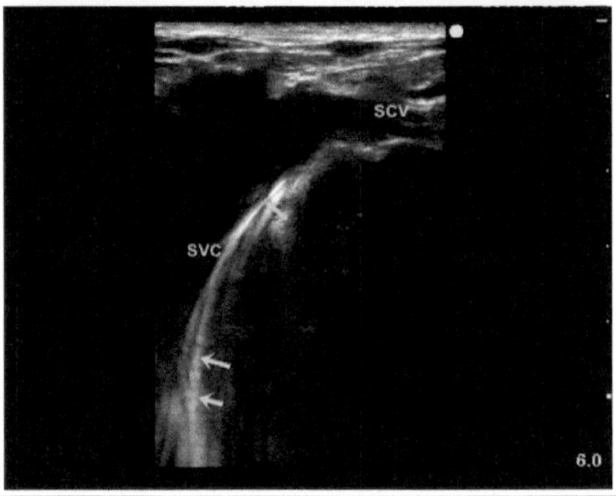

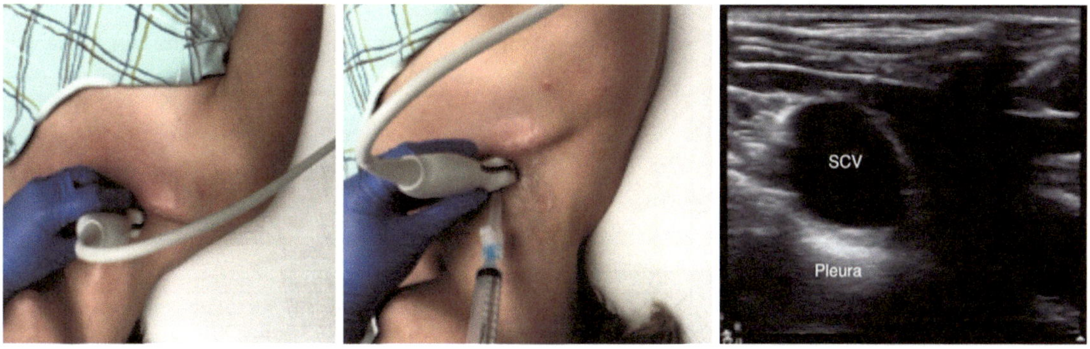

Fig. 2.11 Supraclavicular approach short axis

(Figs. 2.11 and 2.12). Compression with the UST will collapse the veins, allowing the artery to be identified, which lies flanked on both sides by the veins. Color Doppler should be used to confirm the artery. Once the PTA is identified a LAX view is obtained and in-plane cannulation is performed (Fig. 2.12). Out-of-plane cannulation can also be performed, depending on the experience and preference of the proceduralist (Figs. 2.13, 2.14, 2.15, 2.16, 2.17, 2.18, 2.19, and 2.20).

2.6 Recommendations for Ultrasound-Guided Vascular Access [1]

The 2020 practice guidelines from the ASA recommends-.

2.7 Recommendations for Prevention of Mechanical Trauma or Injury

2.7.1 Catheter Insertion Site Selection

- Determine catheter insertion site selection based on clinical need and practitioner judgment, experience, and skill.
- Select an upper body insertion site when possible to minimize the risk of thrombotic complications relative to the femoral site.

2.7.2 Positioning the Patient for Needle Insertion and Catheter Placement

- Perform central venous access in the neck or chest with the patient in the Trendelenburg position when clinically appropriate and feasible.

2.7.3 Needle Insertion, Wire Placement, and Catheter Placement

- Select catheter size (i.e., outside diameter) and type based on the clinical situation and skill/experience of the operator.
- Select the smallest size catheter appropriate for the clinical situation.
- For the subclavian approach select a thin-wall needle (i.e., Seldinger) technique vs a catheter-over-the-needle (i.e., modified Seldinger) technique.
- For the jugular or femoral approach, select a thin-wall needle or catheter-over-the-needle technique based on the clinical situation and the skill/experience of the operator.
- For accessing the vein before threading a dilator or large-bore catheter, base the decision to use a thin-wall needle technique or a catheter-over-the-needle technique at least in part on the method used to confirm that the wire resides in the vein (Fig. 2.21).

Fig. 2.12 IJV cannulation

1. Identify anatomy of the insertion site and localization of the vein

a. Identify the vein, artery and nearby structures
b. Image in SAX and LAX
c. Perform scan before prepping

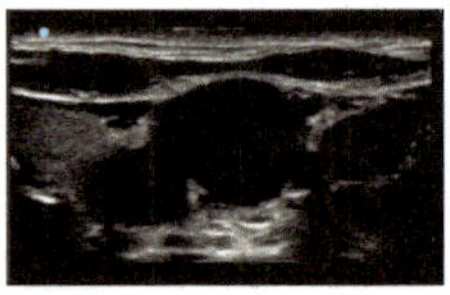
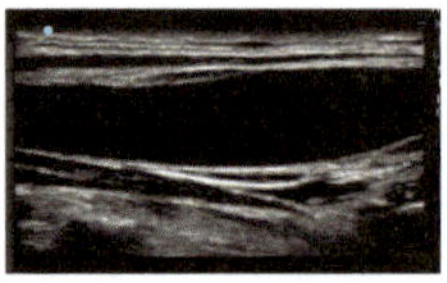

2. Confirm patency of the vein

a. Confirm compressability of the vein
b. Scan up and down to observe blood flow
c. Use colour Doppler

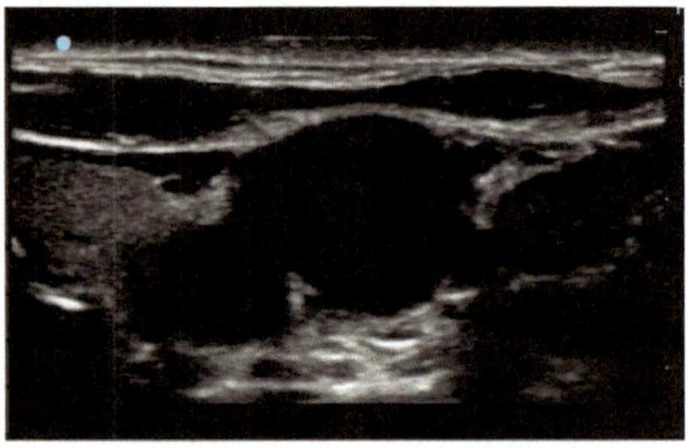

3. Use real time US guidance for puncture of the vein

a. Full sterile precautions
b. Use SAX or LAX or both
c. Keep the needle tip under "vision" all the time.

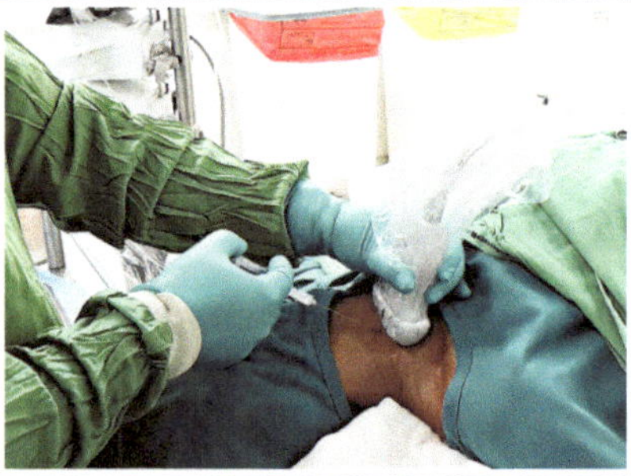

4. Confirm needle position in the vein

a. Confirm that the needle tip is placed centrally in the vein in SAX before inserting the guidewire.
b. Observe the needle in LAX

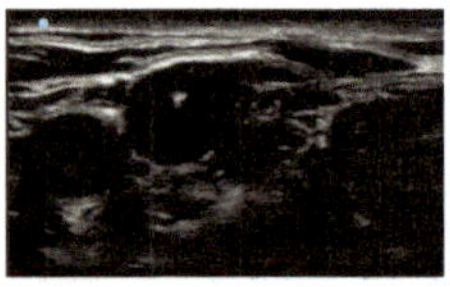
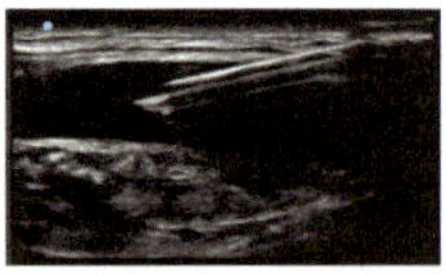

5. Confirm wire position in the vein

a. Confirm position of the guidewire inside the vein.
b. Tilt the probe caudally to notice the guidewire entering the superior vena cava

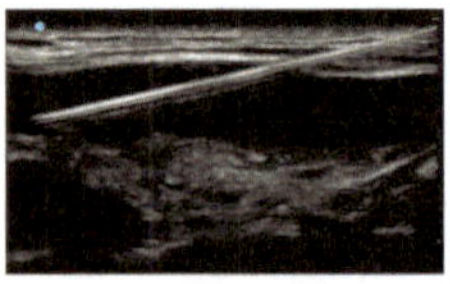
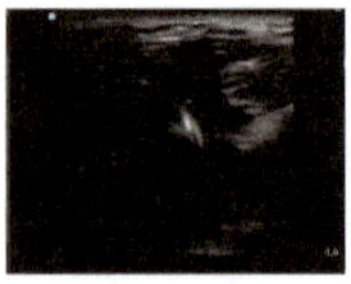

6. Confirm catheter position in the vein

a. Confirm the position of the catheter inside the vein in SAX and LAX
b. Confirm free flow of blood from the hubs

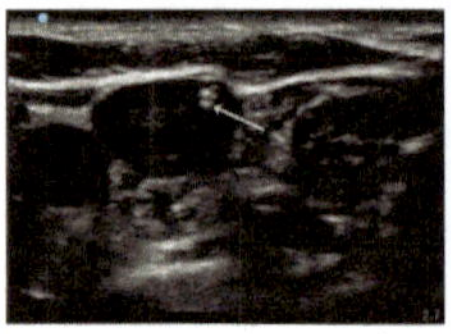
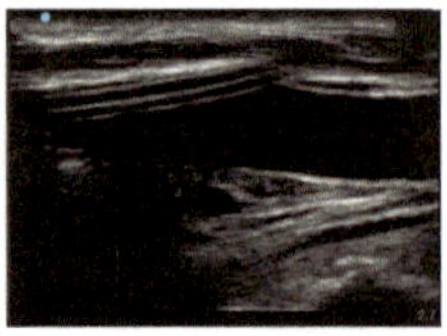

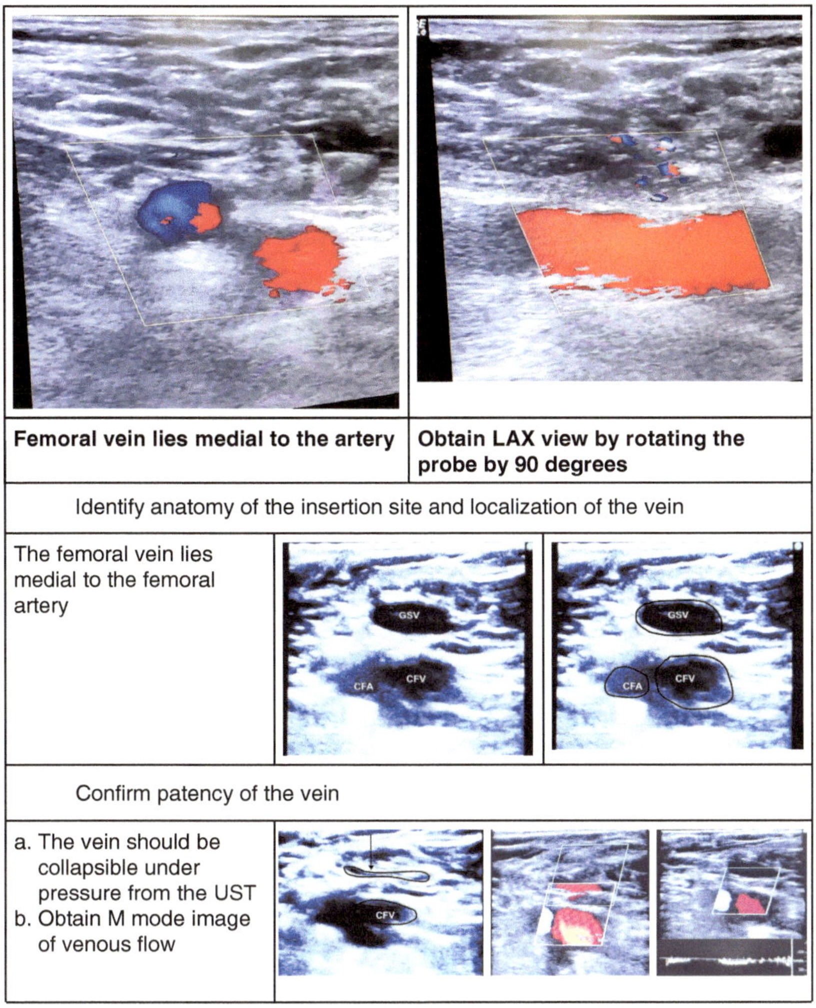

Fig. 2.13 Femoral vein cannulation

Use real time US guidance for puncture of the vein	
a. The FV can be punctured in SAX or LAX view. b. Image the needle tip in the center of the vein (arrows).	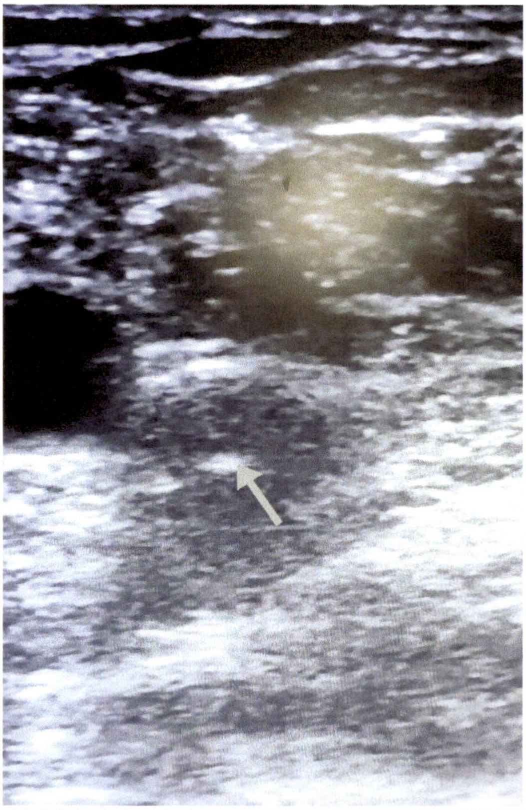
	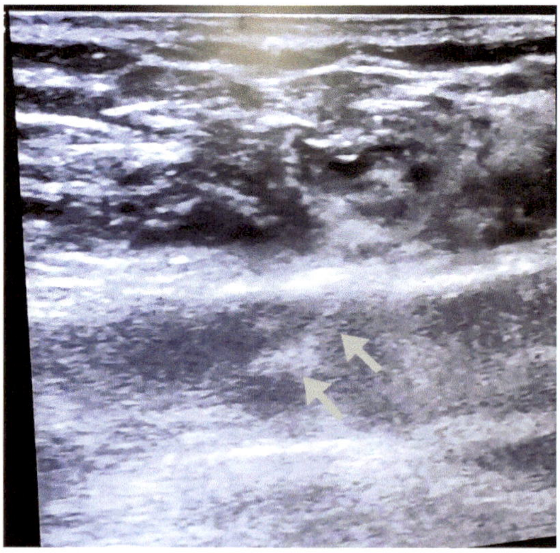

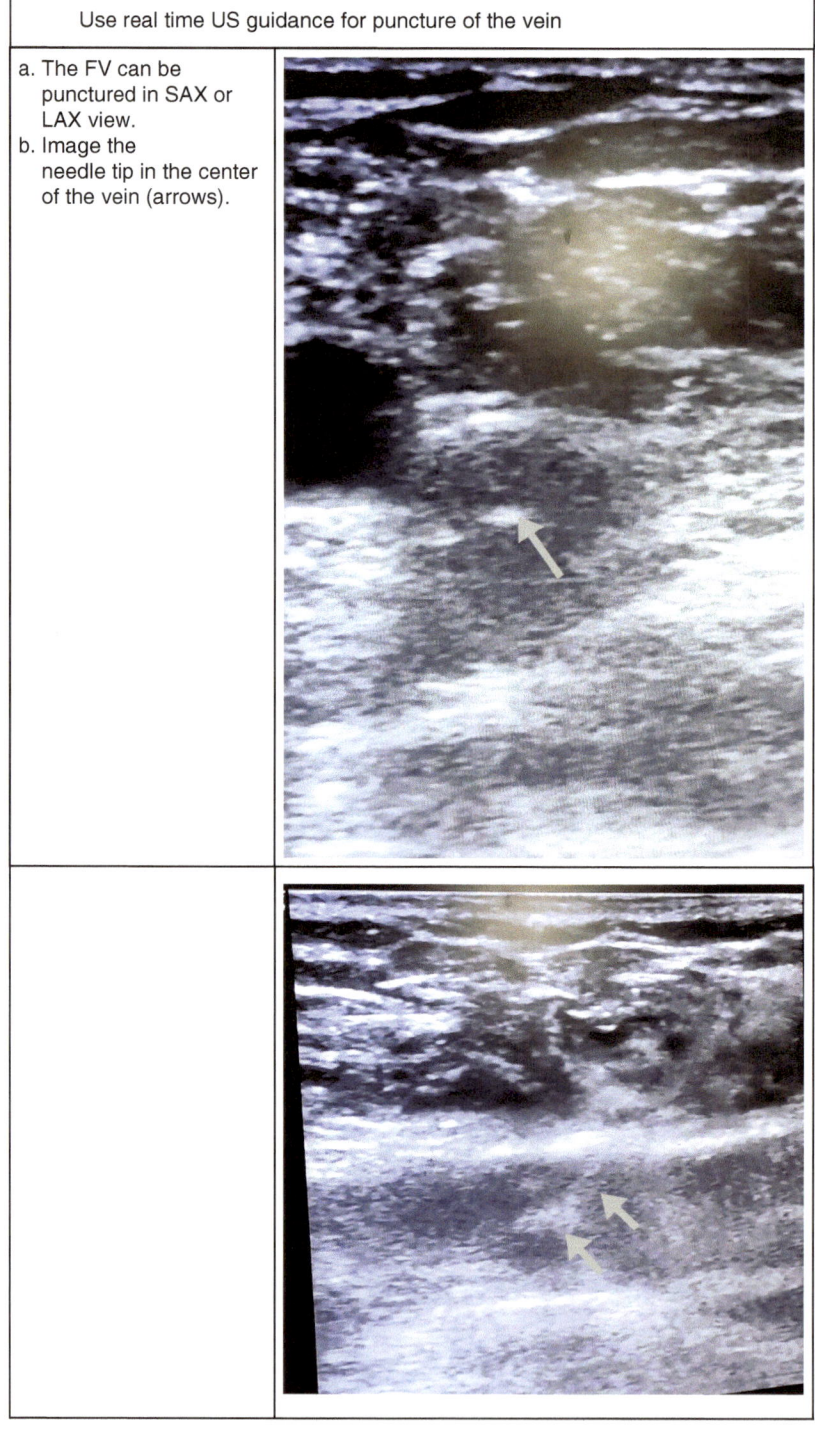

Fig. 2.13 (continued)

Confirm wire position in the vein	
	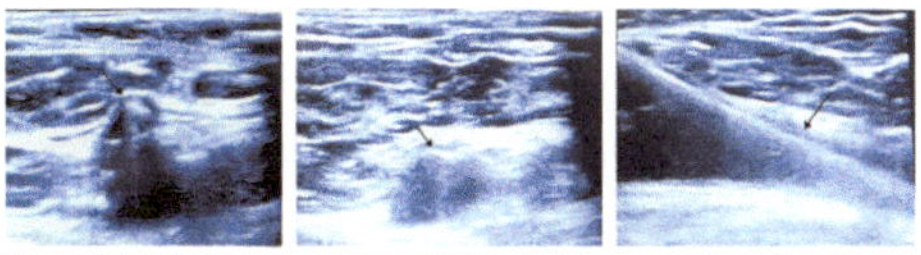
Confirm catheter position in the vein	
The catheter can be imaged inside the vein in LAX or SAX view. In the SAX, a "target" sign can be seen.	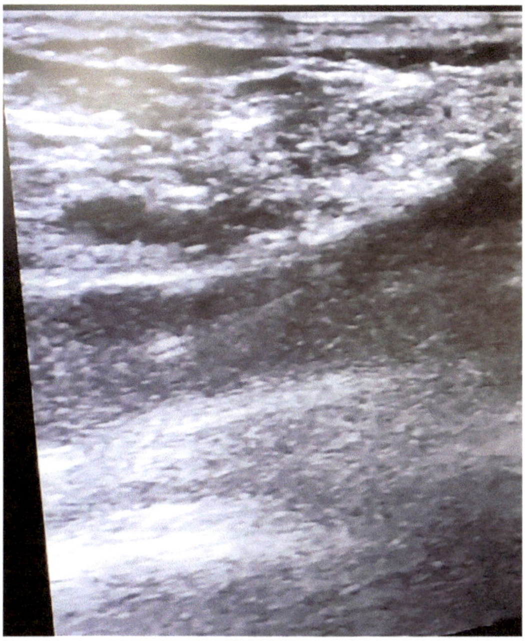

Fig. 2.13 (continued)

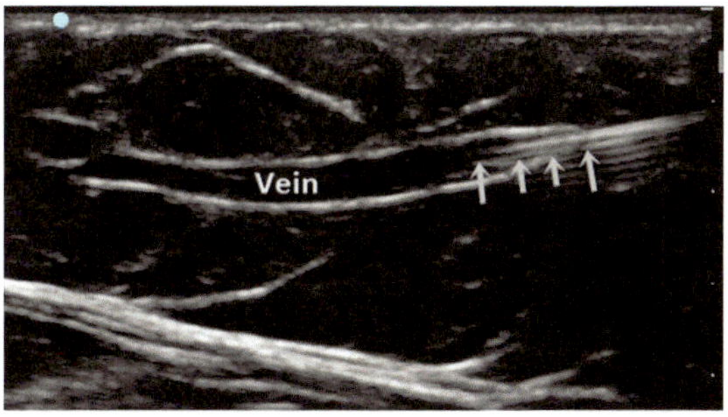

Fig. 2.14 Venous cannulation in the long-axis view and in-plane approach; Arrowheads represent the advancing cannula

- The number of insertion attempts should be based on clinical judgment.
- The decision to place two catheters in a single vein should be made on a case-by-case basis.

2.7.4 Guidance of Needle, Wire, and Catheter Placement

- Use real-time ultrasound guidance for vessel localization and venipuncture when the internal jugular vein is selected for cannulation (Fig. 2.21).

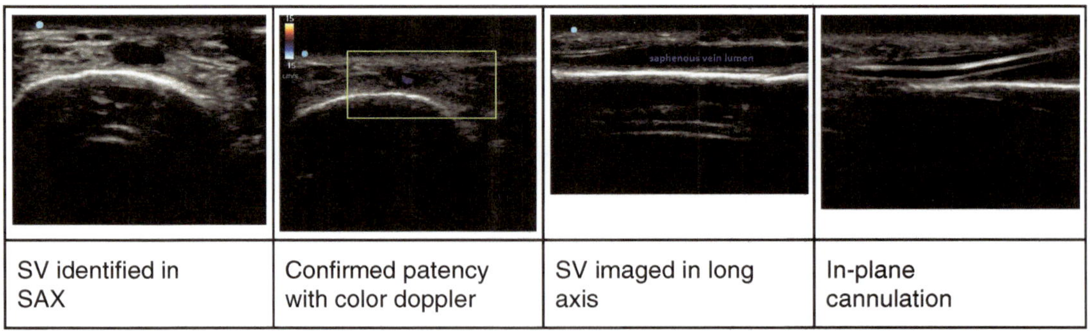

saphenous vein lumen
SV identified in SAX
Confirmed patency with color doppler
SV imaged in long axis
In-plane cannulation

Fig. 2.15 Cannulation of the saphenous vein (SV)

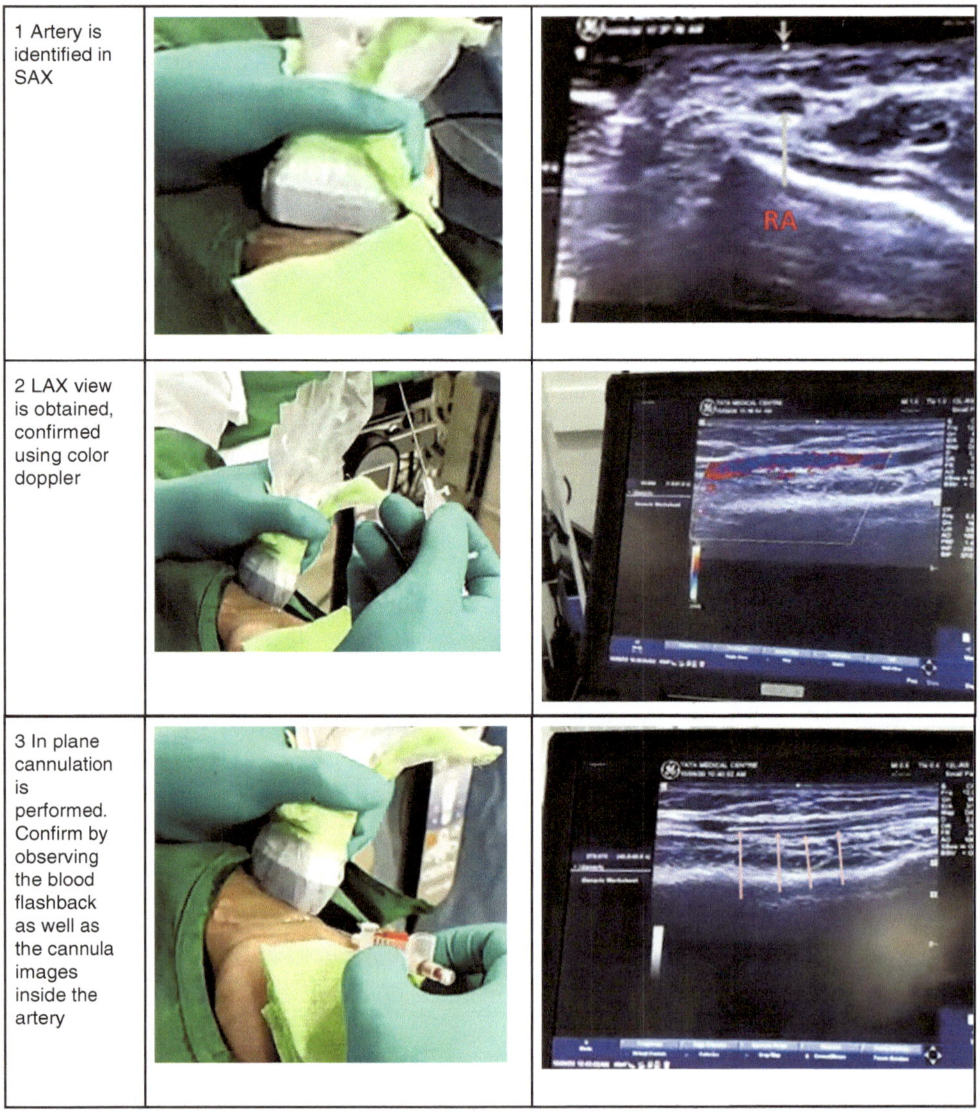

Fig. 2.16 Cannulation of the radial artery in 3 steps: 1. Identification of the artery in the short-axis view, 2. Long-axis view with color Doppler, 3. In-plane cannulation with real-time imaging (note the blood in the hub and the cannula inside the artery—arrows)

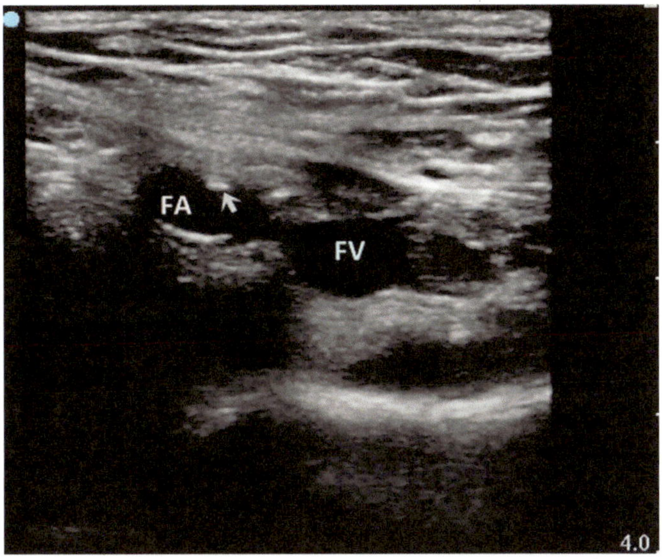

Fig. 2.17 Cannulation of the femoral artery in short-axis view; note the needle tip (Arrow) inside the artery

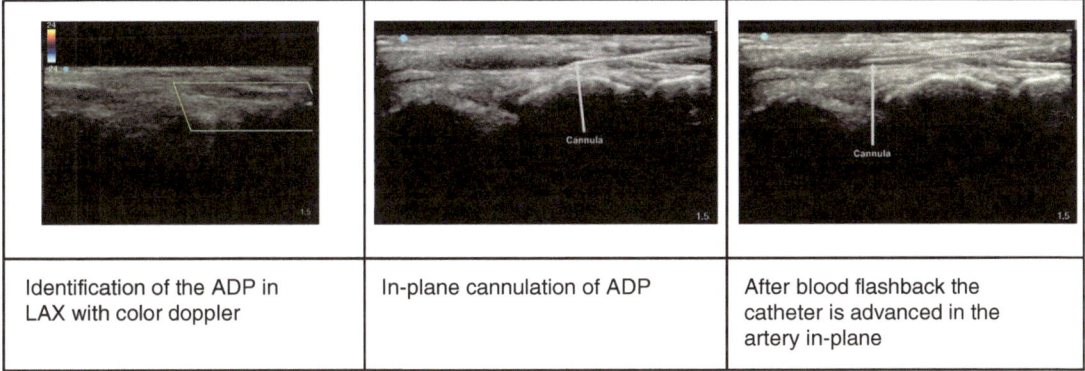

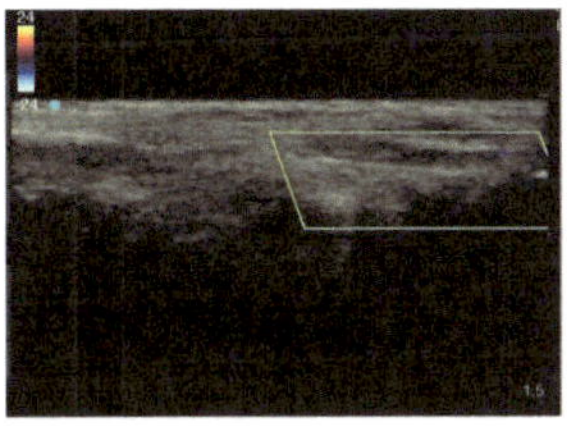	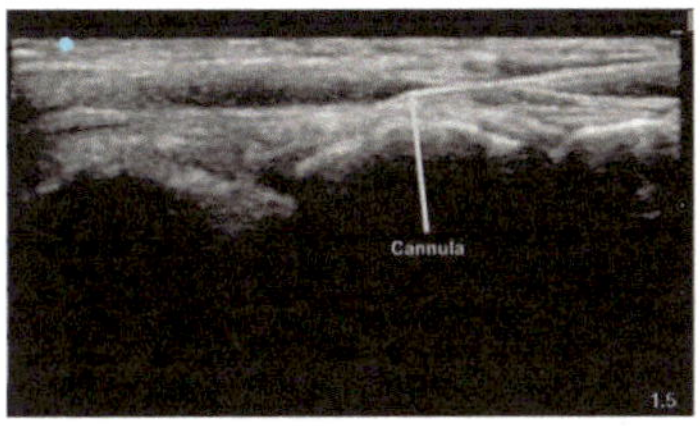	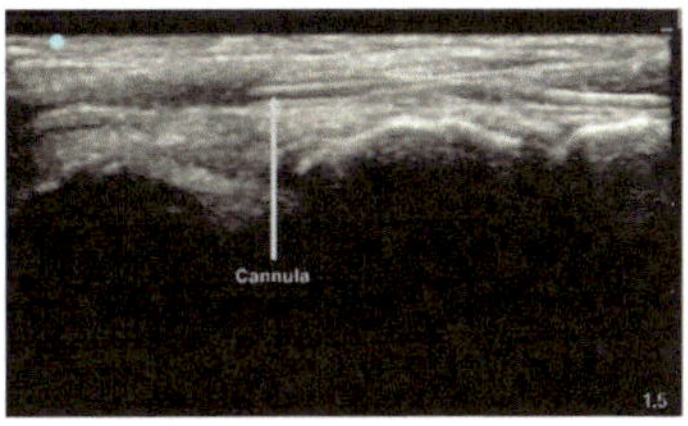
Identification of the ADP in LAX with color doppler	In-plane cannulation of ADP	After blood flashback the catheter is advanced in the artery in-plane

Fig. 2.18 Arteria dorsalis pedis (ADP) cannulation

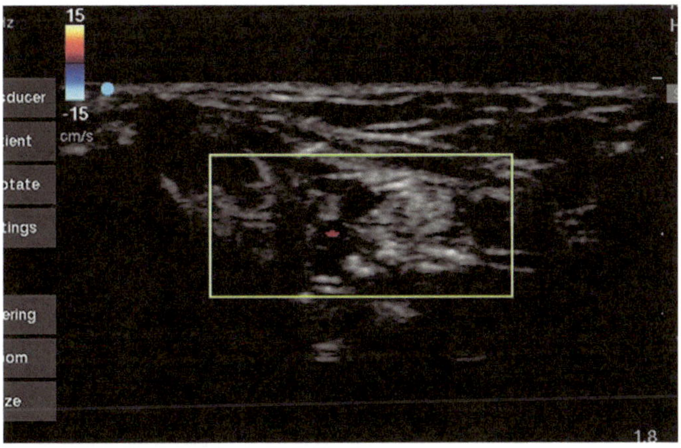

Fig. 2.19 Short-axis view of the posterior tibial artery with color Doppler (note the red color)

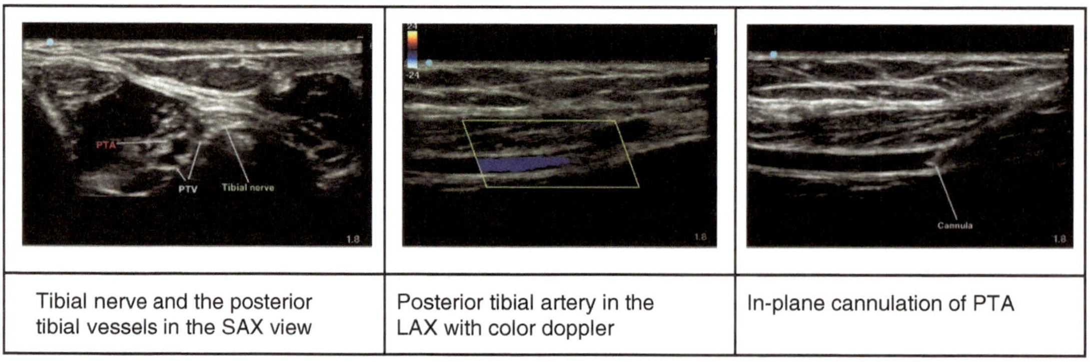

PTA
PTV
Tibial nerve
Cannula
Tibial nerve and the posterior tibial vessels in the SAX view
Posterior tibial artery in the LAX with color doppler
In-plane cannulation of PTA

Fig. 2.20 Cannulation of posterior tibial artery

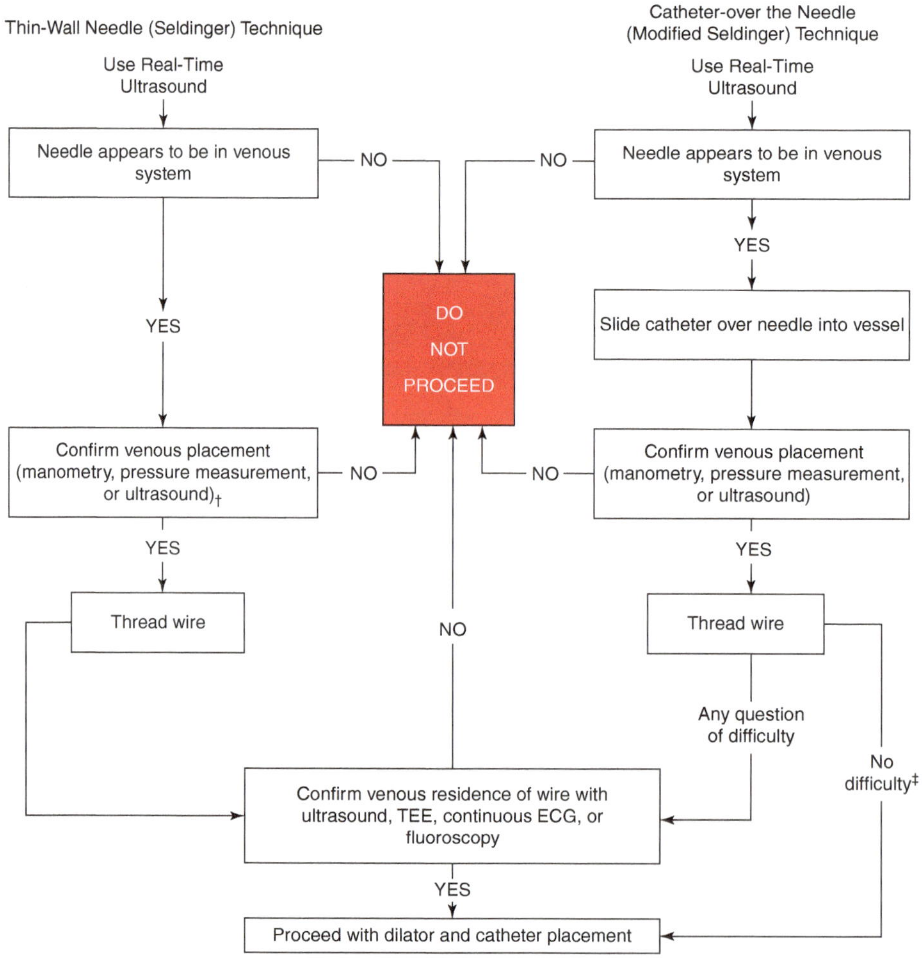

Fig. 2.21 Algorithm for central venous insertion and verification. This algorithm compares the thin-wall needle (i.e., Seldinger) technique vs the catheter-over-the needle (i.e., modified Seldinger) technique in critical safety steps to prevent unintentional arterial placement of a dilator or large-bore catheter. The variation between the two techniques reflects mitigation steps for the risk that the thin-wall needle in the Seldinger technique could move out of the vein and into the wall of an artery between the manometry step and the threading of the wire step. ECG, electrocardiography; TEE, transesophageal echocardiography. †For neonates, infants, and children, confirmation of venous placement may take place after the wire is threaded. ‡Consider confirming venous residence of the wire [1].

- When feasible, real-time ultrasound may be used when the subclavian or femoral vein is selected.
- Use static ultrasound imaging before prepping and draping for prepuncture identification of anatomy to determine vessel localization and patency when the internal jugular vein is selected for cannulation.
  - Static ultrasound may also be used when the subclavian or femoral vein is selected.

2.7.5 Verification of Needle, Wire, and Catheter Placement

- After insertion of a catheter that went over the needle or a thin-wall needle, confirm venous access.
  - Do not rely on blood color or absence of pulsatile flow for confirming that the catheter or thin-wall needle resides in the vein.
- When using the thin-wall needle technique, confirm venous residence of the wire after the wire is threaded.
  - When using the catheter-over-the-needle technique, confirmation that the wire resides in the vein may not be needed (1) when the catheter enters the vein easily and manometry or pressure-waveform measurement provides unambiguous confirmation of venous location of the catheter and (2) when the wire passes through the catheter and enters the vein without difficulty.
  - If there is any uncertainty that the catheter or wire resides in the vein, confirm venous residence of the wire after the wire is threaded; insertion of a dilator or large-bore catheter may then proceed.
- After final catheterization and before use, confirm residence of the catheter in the venous system as soon as clinically appropriate.
- Confirm the final position of the catheter tip as soon as clinically appropriate.
  - For central venous catheters placed in the operating room, perform a chest radiograph no later than the early postoperative period to confirm the position of the catheter tip.
- Verify that the wire has not been retained in the vascular system at the end of the procedure by confirming the presence of the removed wire in the procedural field.
  - If the complete guidewire is not found in the procedural field, order chest radiography to determine whether the guidewire has been retained in the patient's vascular system.

2.8 Recommendations for Management of Arterial Trauma or Injury Arising from Central Venous Access

- When unintended cannulation of an arterial vessel with a dilator or large-bore catheter occurs, leave the dilator or catheter in place and immediately consult a general surgeon, a vascular surgeon, or an interventional radiologist regarding surgical or nonsurgical catheter removal for adults.
- For neonates, infants, and children, determine on a case-by-case basis whether to leave the catheter in place and obtain consultation or to remove the catheter nonsurgically.
- After the injury has been evaluated and a treatment plan has been executed, confer with the surgeon regarding relative risks and benefits of proceeding with the elective surgery vs deferring surgery to allow for a period of patient observation.

2.8.1 Resource Preparation

- Perform central venous catheterization in an environment that permits use of aseptic techniques.
- Ensure that a standardized equipment set is available for central venous access.
- Use a checklist or protocol for placement and maintenance of central venous catheters.
- Use an assistant during placement of a central venous catheter.

2.8.2 Prevention of Infectious Complications

2.8.2.1 Intravenous Antibiotic Prophylaxis

- Do not routinely administer intravenous antibiotic prophylaxis.

2.8.2.2 Aseptic Preparation

- In preparation for the placement of central venous catheters, use aseptic techniques (e.g., hand washing) and maximal barrier precautions (e.g., sterile gowns, sterile gloves, caps, masks covering both mouth and nose, full-body patient drapes, and eye protection).

2.8.2.3 Selection of Antiseptic Solution

- Use a chlorhexidine-containing solution for skin preparation in adults, infants, and children.
  - For neonates, determine the use of chlorhexidine-containing solutions for skin preparation based on clinical judgment and institutional protocol.
- If there is a contraindication to chlorhexidine, povidone–iodine or alcohol may be used.
- Unless contraindicated, use skin preparation solutions containing alcohol.

2.8.2.4 Catheters Containing Antimicrobial Agents

- For selected patients, use catheters coated with antibiotics, a combination of chlorhexidine and silver sulfadiazine, or silver-platinum-carbon–impregnated catheters based on risk of infection and anticipated duration of catheter use.
  - Do not use catheters containing antimicrobial agents as a substitute for additional infection precautions.

2.8.2.5 Catheter Fixation

- Minimize the number of needle punctures on the skin.

2.8.2.6 Insertion Site Dressings

- Use transparent biocclusive dressings to protect the site of central venous catheter insertion from infection.
- Unless contraindicated, dressings containing chlorhexidine may be used in adults, infants, and children.
- For neonates, determine the use of transparent or sponge dressings containing chlorhexidine based on clinical judgment and institutional protocol.
- If a chlorhexidine-containing dressing is used, observe the site daily for signs of irritation, allergy, or necrosis.

2.8.2.7 Catheter Maintenance

- Determine the duration of catheterization based on clinical need.
- Assess the clinical need for keeping the catheter in place on a daily basis.
- Remove catheters promptly when no longer deemed clinically necessary.
- Inspect the catheter insertion site daily for signs of infection.
- Change or remove the catheter when catheter insertion site infection is suspected.
- When a catheter-related infection is suspected, a new insertion site may be used for catheter replacement rather than changing the catheter over a guidewire.

2.9 Aseptic Techniques Using an Existing Central Venous Catheter for Injection or Aspiration

- Clean catheter access ports with an appropriate antiseptic (e.g., alcohol) before each access when using an existing central venous catheter for injection or aspiration.
- Cap central venous catheter stopcocks or access ports when not in use.
- Needleless catheter access ports may be used on a case-by-case basis.

2.10 Recognized Benefits and Concerns about Ultrasound-Guided Vascular Access

2.10.1 Recognized Benefits

Traditionally cannulation of vascular structures are based on palpatory and landmark-based techniques. Ultrasound(US)-guided vascular cannulation has shown to improve success rate in the first attempt, reduce the number of overall attempts, improve patient's satisfaction and reduce overall procedure-related complications [50–54].

US aid leads to increased success rates of catheter placement in the first attempt, both in central venous catheters [55] and arterial catheters, in adults and children [56]. Shiloh et al. [57] reported an increase of 71% in the success rate of radial artery catheterizations.

Estimates of the complication rate of central venous catheterization without the use of US range between 5% and 19% [58, 59]. Us-guided vascular punctures lead to reduced complications associated with traditional techniques, such as failure of catheter placements, arterial puncture, hematoma formation, hemothorax, and pneumothorax. Hind et al. [55] in a meta-analysis compared central venous catheterization using US-guided puncture with those carried out by traditional methods. They reported a reduction of 86% in relative risk of catheter placement failures using ultrasonography, 57% reduction was seen in relative risk of mechanical complications ($p = 0.02$).

In another systematic review, which included cannulation of various central venous structures, it was reported that US aid leads to reduction of 82% of relative risk of failure of catheterization and significantly less occurrence of arterial punctures, local hematomas, pneumothorax, and hemothorax had a reduction of relative risk of 75%, 70%, 79%, and 90%, respectively [60].

US-guided cannulations lead to cost saving. Calvert et al. estimated a saving of 2000 pounds for each thousand venous central catheterization guided by ultrasonography compared with those guided by anatomic parameters [61]. Reduction in the average time spent in the procedure is also reported as fewer attempts are needed to successfully puncture the vessel [56].

US is found to be useful in patients with bleeding diathesis or coagulopathies. Using the traditional method, Fisher et al. [57] reported a rate of 9% of minor complications (hematoma formation and bleeding on puncture site) in patients with abnormal platelet count or coagulation parameters. In another study, no major complications were reported in 133 patients with deranged coagulation. Bleeding on puncture site or formation of small hematomas was observed in 6% of cases [62, 63]. Similar findings were reported while subclavian venous cannulation under US guidance in patients with deranged coagulation parameters [64].

US is useful in patients who are obese, edematous, have hematomas from previous attempts, or have weak or missing arterial pulsations. During cardiopulmonary resuscitation, US can visualize the vascular anatomy without relying on an arterial pulsation [65]. In patients with nonpulsatile ventricular assist device in situ, the peripheral pulses are weak or absent and most of them are anticoagulated, inadvertent arterial puncture during central venous cannulation may lead to serious complications [66].

In addition, US can be used to screen for vessel patency, vascular abnormalities, and anatomical variations, which can be useful in patients having variations in the relationship between the internal jugular vein and carotid artery [67, 68].

There are very few alternatives to using US and obtaining visual feedback during vessel cannulation. Most of them, such as fluoroscopy, are not as readily available, require specialized training and certification, and cost.

2.11 Concerns and Limitations of us-Guided Vascular Access

US itself is noninvasive and does not cause any harm to the patient directly, but it guides an invasive procedure (needle/catheter insertion into a vessel), and, thus, may result in complications. The following concerns can be identified while using US for vascular puncture/cannulation.

The operator is usually busy looking at the US screen searching for the needle, which is always not clearly visible especially during the out-of-plane approach, which can lead to inadvertent carotid puncture. The needle also may exit the posterior wall of the jugular vein and enter the carotid artery [69]. The long-axis approach may not prevent this complication as the carotid artery is not visualized side by side, and a slight oblique needle orientation may not allow proper needle visualization. Therefore, the incidence of carotid puncture during right IJV cannulation can be as high as 4% [70] despite using US [71–73]. Similarly during subclavian vein cannulation, inadvertent puncture of the pleura may result in a pneumothorax.

In patients with shorter neck anatomy, the long-axis US view of the internal jugular vein may be difficult to obtain. The use of US to puncture the subclavian vein results in a puncture site that is usually more lateral compared to the landmark puncture technique. The close proximity of the vessels and the pleura must be kept in mind because the angle of cannulation is usually steeper when using US, it is especially important to align and constantly visualize the needle to avoid pleural injury [74].

US guidance does not necessarily mean correct placement of the guidewire in the vascular lumen, rather the visualization of the guidewire in the venous lumen via peripheral ultrasonography can be misleading as the wire may have punctured the posterior wall and entered the carotid artery [75].

Other concerns of US-guided vascular access are infections if a proper aseptic technique is not applied, procedural delays due to nonavailability of the equipment, and the costs involved with the buying and maintaining the US equipment [76].

Routine US use may result in a "de-skilling" of the landmark-based techniques as they are less taught and practiced nowadays, which might result in higher complication rates when US is not available [76].

To achieve adequate skills for using US skills high-quality care, formal education and training (including simulation) with a structured certification of US skills for vascular access and the development of a consensus standard for these training programs have been suggested.

2.12 Training

2.12.1 Training for Ultrasound-Guided Vascular Cannulations

Vascular cannulation is an important aspect of patient care for the administration of fluids and medications and for monitoring purposes. Due to better safety profile, ultrasound (US)-assisted vascular cannulation is being preferred over classic landmark-based techniques. Literature regarding training, supervision, and competence needed regarding central venous access device (CVAD) insertion is scarce and not fully standardized. No standard didactic or simulation training is required before CVAD insertions by clinicians in training, neither the role, experience, or competence of the supervisor is specified [77].

Ultrasound guidance CVAD insertion needs education and training to ensure patient safety and avoid major complications with the insertion of CVAD [78–82].

Understanding of basic anatomy, ultrasound physics and imaging, and infection prevention strategies are necessary [45, 83].

Multiple training techniques have been described to aid the use of ultrasound for central venous cannulation [45, 84]. All forms of training should lay importance on developing proficiency in both cognitive and psychomotor skill sets and must include image acquisition, interpretation, real-time use of ultrasound for vessel puncture and cannulation, and an experienced instructor who demonstrates to the trainee how to translate 2D imaging to perform a 3D task [85].

In 2013, an international evidence-based consensus task force was established through the World Congress of Vascular Access (WoCoVA) to provide definitions and recommendations for training and insertion of CVADs.

The task force proposed 16 recommendations.

1. Anatomy and physiology of relevant body system.
2. Ultrasound for insertion and assessment.
3. Central venous device tip location.
4. Infection control and sterile technique.
5. Device selection and indications.
6. Insertion procedures, complication prevention, evaluation, and management.
7. Care and maintenance practices.
8. Qualification and competency.
9. Simulation training.
10. Anatomical models.
11. Objective grading and proficiency.
12. Examination and competency.

13. Supervised instruction.
14. Didactic or web-based training.
15. Developing clinical competence.
16. Education for children and neonates.

Simulation-based education has recently emerged as an important learning tool in several areas of surgical expertise [86, 87] and it is particularly useful for teaching invasive procedures such as CVAD insertion, which require eye-hand coordination and ambidextrous maneuvers [88, 89]. Simulation allows residents-in-training to repeatedly practice a procedure prior to performing it on a living patient and also has potential benefits to improve provider performance, to reduce errors, and, ultimately, to enhance patient safety.

Multiple studies have assessed the learning effect of a standardized simulation-based teaching program on ultrasound-guided cannulation in a low-cost cadaver tissue model. Some of them have used avian muscle, chicken or turkey thigh and have inserted fluid-filled latex/elastic tubes, into cadaver tissue to mimic vessels to create a model for central venous catheterization, while others have used latex, gelatin, or silicone rubber models, where plastic structures simulating central vessels are inserted. Successful attempts, number of failed attempts, and insertion times were evaluated as end-points of the training module.

There is a paucity of literature to specifically suggest the number of procedures necessary to develop competence in performing real-time ultrasound cannulation. One has to be mindful of the fact that clinicians acquire knowledge and develop dexterity for the technique at different rates. The opinion among expert users with >10 years of experience with this technique has suggested that training includes a minimum of 10 procedures performed under the guidance of an experienced user.

There are no clear recommendations on the total number of hours that trainees must practice to acquire US-guided CVC skills. In fact, The American College of Emergency Physicians recommends that all US practitioners should undergo initial basic US training varying in length from 1 to 2 days followed by at least 25 documented and reviewed cases of primary applications including US-guided procedures such as central venous cannulations.

There is a need for establishing consistency in the development of training programs and measuring competency through completion of didactic lessons, simulation, examination, and supervised practice. More research is necessary to establish stronger recommendations and clearer directives.

2.13 Conclusion

Using ultrasound for vascular cannulations is an important skill a physician should learn and keep on practicing. Using ultrasound increases success rate, reduces complications, and thereby reduces the cost of health care. In the near future ultrasound is going to become more and more available for all healthcare workers making the skill of ultrasound-guided vascular cannulations essential for a successful physician.

POCUS Pearls

- A shallower angle of the needle is required for cannulating superficial and smaller vessels.
- Deeper vessels are better cannulated with a steep needle angle to facilitate location of the needle tip.
- While cannulating the radial artery, make sure the BP cuff is on the other hand or the automatic cycle timer is off if it is on the same hand.
- Check the BP before arterial cannulation. If the pressure is low, expect difficulty and consider administration of a short acting vasoactive agent such as phenylephrine to increase BP temporarily.

Self Assessment Questions: (Answer Keys at the End of the Chapter)

1. When using ultrasound to assist in cannulation of the radial artery, which of the following techniques are recommended
   A. Artery can be identified by color Doppler
   B. Angle of the entry is usually about 30° or less
   C. Distance from the center of the probe to point of entry varies between individuals
   D. Out-of-plane technique is usually used
   E. All of the above
2. When using ultrasound to identify structures for vascular cannulation, which of the following options can be used to confirm that a blood vessel is vein?
   A. Color Doppler showing blue Doppler flow
   B. Compressibility under the gentle pressure of ultrasound probe
   C. Presence of hypoechoic content within the lumen and posterior wall showing enhancement artifact
   D. Pulsed wave Doppler showing pulsatile waveform
   E. Identifying surrounding structures
3. No flashback is seen in the hub during cannulation of the peripheral vein under ultrasound guidance. What is the most likely reason for this?
   A. Low-frequency ultrasound probe is being used
   B. Patient is hypotensive
   C. The vein is thrombosed
   D. Venous valve is preventing any flashback
   E. Wrong depth is being targeted
4. During internal jugular vein (IJV) cannulation, which of the following steps can be taken to minimize the risk of inadvertent arterial puncture?
   A. Avoid hyperextension and sideway rotation of head at the time of positioning
   B. Identify the lateral and medial wall of the IJV before entering the skin
   C. Note the depth of the needle entering the skin at any time
   D. Scan up and down the IJV to identify the point of puncture where there is minimum overlap with common carotid artery (CCA)
   E. All of the above
5. During cannulation of the femoral vein, which of the following steps should be done to ensure proper placement of the central venous catheter?
   A. Confirm guidewire position on short-axis view (SAX) with the ultrasound probe placed parallel to the inguinal crease
   B. Ensure free flow of blood from the cannula
   C. Place ultrasound probe on the inguinal crease
   D. Slide ultrasound probe up and down to follow the needle tip and advance only when needle is visualized
   E. Visualize the femoral vein to be lateral to the superficial femoral artery
6. When cannulating the IJV, which one of the following statements is true
   A. CCA lies directly posterior to IJV hence when both vessels are observed to be overlapping significantly, cannulation can still occur at that position
   B. In short-axis view (SAX), the echogenic point seen is always the tip of the needle
   C. Long-axis view of the IJV can prevent carotid artery puncture and hence always required prior to cannulation
   D. Once placement of guidewire is confirmed on ultrasound, arterial puncture is unlikely
   E. None of the above
7. During cannulation of the subclavian veins, which one of the following statements is true
   A. In an infraclavicular approach, the ultrasound probe is first placed perpendicular to the clavicles to identify all the vascular structures
   B. In-plane approach is usually taken for cannulation to avoid pleura puncture
   C. Subclavian artery must be visualized prior to cannulation
   D. Subclavian vein lies superior to the subclavian artery

E. All of the above

8. When cannulating radial artery, which of the following statement is true
   A. Ensure the patient is not hypotensive
   B. Blood pressure cuff should not be applied onto the same arm
   C. Needle often enters at a shallow angle
   D. When using needle in catheter technique and flashback is obtained, a few mm more can be inserted to avoid kinking of the catheter during advancement
   E. All of the above
9. After placement of the needle and flashback obtained during cannulation of the central vein, what would be the immediate next step?
   A. Insertion of guidewire through the needle
   B. Confirmation of needle position within the vascular lumen via ultrasound
   C. Dilation of vein to admit the central line catheter
   D. Flush with saline and observe them for bubbles within the lumen on ultrasound
   E. Draw blood to test for blood gas
10. When performing infraclavicular subclavian vein insertion, which of the following complications can be avoided if needle tip is constantly visualized
    I. Central line catheter entry into common carotid artery
    II. Central line catheter entry into IJV
    III. Pleura puncture and pneumothorax
    IV. Subclavian artery puncture
       A. I
       B. I and II
       C. II
       D. III and IV
       E. All of the above
11. When using catheter-over-needle technique, ultrasound confirmation of guidewire in the vein is not necessary when the following occurs:
    A. Blood gas performed through the catheter unambiguously shows venous origin
    B. Guidewire can enter the vein without any difficulty
    C. When transduced, central venous waveforms are shown
    D. When the catheter enters the vein easily with no resistance
    E. All of the above
12. When inadvertent arterial trauma occurs after a dilator or large-bore catheter is introduced during central venous catheter placement, what would be the immediate next step?
    A. Do not proceed further
    B. Flush the large-bore catheter
    C. Put back the guidewire through the dilator
    D. Place patient in Trendelenburg position
    E. Remove the dilator immediately
13. Which of the following methods is the most effective in minimizing central line associated bloodstream infection?
    A. Aseptic placement technique at the time of placement
    B. Assess clinical need for catheter daily and remove catheter promptly when no longer deemed clinically necessary
    C. Clean catheter access ports with an appropriate antiseptic solution before each access
    D. Routine use of intravenous antibiotics prophylaxis
    E. Use of chlorhexidine-containing solution for skin preparation during placement of CVL
14. Which of the following option determines the angle of entry of the needle during ultrasound-guided CVL placement?
    A. Distance from footprint of the ultrasound probe to the point of entry
    B. Depth of the target vein
    C. Location of the CVL
    D. Weight of the patient
    E. All of the above
15. When planning for subclavian vein cannulation, which of the following statement is true with regard to the anatomical relations of the subclavian vein?
    A. Axillary vein can be seen joining the subclavian vein

B. Internal jugular vein can be seen joining the subclavian vein above the clavicle
C. Pleura can be seen inferior to the subclavian vein
D. Subclavian artery lies posterior to the subclavian vein
E. All of the above

16. Difficult cannulation is expected for an obese individual who requires CVL placement. Which of the following should be considered during the preparation?
A. High-frequency linear transducer with a large footprint
B. Low-frequency curvilinear probe with a large footprint
C. Hockey stick transducer with a small footprint
D. High-frequency linear transducer with a small footprint
E. None of the above

17. When cannulating the femoral for CVL placement, which of the following statement is true with regard to the anatomical relations of the femoral vein?
A. Femoral artery is the most medial structure
B. Femoral vein lies lateral to the femoral artery
C. Femoral vein lies medial to the femoral artery
D. Femoral vein lies next to the femoral nerve
E. None of the above

18. Which of the following options can accurately assess IJV CVL position tip?
I. Chest radiography
II. Vascular ultrasound imaging
III. Intracavitary electrocardiography
IV. Transthoracic echocardiography
A. III
B. I and II
C. II and IV
D. II, III, and IV
E. I, II, III, and IV

19. Which of the following statement is true with regard to long-axis (LAX) in-plane and short-axis (SAX) out-of-plane approach to ultrasound-guided CVL insertion?
A. LAX in-plane approach is preferred as the depth of the needle tip can be seen and hence reducing the risk of arterial puncture
B. LAX in-plane approach allows the entire needle to be visualized and hence success rate is higher
C. SAX out-of-plane approach allows better visualization of vein in relation to the artery and helps to avoid accidental arterial puncture
D. SAX out-of-plane approach allows the entire needle to be visualized and hence reducing the risk of arterial puncture
E. SAX out-of-plane approach allows needle tip to be visualized and can help to minimize the risk of posterior wall puncture

20. Which of the following statement is true with regard to limitations of US-guided CVL insertion
A. Arterial puncture is not possible if CVL is inserted under US guidance
B. Central line infection rate is higher when US is used for CVL insertion
C. In obese patients with short neck, the use of linear probe and long-axis view is necessary in order to increase change of successful puncture
D. When using US in CVL insertion, an inexperienced user might focus on the US images and neglect traditional principles with regard to needle direction
E. None of the above

References

1. Practice Guidelines for Central Venous Access. An Updated Report by the American Society of Anesthesiologists Task Force on Central Venous Access. Anesthesiology. 2020;2020(132):8–43. https://doi.org/10.1097/ALN.0000000000002864.
2. Bansal R, Agarwal SK, Tiwari SC, Dash SC. A prospective randomized study to compare ultrasound-guided with nonultrasound-guided double lumen internal jugular catheter insertion as a temporary hemodialysis access. Ren Fail. 2005;27:561–4.
3. Cajozzo M, Quintini G, Cocchiera G, Greco G, Vaglica R, Pezzano G, Barbera V, Modica G. Comparison of

central venous catheterization with and without ultrasound guide. Transfus Apher Sci. 2004;31:199–202.
4. Dolu H, Goksu S, Sahin L, Ozen O, Eken L. Comparison of an ultrasound-guided technique versus a landmark-guided technique for internal jugular vein cannulation. J Clin Monit Comput. 2015;29:177–82.
5. Mallory DL, McGee WT, Shawker TH, Brenner M, Bailey KR, Evans RG, Parker MM, Farmer JC, Parillo JE. Ultrasound guidance improves the success rate of internal jugular vein cannulation: a prospective, randomized trial. Chest. 1990;98:157–60.
6. Milling TJ Jr, Rose J, Briggs WM, Birkhahn R, Gaeta TJ, Bove JJ, Melniker LA. Randomized, controlled clinical trial of point-of-care limited ultrasonography assistance of central venous cannulation: the third sonography outcomes assessment program (SOAP-3) trial. Crit Care Med. 2005;33:1764–9.
7. Shrestha BR, Gautam B. Ultrasound versus the landmark technique: a prospective randomized comparative study of internal jugular vein cannulation in an intensive care unit. JNMA J Nepal Med Assoc. 2011;51:56–61.
8. Slama M, Novara A, Safavian A, Ossart M, Safar M, Fagon JY. Improvement of internal jugular vein cannulation using an ultrasound-guided technique. Intensive Care Med. 1997;23:916–9.
9. Teichgräber UK, Benter T, Gebel M, Manns MP. A sonographically guided technique for central venous access. AJR Am J Roentgenol. 1997;169:731–3.
10. Troianos CA, Jobes DR, Ellison N. Ultrasound-guided cannulation of the internal jugular vein: a prospective, randomized study. Anesth Analg. 1991;72:823–6.
11. Agarwal A, Singh DK, Singh AP. Ultrasonography: a novel approach to central venous cannulation. Indian J Crit Care Med. 2009;13:213–6.
12. Denys BG, Uretsky BF, Reddy PS. Ultrasound-assisted cannulation of the internal jugular vein: a prospective comparison to the external landmark-guided technique. Circulation. 1993;87:1557–62.
13. Palepu GB, Deven J, Subrahmanyam M, Mohan S. Impact of ultrasonography on central venous catheter insertion in intensive care. Indian J Radiol Imaging. 2009;19:191–8.
14. Verghese ST, McGill WA, Patel RI, Sell JE, Midgley FM, Ruttimann UE. Comparison of three techniques for internal jugular vein cannulation in infants. Paediatr Anaesth. 2000;10:505–11.
15. Verghese ST, McGill WA, Patel RI, Sell JE, Midgley FM, Ruttimann UE. Ultrasound-guided internal jugular venous cannulation in infants: a prospective comparison with the traditional palpation method. Anesthesiology. 1999;91:71–7.
16. Karakitsos D, Labropoulos N, De Groot E, Patrianakos AP, Kouraklis G, Poularas J, Samonis G, Tsoutsos DA, Konstadoulakis MM, Karabinis A. Real-time ultrasound-guided catheterisation of the internal jugular vein: a prospective comparison with the landmark technique in critical care patients. Crit Care. 2006;10:R162.
17. Grebenik CR, Boyce A, Sinclair ME, Evans RD, Mason DG, Martin B. NICE guidelines for central venous catheterization in children: is the evidence base sufficient? Br J Anaesth. 2004;92:827–30.
18. Airapetian N, Maizel J, Langelle F, Modeliar SS, Karakitsos D, Dupont H, Slama M. Ultrasound-guided central venous cannulation is superior to quick-look ultrasound and landmark methods among inexperienced operators: a prospective randomized study. Intensive Care Med. 2013;39:1938–44.
19. Turker G, Kaya FN, Gurbet A, Aksu H, Erdogan C, Atlas A. Internal jugular vein cannulation: an ultrasound-guided technique versus a landmark-guided technique. Clinics (Sao Paulo). 2009;64:989–92.
20. Zanolla GR, Baldisserotto M, Piva J. How useful is ultrasound guidance for internal jugular venous access in children? J Pediatr Surg. 2018;53:789–93.
21. Sulek CA, Blas ML, Lobato EB. A randomized study of left versus right internal jugular vein cannulation in adults. J Clin Anesth. 2000;12:142–5.
22. Gualtieri E, Deppe SA, Sipperly ME, Thompson DR. Subclavian venous catheterization: greater success rate for less experienced operators using ultrasound guidance. Crit Care Med. 1995;23:692–7.
23. Fragou M, Gravvanis A, Dimitriou V, Papalois A, Kouraklis G, Karabinis A, Saranteas T, Poularas J, Papanikolaou J, Davlouros P, Labropoulos N, Karakitsos D. Real-time ultrasound-guided subclavian vein cannulation versus the landmark method in critical care patients: a prospective randomized study. Crit Care Med. 2011;39:1607–12.
24. Oh AY, Jeon YT, Choi EJ, Ryu JH, Hwang JW, Park HP, Do SH. The influence of the direction of J-tip on the placement of a subclavian catheter: real time ultrasound-guided cannulation versus landmark method: a randomized controlled trial. BMC Anesthesiol. 2014;14:11.
25. Aouad MT, Kanazi GE, Abdallah FW, Moukaddem FH, Turbay MJ, Obeid MY, Siddik-Sayyid SM. Femoral vein cannulation performed by residents: a comparison between ultrasound-guided and landmark technique in infants and children undergoing cardiac surgery. Anesth Analg. 2010;111:724–8.
26. Kusminsky RE. Complications of central venous catheterization. J Am Coll Surg. 2007;204(4):681–96.
27. Jenssen C, Brkljacic B, Hocke M, Ignee A, Piscaglia F, Radzina M, Sidhu PS, Dietrich CF. EFSUMB guidelines on interventional ultrasound (INVUS), part VI - ultrasound-guided vascular interventions. Ultraschall Med. 2016;37(5):473–6.
28. Bhutta ST, Culp WC. Evaluation and management of central venous access complications. Tech Vasc Interv Radiol. 2011;14(4):217–24.
29. Brass P, Hellmich M, Kolodziej L, Schick G, Smith AF. Ultrasound guidance versus anatomical landmarks for internal jugular vein catheterization. Cochrane Database Syst Rev. 2015;1(1):CD006962.
30. Lamperti M, Bodenham AR, Pittiruti M, Blaivas M, Augoustides JG, Elbarbary M, Pirotte T, Karakitsos

D, Ledonne J, Doniger S, Scoppettuolo G, Feller-Kopman D, Schummer W, Biffi R, Desruennes E, Melniker LA, Verghese ST. International evidence-based recommendations on ultrasound-guided vascular access. Intensive Care Med. 2012;38:1105–17.
31. Dietrich CF, Horn R, Morf S, Chiorean L, Dong Y, Cui XW, Atkinson NS, Jenssen C. Ultrasound-guided central vascular interventions, comments on the European Federation of Societies for Ultrasound in Medicine and Biology guidelines on Interventional Ultrasound. J Thorac Dis. 2016;8:E851–68.
32. Wilson JG, Berona KM, Stein JC, Wang R. Oblique-axis vs. short-axis view in ultrasound-guided central venous catheterization. J Emerg Med. 2014;47:45–50.
33. Troianos CA, Hartman GS, Glas KE, Skubas NJ, Eberhardt RT, Walker JD, Reeves ST. Special articles: guidelines for performing ultrasound guided vascular cannulation: recommendations of the American Society of Echocardiography and the Society of Cardiovascular Anesthesiologists. Anesth Analg. 2012;114:46–72.
34. Aithal G, Muthuswamy G, Latif Z, Bhaskaran V, Haji Sani HS, Shindhe S, Manap NBA, Vadaje KS, Dato Paduka Buntar WS, Daiwajna RG. An alternate in-plane technique of ultrasound-guided internal jugular vein cannulation. J Emerg Med. 2019;57(6):852–8.
35. Blaivas M, Brannam L, Fernandez E. Short-axis versus long-axis approaches for teaching ultrasound-guided vascular access on a new inanimate model. Acad Emerg Med. 2003;10:1307–11.
36. Chittoodan S, Breen D, O'Donnell BD, Iohom G. Long versus short axis ultrasound guided approach for internal jugular vein cannulation: a prospective randomised controlled trial. Med Ultrason. 2011;13:21–5.
37. Stone MB, Moon C, Sutijono D, Blaivas M. Needle tip visualization during ultrasound-guided vascular access: short-axis vs long-axis approach. Am J Emerg Med. 2010;28:343–7.
38. Brass P, Hellmich M, Kolodziej L, Schick G, Smith AF. Ultrasound guidance versus anatomical landmarks for subclavian or femoral vein catheterization. Cochrane Database Syst Rev. 2015;1:Cd011447.
39. Lalu MM, Fayad A, Ahmed O, Bryson GL, Fergusson DA, Barron CC, Sullivan P, Thompson C. Ultrasound-guided subclavian vein catheterization: a systematic review and meta-analysis. Crit Care Med. 2015;43:1498–507.
40. Lamperti M, Biasucci DG, Disma N, Pittiruti M, Breschan C, Vailati D, Subert M, Traškaitė V, Macas A, Estebe JP, Fuzier R, Boselli E, Hopkins P. European Society of Anaesthesiology guidelines on peri-operative use of ultrasound-guided for vascular access (PERSEUS vascular access). Eur J Anaesthesiol. 2020;37(5):344–76. https://doi.org/10.1097/EJA.0000000000001180. Erratum in: Eur J Anaesthesiol 2020;37(7):623
41. Keyes LE, Frazee BW, Snoey ER, et-al. Ultrasound-guided brachial and basilic vein cannulation in emergency department patients with difficult intravenous access. Ann Emerg Med. 1999;34(6):711–4.
42. Costantino TG, Parikh AK, Satz WA, et-al. Ultrasonography-guided peripheral intravenous access versus traditional approaches in patients with difficult intravenous access. Ann Emerg Med. 2005;46(5):456–61. https://doi.org/10.1016/j.annemergmed.2004.12.026.
43. Panebianco NL, Fredette JM, Szyld D, Sagalyn EB, Pines JM, Dean AJ. What you see (sonographically) is what you get: vein and patient characteristics associated with successful ultrasound-guided peripheral intravenous placement in patients with difficult access. Acad Emerg Med Off J Soc Acad Emerg Med. 2009;16(12):1298–303. https://doi.org/10.1111/j.1553-2712.2009.00520.x.
44. Gottlieb M, Sundaram T, Holladay D, Nakitende D. Ultrasound-guided peripheral intravenous line placement: a narrative review of evidence-based best practices. West J Emerg Med. 2017;18(6):1047–54. https://doi.org/10.5811/westjem.2017.7.34610.
45. Lamperti M, Bodenham AR, Pittiruti M, Blaivas M, Augoustides JG, Elbarbary M, et al. International evidence-based recommendations on ultrasound-guided vascular access. Intensive Care Med. 2012;38(7):1105–17.
46. Troianos CA, Hartman GS, Glas KE, Skubas NJ, Eberhardt RT, Walker JD, et al. Special articles: guidelines for performing ultrasound guided vascular cannulation: recommendations of the American Society of Echocardiography and the Society of Cardiovascular Anesthesiologists. Anesth Analg. 2012;114(1):46–72.
47. Costantino TG, Parikh AK, Satz WA, Fojtik JP. Ultrasonography-guided peripheral intravenous access versus traditional approaches in patients with difficult intravenous access. Ann Emerg Med. 2005;46(5):456–61.
48. Keyes LE, Frazee BW, Snoey ER, Simon BC, Christy D. Ultrasound-guided brachial and basilic vein cannulation in emergency department patients with difficult intravenous access. Ann Emerg Med. 1999;34(6):711–4.
49. Kim E-H, Lee J-H, Song I-K, Kim J-T, Lee W-J, Kim H-S. Posterior tibial artery as an alternative to the radial artery for arterial cannulation site in small children: a randomized controlled study. Anesthesiology. 2017;127:423–31. https://doi.org/10.1097/ALN.0000000000001774.
50. Hind D, Calvert N, McWilliams R, Davidson A, Paisley S, Beverley C, et al. Ultrasonic locating devices for central venous cannulation: meta-analysis. BMJ. 2003;327(7411):361.
51. Schindler E, Schears GJ, Hall SR, Yamamoto T. Ultrasound for vascular access in pediatric patients. Paediatr Anaesth. 2012;22(10):1002–7.
52. Shiloh AL, Savel RH, Paulin LM, Eisen LA. Ultrasound-guided catheterization of the radial artery: a systematic review and meta-analysis of randomized controlled trials. Chest. 2011;139(3):524–9.

53. McGee DC, Gould MK. Preventing complications of central venous catheterization. N Engl J Med. 2003;348(12):1123–33.
54. Merrer J, De Jonghe B, Golliot F, Lefrant JY, Raffy B, Barre E, et al. Complications of femoral and subclavian venous catheterization in critically ill patients: a randomized controlled trial. JAMA. 2001;286(6):700–7.
55. Wu S, Ling Q, Cao L, Wang J, Xu M, Zeng W. Real-time two-dimensional ultrasound guidance for central venous cannulation: a meta-analysis. Anesthesiology. 2013;118(2):361–75.
56. Calvert N, Hind D, McWilliams RG, Thomas SM, Beverley C, Davidson A. The effectiveness and cost-effectiveness of ultrasound locating devices for central venous access: a systematic review and economic evaluation. Health Technol Assess Winch Engl. 2003;7(12):1–84.
57. Fisher NC, Mutimer DJ. Central venous cannulation in patients with liver disease and coagulopathy—a prospective audit. Intensive Care Med. 1999;25(5):481–5.
58. Tercan F, Ozkan U, Oguzkurt L. US-guided placement of central vein catheters in patients with disorders of hemostasis. Eur J Radiol. 2008;65(2):253–6.
59. Della Vigna P, Monfardini L, Bonomo G, Curigliano G, Agazzi A, Bellomi M, et al. Coagulation disorders in patients with cancer: nontunneled central venous catheter placement with US guidance—a single-institution retrospective analysis. Radiology. 2009;253(1):249–52.
60. Hilty WM, Hudson PA, Levitt MA, Hall JB. Real-time ultrasound-guided femoral vein catheterization during cardiopulmonary resuscitation. Ann Emerg Med. 1997;29(3):331–6. discussion 337
61. Weiner MM, Geldard P, Mittnacht AJC. Ultrasound-guided vascular access: a comprehensive review. J Cardiothorac Vasc Anesth. 2013;27(2):345–60.
62. Gordon AC, Saliken JC, Johns D, Owen R, Gray RR. US-guided puncture of the internal jugular vein: complications and anatomic considerations. J Vasc Interv Radiol JVIR. 1998;9(2):333–8.
63. Alderson PJ, Burrows FA, Stemp LI, Holtby HM. Use of ultrasound to evaluate internal jugular vein anatomy and to facilitate central venous cannulation in paediatric patients. Br J Anaesth. 1993;70(2):145–8.
64. Parsons AJ, Alfa J. Carotid dissection: a complication of internal jugular vein cannulation with the use of ultrasound. Anesth Analg. 2009;109(1):135–6.
65. Augoustides JG, Horak J, Ochroch AE, Vernick WJ, Gambone AJ, Weiner J, et al. A randomized controlled clinical trial of real-time needle-guided ultrasound for internal jugular venous cannulation in a large university anesthesia department. J Cardiothorac Vasc Anesth. 2005;19(3):310–5.
66. Adachi YU, Sato S. Four cases of inadvertent arterial cannulation despite ultrasound guidance. Am J Emerg Med. 2010;28(4):533.
67. Stone MB, Hern HG. Inadvertent carotid artery cannulation during ultrasound guided central venous catheterization. Ann Emerg Med. 2007;49(5):720.
68. Blaivas M, Adhikari S. An unseen danger: frequency of posterior vessel wall penetration by needles during attempts to place internal jugular vein central catheters using ultrasound guidance. Crit Care Med. 2009;37(8):2345–9. quiz 2359
69. Saugel B, Scheeren TWL, Teboul J-L. Ultrasound-guided central venous catheter placement: a structured review and recommendations for clinical practice. Crit Care Lond Engl. 2017;21(1):225.
70. Mahmood F, Sundar S, Khabbaz K. Misplacement of a guidewire diagnosed by transesophageal echocardiography. J Cardiothorac Vasc Anesth. 2007;21(3):420–1.
71. Hessel EA. Con: we should not enforce the use of ultrasound as a standard of care for obtaining central venous access. J Cardiothorac Vasc Anesth. 2009;23(5):725–8.
72. Moureau N, Lamperti M, Kelly LJ, Dawson R, Elbarbary M, van Boxtel AJH, et al. Evidence-based consensus on the insertion of central venous access devices: definition of minimal requirements for training. Br J Anaesth. 2013;110(3):347–56.
73. Overview I Guidance on the use of ultrasound locating devices for placing central venous catheters I Guidance I NICE [Internet]. NICE; [cited 2021 May 30]. https://www.nice.org.uk/guidance/ta49
74. O'Grady NP, Alexander M, Burns LA, Dellinger EP, Garland J, Heard SO, Lipsett PA, Masur H, Mermel LA, Pearson ML, Raad II. Guidelines for the prevention of intravascular catheter-related infections. Clin Infect Dis. 2011;52(9):e162–93.
75. Marschall J, Mermel LA, Classen D, Arias KM, Podgorny K, Anderson DJ, et al. Strategies to prevent central line-associated bloodstream infections in acute care hospitals. Infect Control Hosp Epidemiol. 2008;29(Suppl 1):S22–30.
76. Eisen LA, Narasimhan M, Berger JS, Mayo PH, Rosen MJ, Schneider RF. Mechanical complications of central venous catheters. J Intensive Care Med. 2006;21(1):40–6.
77. Feller-Kopman D. Ultrasound-guided internal jugular access: a proposed standardized approach and implications for training and practice. Chest. 2007;132(1):302–9.
78. Bodenham AR. Editorial II: ultrasound imaging by anaesthetists: training and accreditation issues. Br J Anaesth. 2006;96(4):414–7.
79. Skippen P, Kissoon N. Ultrasound guidance for central vascular access in the pediatric emergency department. Pediatr Emerg Care. 2007;23(3):203–7.
80. Chenkin J, Lee S, Huynh T, Bandiera G. Procedures can be learned on the web: a randomized study of ultrasound-guided vascular access training. Acad Emerg Med Off J Soc Acad Emerg Med. 2008;15(10):949–54.

81. Troianos CA, Hartman GS, Glas KE, Skubas NJ, Eberhardt RT, Walker JD, et al. Guidelines for performing ultrasound guided vascular cannulation: recommendations of the American Society of Echocardiography and the Society of Cardiovascular Anesthesiologists. J Am Soc Echocardiogr Off Publ Am Soc Echocardiogr. 2011;24(12):1291–318.
82. Reznick RK, MacRae H. Teaching surgical skills—changes in the wind. N Engl J Med. 2006;355(25):2664–9.
83. Bastos EM, Silva RDP. Proposal of a synthetic ethylene-vinyl acetate bench model for surgical foundations learning: suture training. Acta Cir Bras. 2011;26(2):149–52.
84. Evans LV, Dodge KL, Shah TD, Kaplan LJ, Siegel MD, Moore CL, et al. Simulation training in central venous catheter insertion: improved performance in clinical practice. Acad Med J Assoc Am Med Coll. 2010;85(9):1462–9.
85. Ault MJ, Rosen BT, Ault B. The use of tissue models for vascular access training. Phase I of the procedural patient safety initiative. J Gen Intern Med. 2006;21(5):514–7.
86. Eason MP, Goodrow MS, Gillespie JE. A device to stimulate central venous cannulation in the human patient simulator. Anesthesiology. 2003;99(5):1245–6.
87. Pérez-Quevedo O, López-Álvarez JM, Limiñana-Cañal JM, Loro-Ferrer JF. Design and application of model for training ultrasound-guided vascular cannulation in pediatric patients. Med Intensiva. 2016;40(6):364–70.
88. Kendall JL, Faragher JP. Ultrasound-guided central venous access: a homemade phantom for simulation. CJEM. 2007;9(5):371–3.
89. Denadai R, Toledo AP, Bernades DM, Diniz FD, Eid FB, de Moura Lanfranchi LMM, et al. Simulation-based ultrasound-guided central venous cannulation training program1. Acta Cirúrgica Bras. 2014;29:132–44.

Point of Care Ultrasound of the Airway

3

Deborah Khoo

Abbreviations

CTM	Cricothyroid membrane
DLT	Double lumen tube
ETT	Endotracheal tube
FONA	Front of neck access
PDT	Percutaneous dilatational tracheostomy
SGA	Supraglottic airway

3.1 Indications

Point of Care Ultrasound of the airway is a valuable tool that has the following uses:

(a) Pre-intubation screening—especially for predicted difficult intubations. Used to select endotracheal tube (ETT) size, assess submandibular soft tissue, evaluate vocal cord movement and examine airway integrity.
(b) Tracheal intubation—Confirm ETT placement and depth.
(c) Supraglottic Airway (SGA)—to detect laryngeal mask malrotation.
(d) Front of neck access—cricothyroidotomy, percutaneous dilatational tracheostomy (PDT).
(e) Airway nerve blocks—superior laryngeal nerve block.
(f) Extubation—leak test, predicting post-extubation stridor, successful extubation.

3.2 Normal Anatomy

3.2.1 Ultrasound Appearance of Airway Structures

Air conducts ultrasound waves poorly hence the clinician must bear in mind that structures deep into the air-filled structures will not be well visualized. The linear ultrasound probe (13–6 MHz) is usually used in adult patients. The air within the airway also causes reverberation artifacts. The air-mucosa interface is delineated by a bright, hyperechoic appearance. The thyroid and cricoid cartilage appear homogeneously hypoechoic, compared to muscle and connective tissue which are hypoechoic but heterogeneous. As with anywhere else in the body, bony structures (mentum, mandible rami, hyoid, and sternum) appear hyperechoic and bright, with a hypoechoic acoustic shadow below. Fluid-filled spaces are anechoic and cast a posterior acoustic enhancement. The esophagus is seen as a multilayered structure lying to the left of the trachea (Fig. 3.1).

D. Khoo (✉)
Department of Anaesthesia, National University Hospital, Singapore, Singapore
e-mail: Deborah_khoo@nuhs.edu.sg

A. Chakraborty, B. Ashokka (eds.), *A Practical Guide to Point of Care Ultrasound (POCUS)*,
https://doi.org/10.1007/978-981-16-7687-1_3

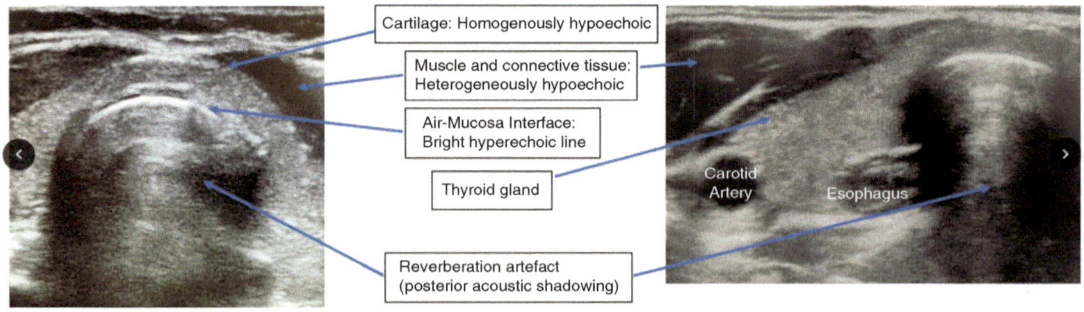

Fig. 3.1 Pattern recognition in airway ultrasound

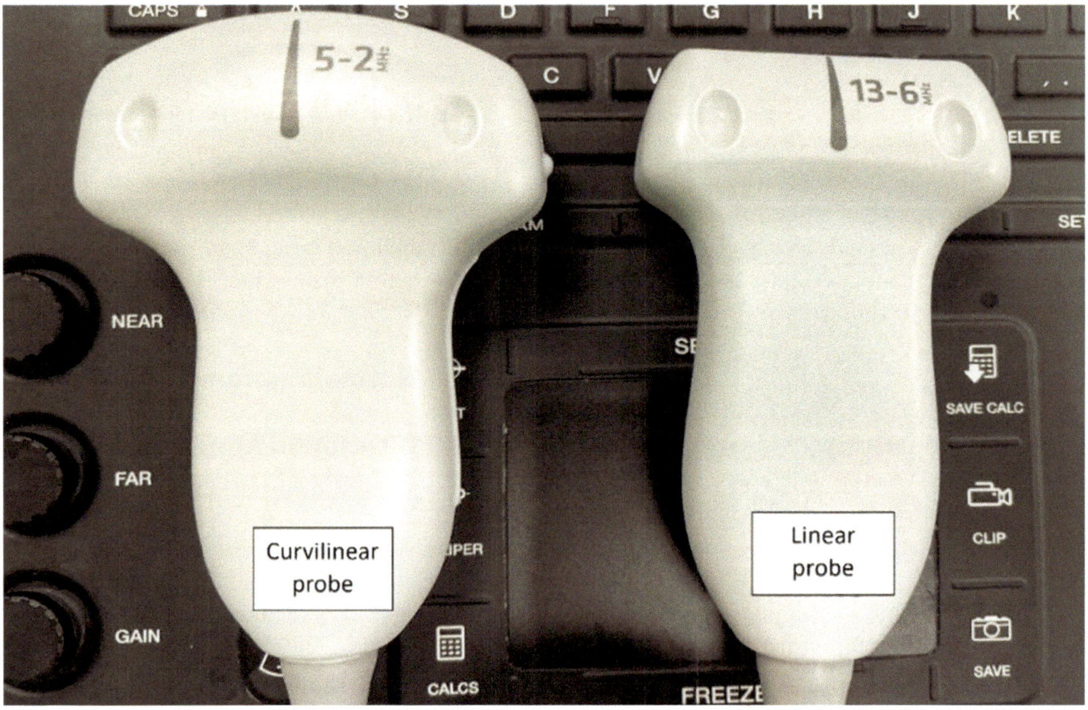

Fig. 3.2 Transducers commonly used for airway ultrasound

3.2.2 Normal Ultrasound Appearance of the Airway

3.2.2.1 Transducer Selection

- The medium to high-frequency linear probe is suitable for visualizing structures close to the skin, usually to a depth of less than ~4 cm.
- The low-frequency curvilinear probe is used for investigating deeper structures, such as the tongue and floor of mouth.

Given the uneven and relatively unyielding nature of the anterior neck surface, usage of sufficient ultrasound gel is important to obtaining a good image. In a spontaneously breathing patient, the breathing movements may result in intermittent visualization of the desired structures. In an awake patient, a gentle yet steady technique is beneficial to the patient's comfort and cooperation (Fig. 3.2).

Normal ultrasound appearances of the airway at various levels are summarized in the table below [1–3] (Table 3.1).

Table 3.1 Normal airway anatomy and views

	Level of airway that probe beam will be traversing	Appropriate manner of holding ultrasound to obtain view	Normal ultrasound appearance	Application
Oropharynx—Submentum	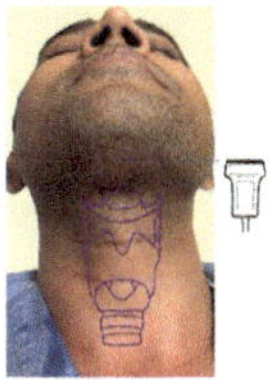 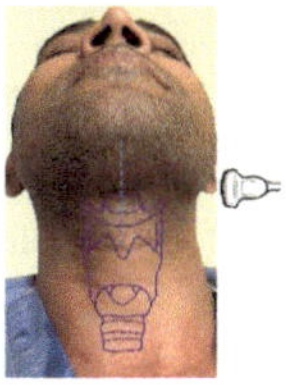	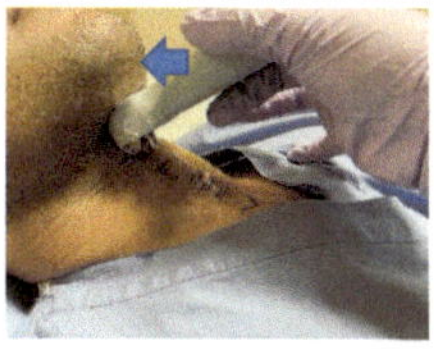 Blue arrow shows the direction of ultrasound probe beam 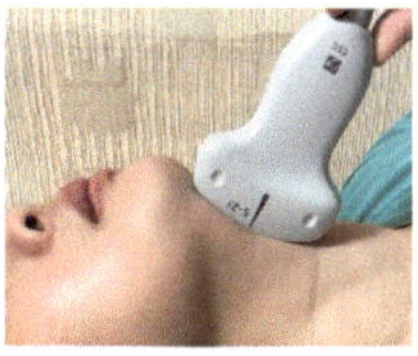 Position of curvilinear probe to examine tongue and submental structures 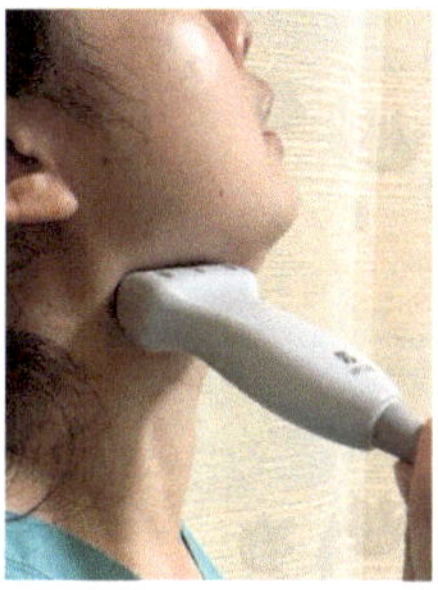 Position of probe (slightly off-midline) for evaluation of retropharyngeal space	A. 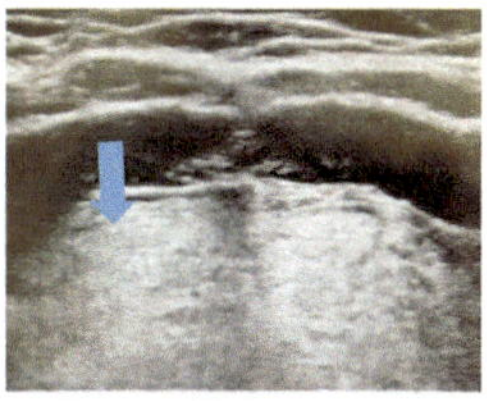 B. 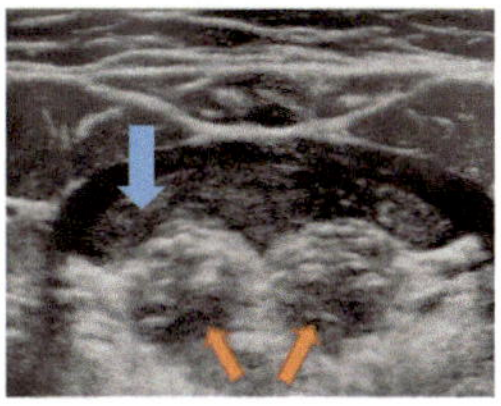 C. 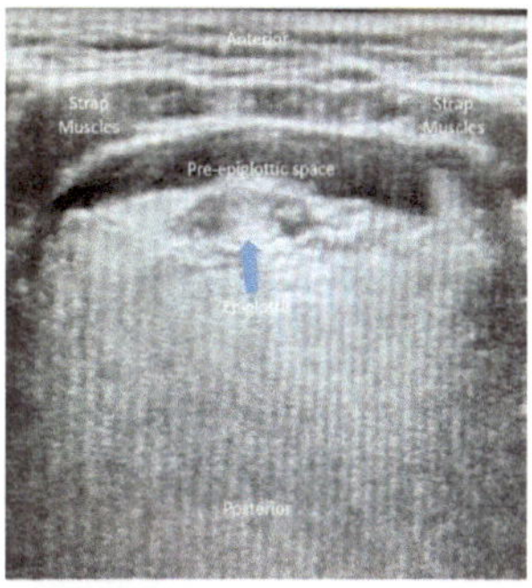 D. 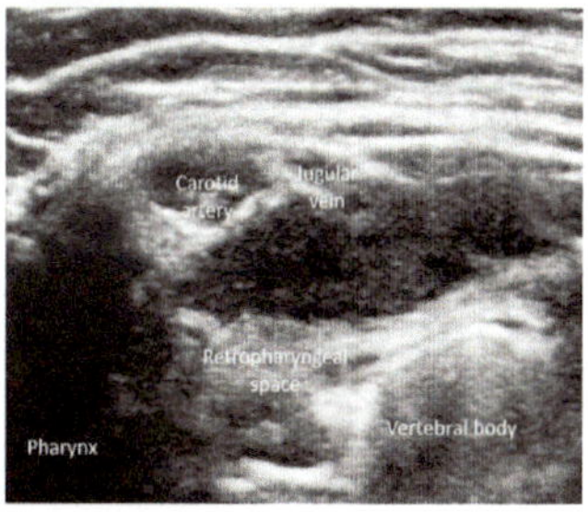	A. Tongue (blue arrow): Look for size, movement, and lesions B. Tonsils (Orange arrows): Size, abscess. Best seen by asking patient to press tongue (blue arrow) against hard palate C. Epiglottis (blue arrow): Assess for inflammation and masses D. Retropharyngeal space: Evaluate for retropharyngeal abscess and patency of airway
Larynx—Hyoid	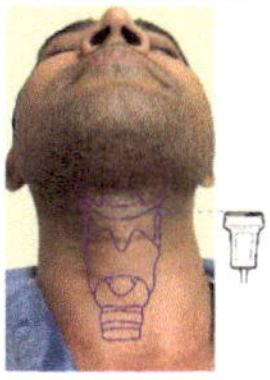	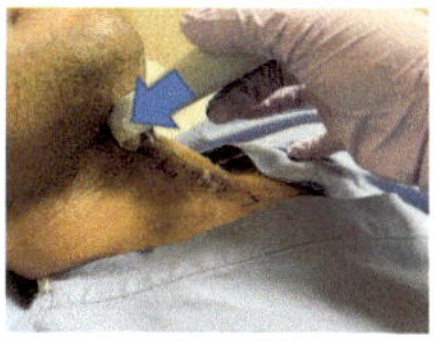 Blue arrow shows the direction of ultrasound probe beam	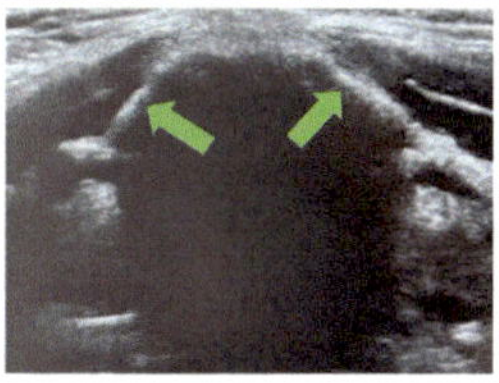	Thin, bright line due to bony nature of hyoid. (green arrows) Aids administration of the superior laryngeal nerve block

(continued)

Table 3.1 (continued)

	Level of airway that probe beam will be traversing	Appropriate manner of holding ultrasound to obtain view	Normal ultrasound appearance	Application
Larynx—Thyroid cartilage and vocal cords	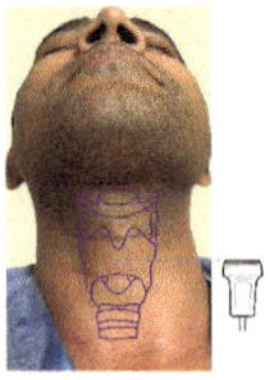	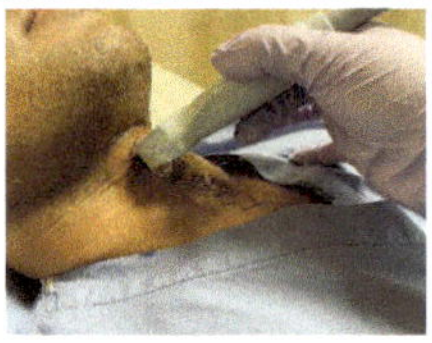	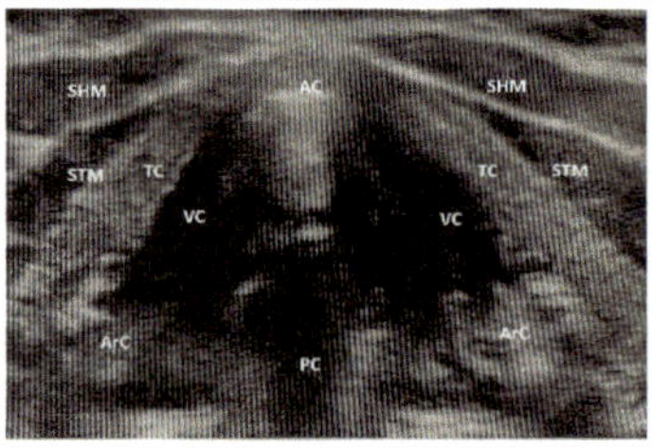 Transverse view of the airway at the level of the thyroid cartilage: AC = anterior commissure; PC = posterior commissure; VC = vocal cords; SHM = sternohyoid muscle; STM = sternothyroid muscle; ArC = arytenoid cartilage; TC = thyroid cartilage 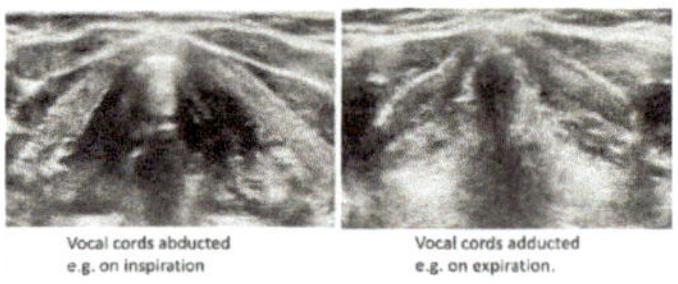	The thyroid cartilage is pyramidal in shape and is the largest cartilaginous structure in the airway ultrasound exam. May be more prominent in males and calcified in the elderly The vocal cords can also be seen at this level. Look for vocal cord asymmetry (indicating vocal cord palsy), lesions, and cysts Extubation—Air column width difference at the level of the vocal cords before and after ETT cuff deflation helps to establish the presence of air leak and minimize the risk of post-extubation stridor
Larynx—Cricothyroid membrane	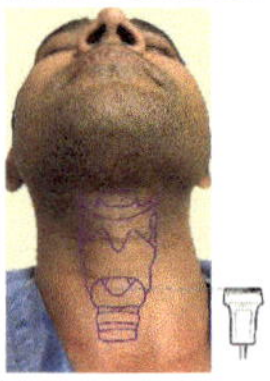	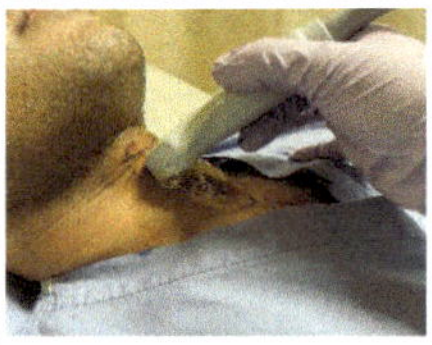	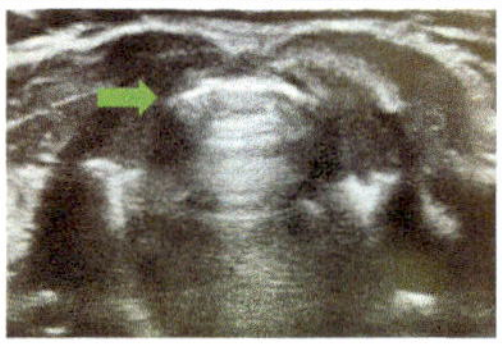	The cricothyroid membrane (CTM) is seen as a bright hyperechoic line (green arrow). Locating and marking out of the CTM can be done rapidly and with more accuracy than by the palpation method, especially in patients who are obese or have impalpable structures Pre-procedural or real-time ultrasound guidance for cricothyroidotomy is also useful for avoidance of unintended airway injury. Look out for vessels (e.g., thyroid artery) crossing the intended puncture site

Table 3.1 (continued)

	Level of airway that probe beam will be traversing	Appropriate manner of holding ultrasound to obtain view	Normal ultrasound appearance	Application
Larynx—Cricoid cartilage	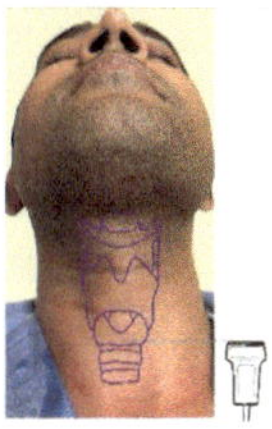	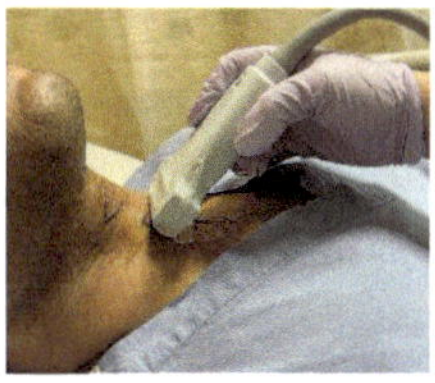	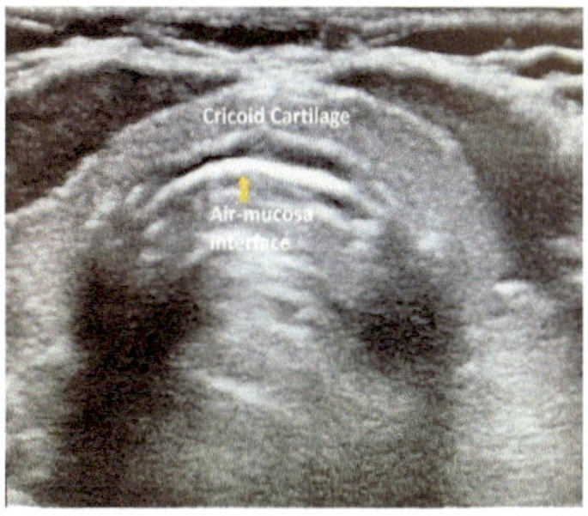 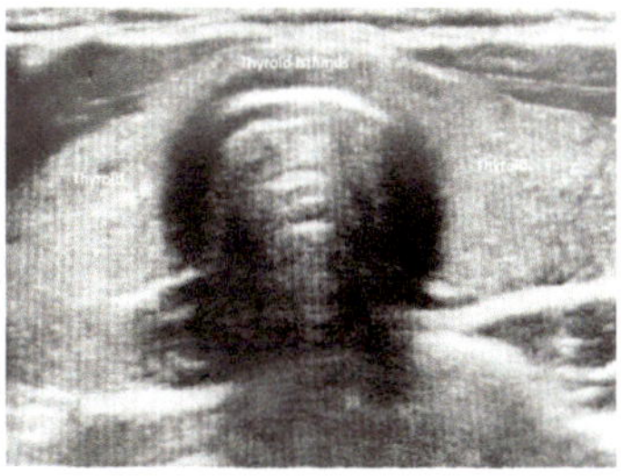	The airway at the level of the cricoid cartilage is the narrowest part of the larynx in pediatric patients. In both adults and paediatric patients, measurement of the diameter of airway (orange arrow) can be used to assist endotracheal tube (ETT) sizing according to the external diameter of the ETT Air creates a bright white air-mucosa interface with a posterior acoustic shadow The thyroid gland and thyroid isthmus may be seen here or at the level of the tracheal rings
Trachea rings—Transverse view	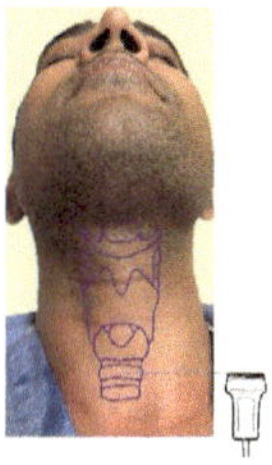	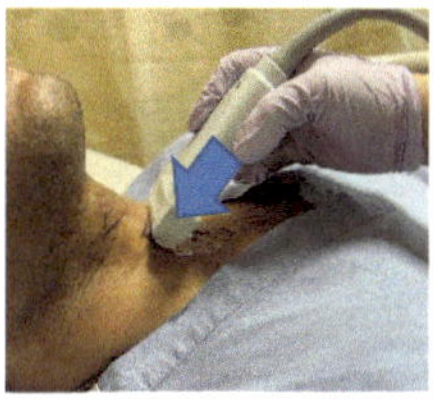	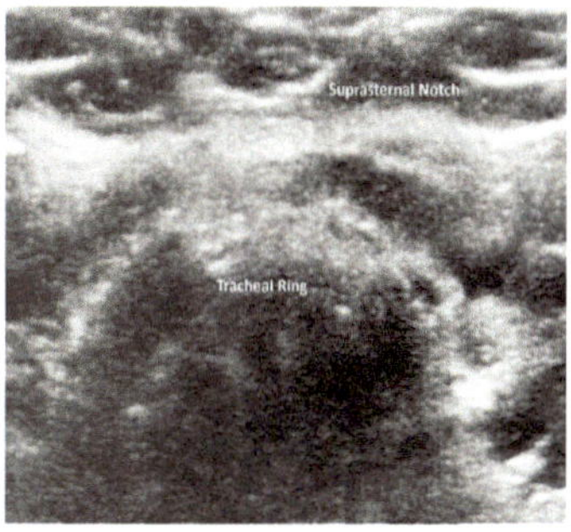	Tracheal rings are less prominent and less superficial compared to the cricoid cartilage Use of color doppler at this level is useful to check for vascular structures (e.g., a high-riding innominate artery) that may be crossing the intended site of a tracheostomy, as well as to assess the optimal site and spacing between tracheal rings for a tracheostomy
Suprasternal notch	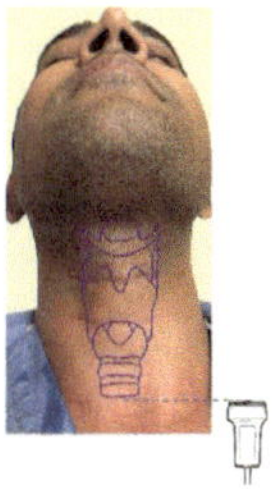	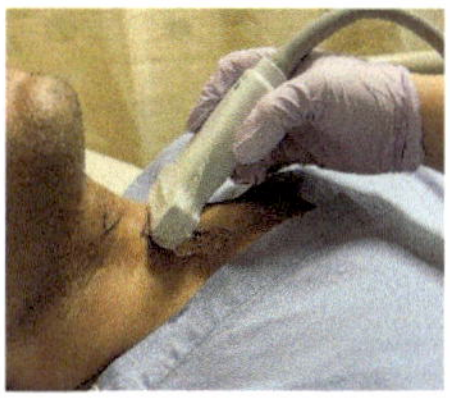	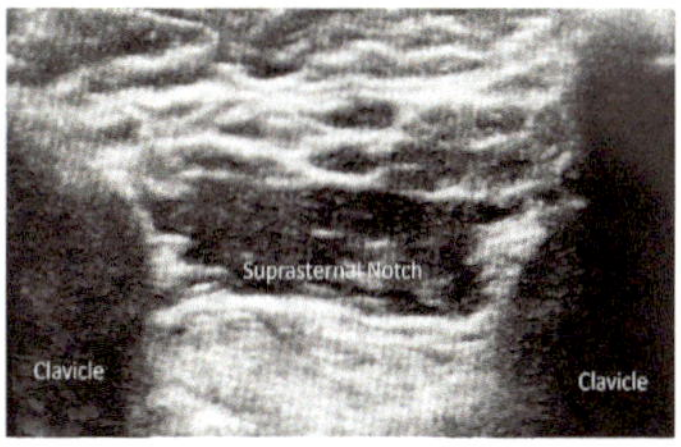	Correlates to sizing of double lumen tubes. Blood vessels may also be seen in this area

(continued)

Table 3.1 (continued)

	Level of airway that probe beam will be traversing	Appropriate manner of holding ultrasound to obtain view	Normal ultrasound appearance	Application
Trachea—Longitudinal view	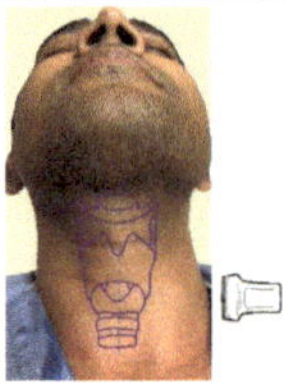	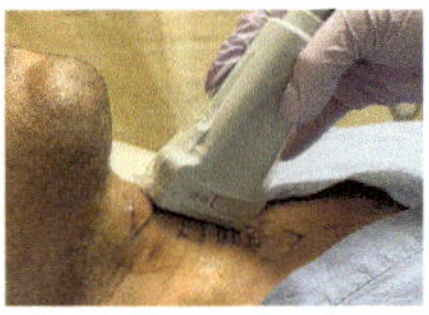	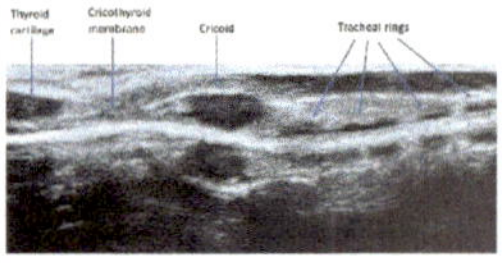	Longitudinal midline ultrasound view of the trachea The hypoechoic tracheal rings give the classic "string of pearls" appearance. The CTM can again be identified between the thyroid and cricoid cartilage

3.3 Airway Devices

3.3.1 Endotracheal Tube (ETT)

Selection of ETT size (according to the outer diameter) can be performed by measuring the transverse diameter of the trachea along the level of the cricoid cartilage to the suprasternal notch (Fig. 3.3). Correct sizing of the ETT can help to avoid airway leaks and insufficient ventilation if too small, and pressure necrosis and subglottic stenosis (Fig. 3.4) if too large, particularly in the pediatric population. This method has been shown to be more accurate than height or weight-based methods of ETT sizing [1, 4]. In smaller sized adult patients and patients with known subglottic stenosis, careful examination of the entire airway to determine the narrowest point can help avoid intubation, ventilation, and even extubation difficulties.

The mid-tracheal level (between the cricoid cartilage and suprasternal notch) may be identified in the longitudinal view and is useful in ensuring appropriate insertion depth placement of an endotracheal tube. This helps to avoid endobronchial intubation if too deep or accidental extubation if too shallow [5].

Successful placement of an ETT can be documented, either in real time or after intubation. The air column within the ETT will cause posterior acoustic shadowing. The ETT may appear as a rounded structure within the trachea, or a "dou-

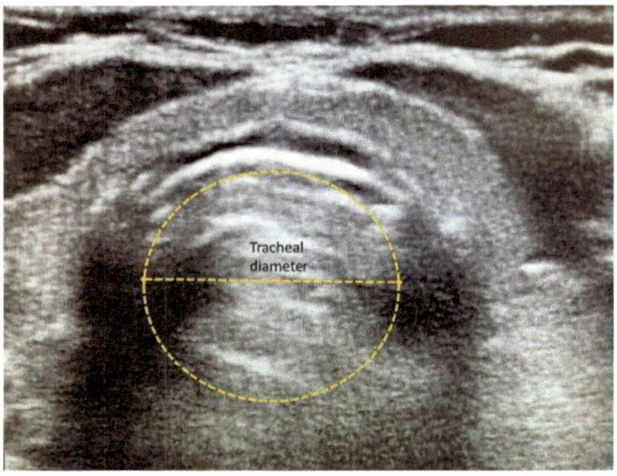

Fig. 3.3 Transverse diameter of trachea

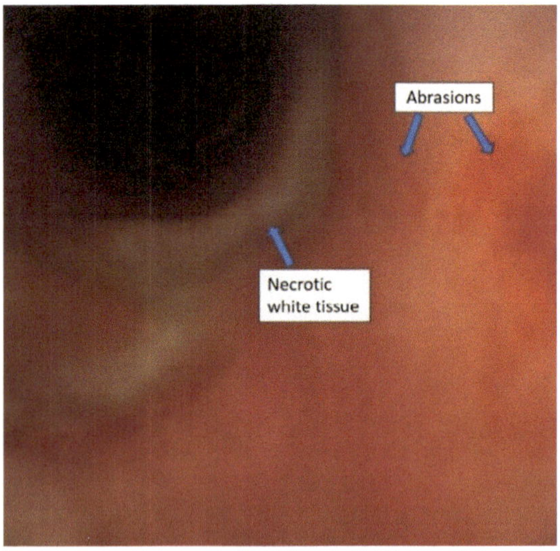

Fig. 3.4 Airway abrasion and necrosis from a larger than required ETT, which may lead to subglottic stenosis

ble track" appearance parallel to the air-mucosa interface (Figs. 3.5 and 3.6) [6].

3.3.1.1 Extubation

Post-extubation stridor (PES) is a concern in patients who have been intubated for an extended period, or who may have airway edema for various reasons. Cuff-leak tests are widely used to predict if the patient may be successfully extubated, and have good specificity, but low sensitivity, as well as inter-individual variability. This means that even if a leak is present, the patient must be closely monitored for PES post-extubation [7, 8]. PES often results in reintubations, prolonged intubation, and its associated comorbidities.

Pre-extubation ultrasound can allow for assessment of the vocal cords, larynx, and ease of airflow. The ratio of the air column width (Fig. 3.7) pre-extubation (with cuff deflated) to the air column width immediately post-intubation, is a potential predictor of post-extubation stridor. A ratio of <0.8 is predictive of post-extubation stridor [8, 9]. If the immediate post-intubation air column width is not available, the difference in the air column width with the cuff inflated and deflated may be a possible predictor, although cut-off values in adults have not yet been established [10].

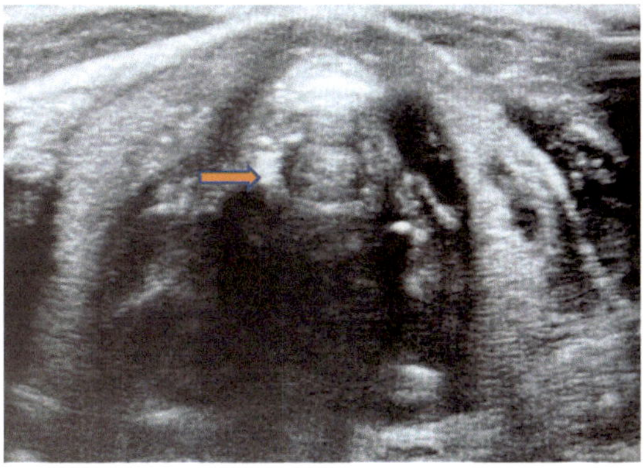

Fig. 3.5 Rounded ETT appearing in airway (orange arrow)

3.3.2 Supraglottic Airway (SGA)

Supraglottic airways may be visualized in the transverse orientation, at the submental level. Appearance may differ depending on the make and model of the SGA, but generally would have a rounded, spade-like shape. Ultrasound may help in troubleshooting a mispositioned SGA. Ultrasound may also be used to confirm intraesophageal position of a gastric tube inserted via the gastric port of second-generation SGAs (Fig. 3.8).

3.3.3 Double Lumen Endotracheal Tube (DLT)

Sizing of a left-sided double lumen tube can be performed by measuring the transverse diameter of the trachea at the level of the suprasternal

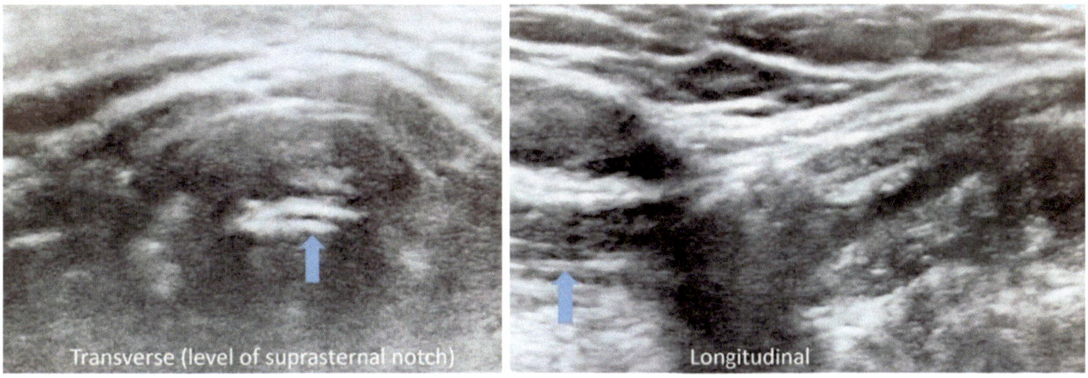

Fig. 3.6 Double track lines (blue arrows) can also help to confirm endotracheal ETT placement

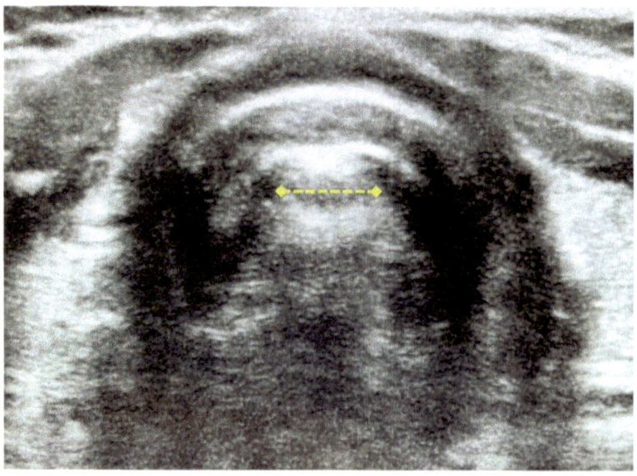

Fig. 3.7 Air column width (dotted yellow line) in an intubated patient with cuff deflated

notch [11]. This is particularly useful in smaller sized patients or patients who have had previous airway surgery or injury. The double lumen tube exhibits the same "double track" sign as a single lumen ETT, but with slight midline depression in transverse and parallel lines in the longitudinal orientation (Fig. 3.9).

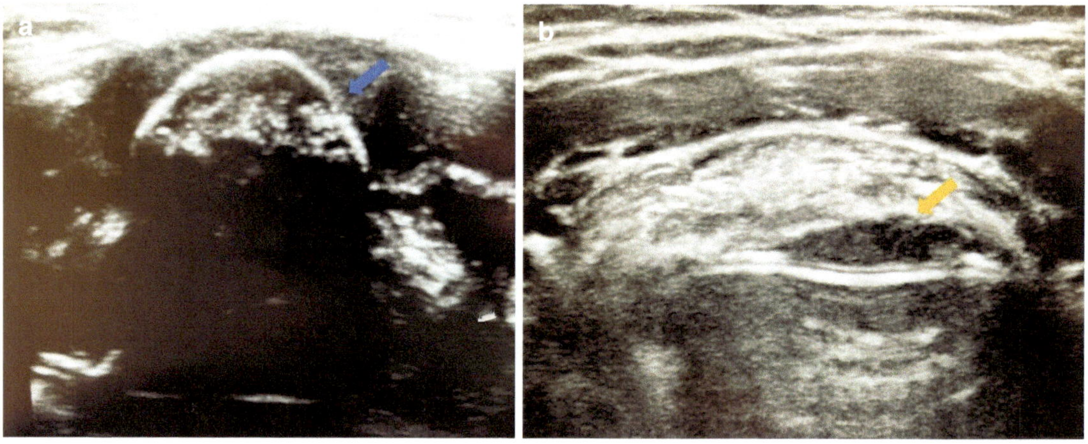

Fig. 3.8 (**a**) Central, well-positioned SGA (blue arrow), seen in the transverse view at the submentum level. (**b**) SGA tip folded and off-midline (orange arrow)

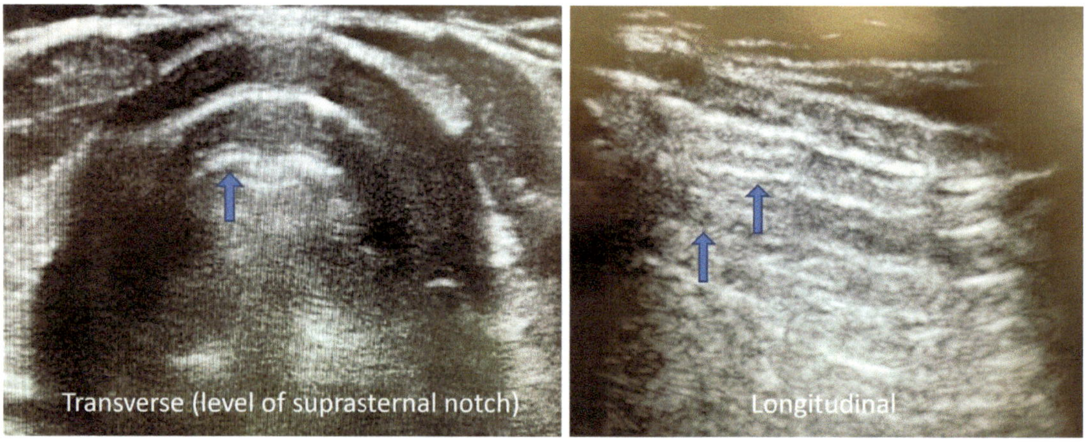

Fig. 3.9 Ultrasound appearance of a double lumen tube (blue arrows) in the trachea

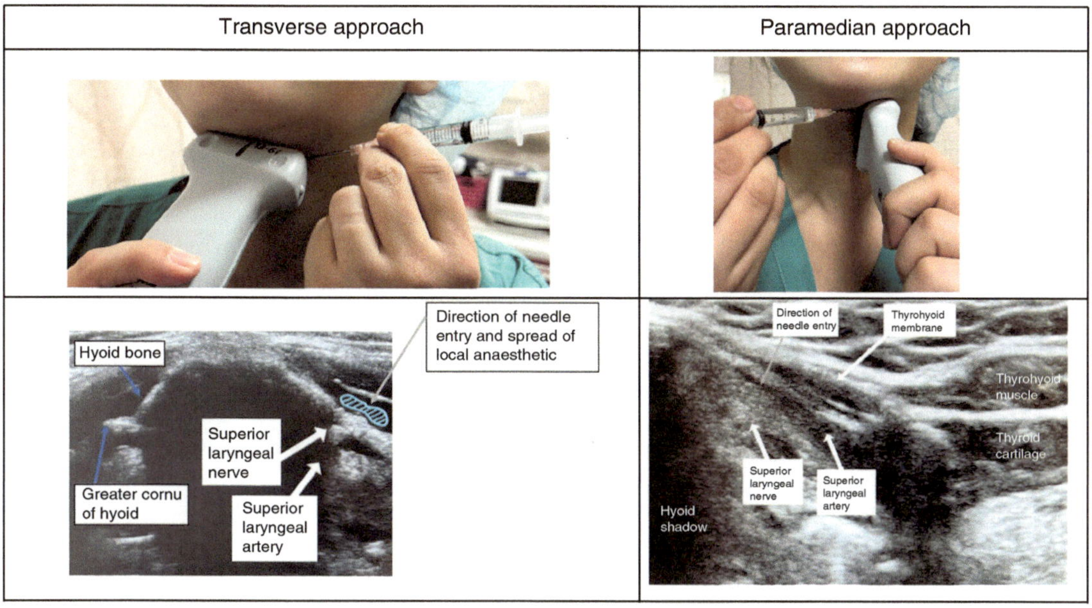

Fig. 3.10 Ultrasound visualization and techniques for superior laryngeal nerve blocks

3.4 Airway Nerve Block

The superior laryngeal nerve (SLN) block is a useful adjunct to facilitate awake intubations or rigid bronchoscopy. The internal branch of the SLN runs beneath or lateral to the greater horn of the hyoid, before penetrating the thyrohyoid membrane to provide innervation to the larynx. Ultrasound-guided superior laryngeal nerve blocks allow for target visualization, as well as ensuring spread of local anesthetic and avoidance of vascular (e.g., the superior laryngeal artery) and other anterior neck structures (Fig. 3.10) [12, 13].

3.5 Clinical Pearls and Applications

3.5.1 Focused Rapid Ultrasound Review of the Upper Airway

3.5.1.1 Goals

- To inform of obstructions to securing the airway in potentially difficult airways.
- To check for injuries to the airway, especially in patients who have sustained trauma.
- Identify and mark out the CTM—in preparation for emergency front of neck access if it becomes necessary. Recommended to do before undertaking potentially difficult airways such as awake intubations, trauma, or obese airways [1, 14, 15].
- Identify the location of airway structures in patients who may have tracheal deviation or limited neck mobility, e.g., previous radiotherapy or surgery to the neck, cervical spine contractures, neck masses, and thoracic and spine deformities.
- Right-sizing of airway device and selection of a safe tracheal interspace or location of CTM for front of neck access.

Stepwise approach to focused rapid ultrasound of the upper airway.

1. Identify the mentum and sternal notch as the cephalad and caudal ends of the airway, respectively.
2. Holding the ultrasound probe in a transverse manner, begin from the mentum and move the ultrasound probe in a caudal direction.
3. Identify the thin, bright line of the hyoid bone, looking for continuity of the bone and presence of soft tissue swelling.

4. Move the probe in a caudal direction and identify the triangular thyroid cartilage and vocal folds. In a spontaneously breathing patient, look for symmetry of vocal cord shape and movement. If trauma is suspected, look for discontinuity on the external surface of the cartilage as well as soft tissue swelling.
5. Sliding the probe caudally, identify the bright white line that denotes the air-mucosa interface of the cricothyroid membrane (CTM).
6. Confirm the position of the CTM by continuing to slide the probe caudally in a transverse orientation, seeing the change to the homogeneously hypoechoic cricoid cartilage.
7. Return the probe to the level of the CTM and mark its position, as well as that of the midline, on the patient.
8. Continue to scan caudally, observing the change from the cricoid cartilage to the tracheal rings until it reaches the suprasternal notch. Observe for pulsatile arterial structures in this area.
9. To obtain the longitudinal midline view of the trachea, slide the ultrasound probe laterally until medial edge of the probe is positioned such that only half of the trachea is in view at the edge of the ultrasound screen. Rotate the ultrasound probe so that the lateral edge is now cephalad in the sagittal plane. Identify the thyroid and cricoid cartilages, and the CTM in between. Mark out the CTM as well as the midline of the airway.

3.5.2 Potential Ultrasound Predictors of Laryngoscopy

Airway ultrasound is being increasingly used to identify potentially difficult airways, alongside clinical examination and patient history [2]. It is important to note that no single criteria predict airway difficulty in totality, and greater accuracy can be achieved with combination of predictors and tailoring to the patient's history and anatomy. Figure 3.11 and Table 3.2 summarize the parameters [4, 16–19].

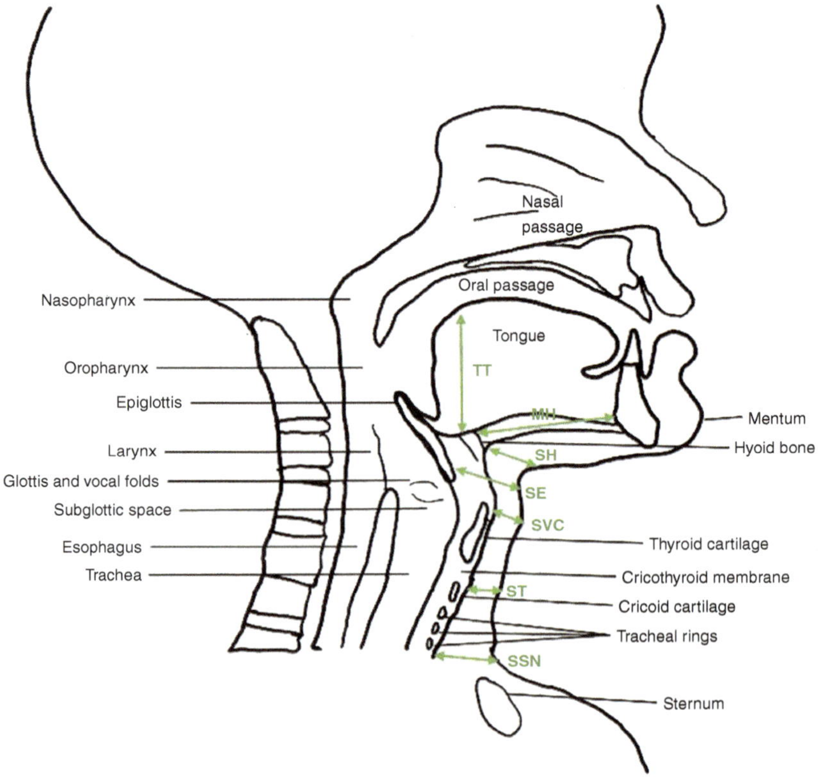

Fig. 3.11 Levels at which measurement of airway parameters may predict difficult laryngoscopy. *TT* tongue thickness, *MH* mentohyoid distance, *SH* skin to hyoid distance, *SE* skin to epiglottis distance, *SVC* skin to anterior commissure of vocal cords distance, *ST* skin to thyroid isthmus distance, *SSN* skin to suprasternal notch distance

Table 3.2 Summary of ultrasound airway parameters that may predict a difficult airway

Tongue width: How to obtain image: Linear probe in transverse orientation at submental level Interpretation: A width of >28 mm corresponds to a higher probability of obstructive sleep apnoea and difficult laryngoscopy	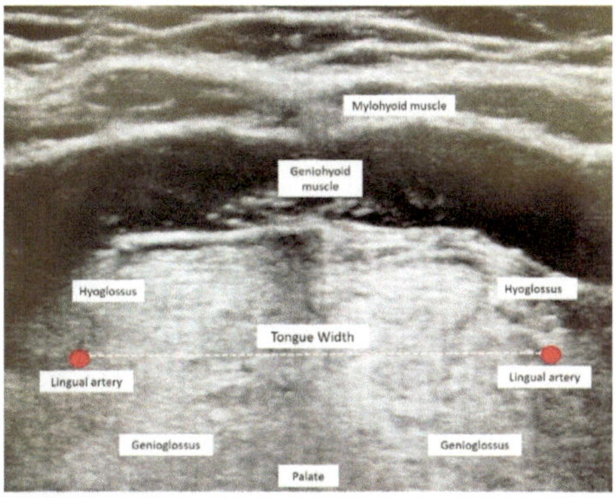
Mentohyoid distance and tongue thickness: How to obtain image: Curvilinear probe in sagittal orientation between mentum and hyoid **Mentohyoid (MH) distance:** Interpretation: 1. An MH distance of <52 ± 6 mm indicates a possible difficult airway, while >65 ± 4 mm indicates easy intubations 2. Calculate the ratio of the MH distance with the patient's head in hyperextension to that in neutral position. A ratio of <1.1 is predictive of difficult laryngoscopy and intubation These measurements also give an indication of the degree of cervical spine mobility **Tongue thickness (TT):** Interpretation: Measure the maximal thickness of the tongue between the floor of mouth and hard palate. A distance of more than 60 mm is indicative of macroglossia and may be suggestive of obstructive sleep apnoea (OSA)	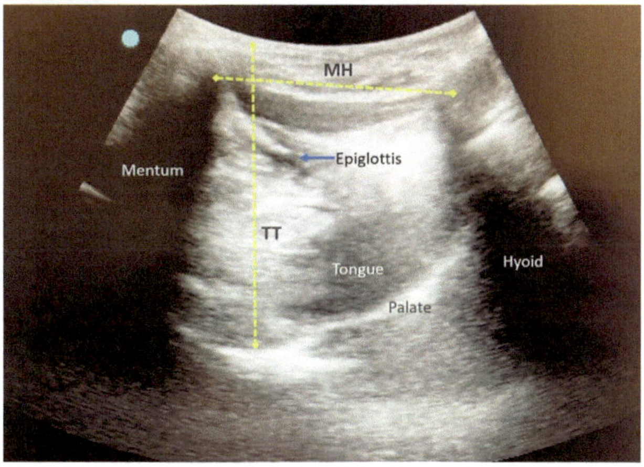
Skin to hyoid (SH) distance: How to obtain image: Linear probe in transverse orientation at level of hyoid bone Interpretation: An SH distance of >16.9 mm may predict a difficult airway	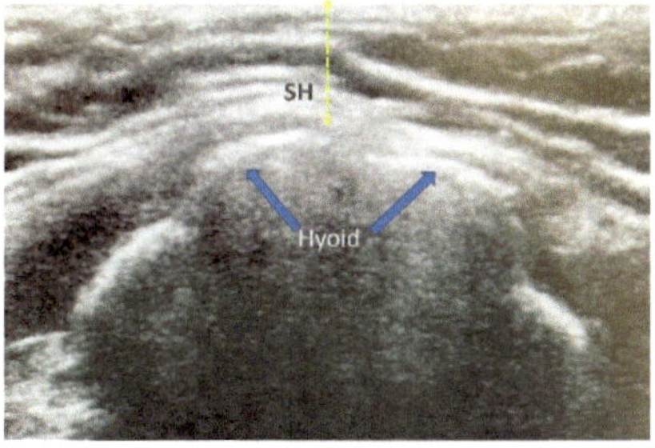

(continued)

Table 3.2 (continued)

Skin to epiglottis (SE) distance: How to obtain image: Linear probe in transverse orientation just below level of hyoid bone Interpretation: An SE distance of >24 mm may indicate a difficult airway	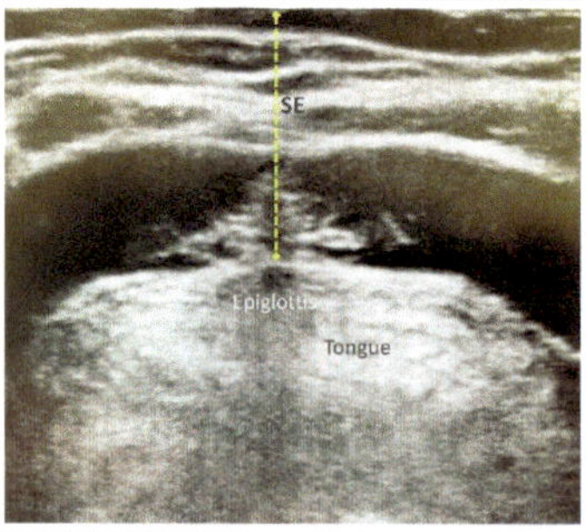
Skin to anterior commissure of vocal cords (SVC) distance: How to obtain image: Linear probe in transverse orientation at level of thyroid cartilage Interpretation: An SVC distance of >28 mm may indicate a difficult airway	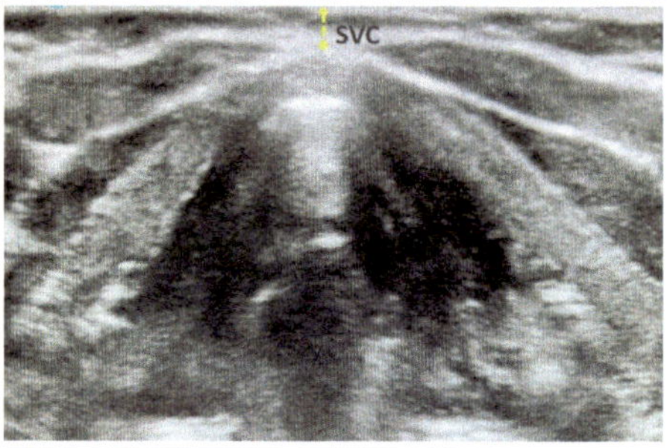
Skin to thyroid isthmus (ST) distance: How to obtain image: Linear probe in transverse orientation at level of the cricoid, looking for the point where the thyroid gland isthmus is maximally seen Interpretation: An ST distance of >34.7 mm may indicate a difficult airway	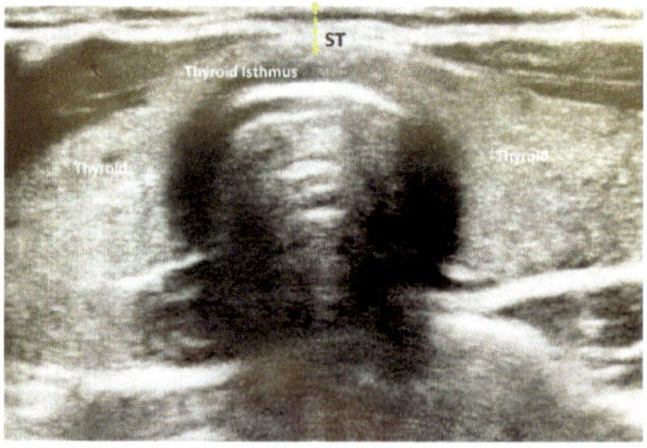
Skin to suprasternal notch distance: How to obtain image: Linear probe in transverse orientation at level of the suprasternal notch Interpretation: Not a proven predictor, but may be useful as a screening tool to predict a difficult airway [20, 21]	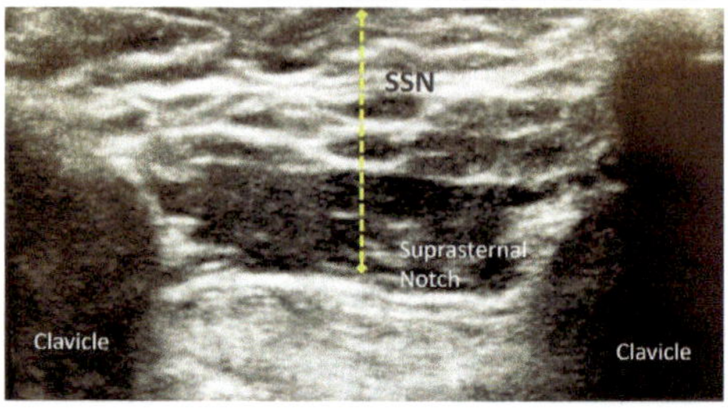 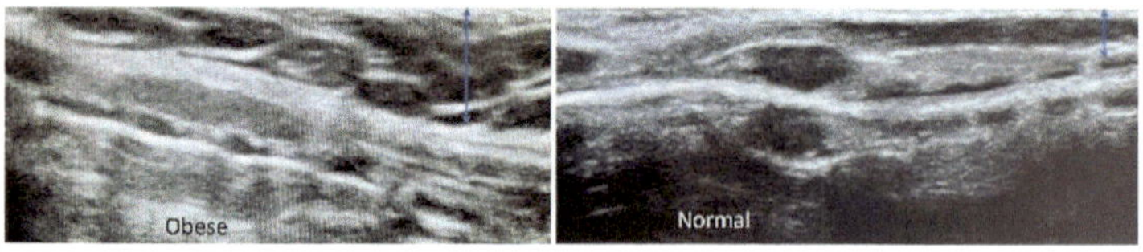 Blue arrows show skin to SSN distance in obese vs normal patients in longitudinal orientation

3.6 Summary

Ultrasound of the airway is a very useful skill to incorporate into airway evaluation and management. While not yet standard of care, it is gaining increasing acceptance and use in both adults and pediatric patients [4, 22]. Consistent practice on a wide range of patients will enable the user to recognize common and abnormal morphology, as well as to add to current knowledge and practice.

MCQs: Chose the Single Best Answer

(Read the questions with a book or a paper covering the answer side, try to answer on your own, and then check with the answer)

<table>
<tr><th>Questions</th><th>Answers</th></tr>
<tr><td>1. A pre-scan prior to performance of a cricothyroidotomy reveals the following structures
Which of the following accurately labels structures 1, 2, and 3?
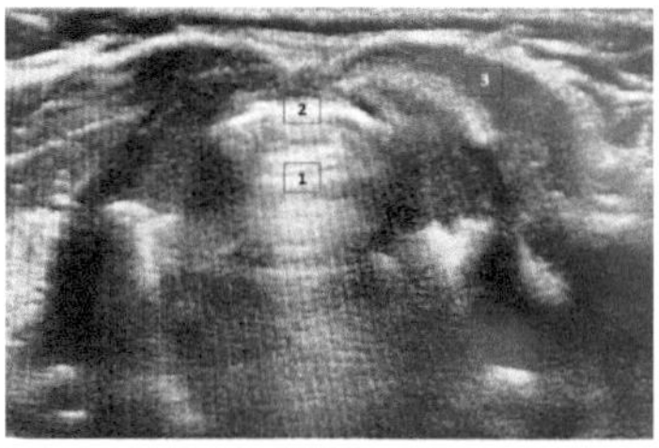
<table>
<tr><th></th><th>1</th><th>2</th><th>3</th></tr>
<tr><td>A</td><td>Cricothyroid membrane</td><td>Reverberation artifact</td><td>Sternohyoid muscle</td></tr>
<tr><td>B</td><td>Cricoid cartilage</td><td>Reverberation artifact</td><td>Thyroid gland</td></tr>
<tr><td>C</td><td>Thyroid cartilage</td><td>Endotracheal tube</td><td>Sternocleido-mastoid muscle</td></tr>
<tr><td>D</td><td>Cricothyroid membrane</td><td>Endotracheal tube</td><td>Sternothyroid muscle</td></tr>
</table></td><td>Answer: A. The cricothyroid membrane (CTM) appears as a bright white line due to the air-mucosa interface, with a reverberation artifact posteriorly. The CTM is 13–15 mm long in adults. In the transverse orientation, scanning from the thyroid cartilage, then to the CTM, followed by the cricoid, and finally back to the CTM helps to visualize the transition and ascertain the identity of the CTM [23]</td></tr>
<tr><td>2. A patient who has sustained a penetrating head and neck trauma develops difficulty breathing and is desaturating. Ultrasound of his airway reveals subcutaneous emphysema. Appropriate management includes
A. Monitor the patient closely but do not manipulate the airway at this point as it may worsen the situation
B. Support the patient with bag-mask ventilation
C. Intubate the patient via the oral or nasal route
D. Identify the level of injury and proceed to secure the airway</td><td>Answer: D. Subcutaneous emphysema indicates discontinuity in the airway or aerodigestive tract. Nonintervention may miss the window of opportunity for management before the patient becomes more unstable. Positive pressure ventilation should be minimized until the airway is secured. Careful ultrasound examination of the airway is useful to rapidly delineate distorted anatomy and formulate the safest location to secure the patient's airway, whether by intubation or front of neck access. Bronchoscopy evaluation is indicated as well where possible. Cervical spine immobility is likely to add to the complexity</td></tr>
</table>

Questions	Answers
3. After a difficult intubation, this image is seen on ultrasound of the airway. Appropriate immediate management should include: 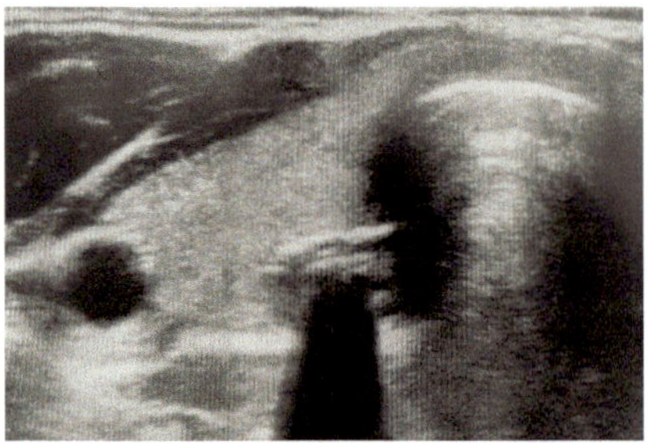 A Ventilate the patient with appropriate tidal volumes B Remove and reinsert the endotracheal tube (ETT) C Check for $ETCO_2$ using a colorimeter or capnograph D Deepen the patient using inhalational or intravenous agents	Answer: B. This ultrasound image shows an oesophageal intubation. The air column in the ETT produces a "drop-out" dark area below the air-ETT interface. Stylets or bougies may produce the same, albeit smaller, effect. Monitoring of an intubation in real time using ultrasound allows for immediate identification of esophageal intubation
4. Prior to performing a percutaneous dilatational tracheostomy (PDT), a vascular structure is seen at the level of the fourth tracheal ring. This vascular structure is likely to be the: A. Thyroid artery B. Superior laryngeal artery C. Innominate artery D. Tonsillar artery 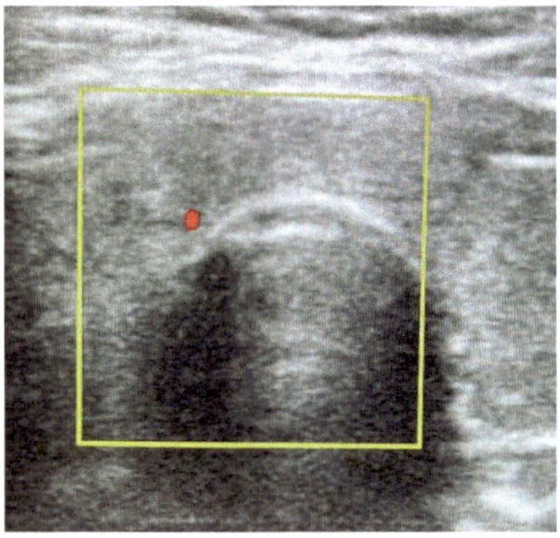	Answer: C. The innominate artery is also known as the brachiocephalic artery. It is the most proximal branch of the aortic arch, originating medial and anterior to the left common carotid artery. This short artery courses superiorly posterior to the aortic arch, bifurcating into the right subclavian artery and right common carotid artery at the level of the sternoclavicular joint. It crosses from left to right anterior to the trachea, usually around the ninth tracheal ring. However, it has a very variable location, and can sometimes be observed at or above the suprasternal notch as a pulsatile structure Avoidance of this artery is paramount as cases of fatal bleeding, or trachea-innominate artery fistulas post tracheostomy, have been described. It should be located prior to both surgical and percutaneous dilatational tracheostomies

Questions	Answers
5. In a preoperative assessment for an elective surgery, you note that your patient has a hoarse voice. Ultrasound examination reveals the following 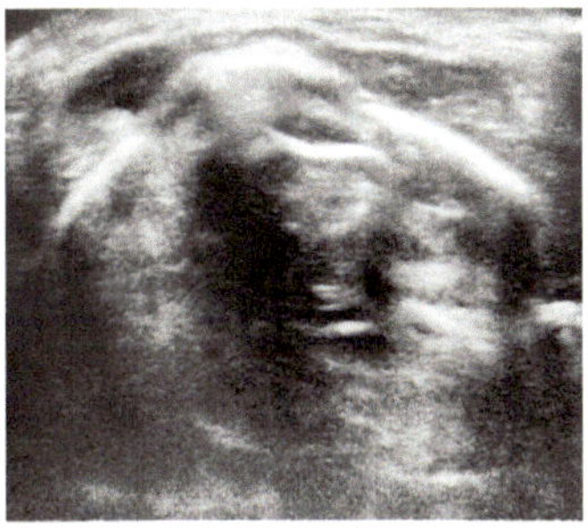 Appropriate management includes: A. Continue with surgery with careful intubation technique B. Assure patient and document voice hoarseness before proceeding with surgery C. Referral to otolaryngologist for further evaluation D. Investigate the patient for left recurrent laryngeal nerve palsy	Answer: C. There is a vocal cord cyst at the anterior commissure. On the ultrasound, posterior acoustic enhancement of the area below the fluid cyst hints at its nature. Careful documentation and preoperative evaluation, as well as counselling of patient for potential worsening of voice hoarseness is indicated. The vocal cords are abducted hence vocal cord paralysis is unlikely. Depending on how time-sensitive the surgery is, investigation into the cause of the patient's hoarse voice is useful but should not prohibit urgent surgery from proceeding 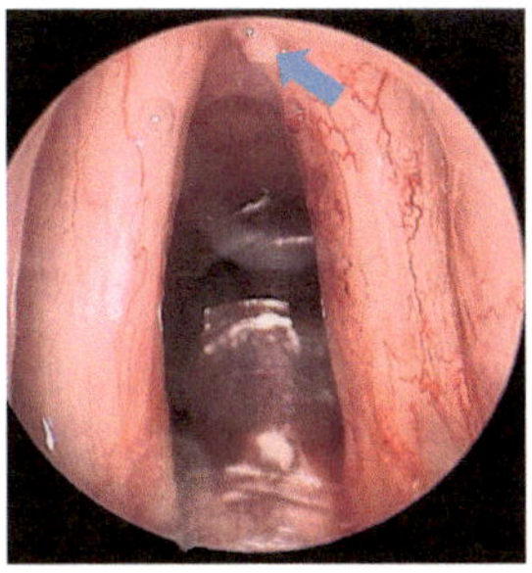
6. A patient is noted to have a left-sided neck fullness just below his chin. Bedside ultrasound revealed the following: 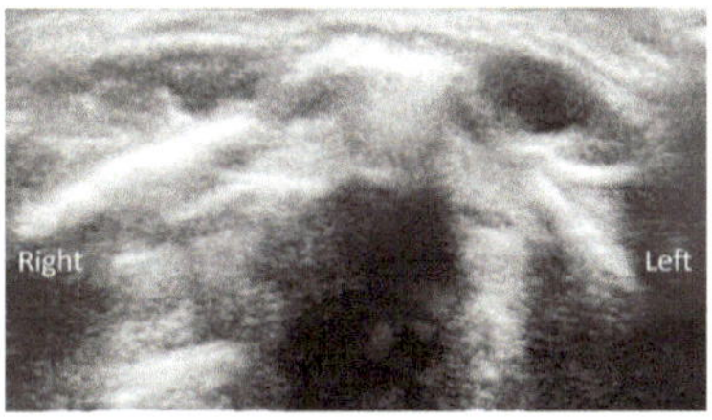 The lesion shown is most likely to be: A. A thyroglossal duct cyst B. Ectopic thyroid tissue C. A vocal cord cyst D. A branchial cleft cyst	Answer: A. Thyroglossal duct cysts are the most common congenital neck mass. They are thin-walled, fluid-filled, usually close to the midline, anterior to the thyroid cartilage, and splaying the strap muscles. They are generally close to the hyoid bone and can be traced to a tail diving under the hyoid. On ultrasound, they appear anechoic, with posterior acoustic enhancement. Stranding within the cyst or thickened walls may indicate inflammation. Thyroid tissue would exhibit a homogenously hypoechoic appearance but can be found in very variable locations. A vocal cord cyst would appear posterior to the thyroid cartilage and branchial cleft cysts tend to be located more laterally. Ultrasound is a useful initial investigation modality due to its noninvasiveness, accessibility, relatively low cost, and avoidance of exposure to radiation
7. Ultrasound features that correlate to a higher likelihood of obstructive sleep apnoea (OSA) include all EXCEPT: A. Tongue thickness > 60 mm B. Tongue width > 28 mm C. Thickened lateral pharyngeal walls D. Mentohyoid distance < 52 mm	Answer: D. Together with patient history and physical examination, airway ultrasound can help improve the accuracy of OSA screening. Airway ultrasound features include the tongue thickness and width, as well as thickening of the lateral pharyngeal wall. Non-airway parameters include carotid plaque formation and carotid intimal thickening as surrogate markers [24]

<table>
<tr><th>Questions</th><th>Answers</th></tr>
<tr><td>8. In a patient with known right recurrent laryngeal nerve palsy, you would expect to see the following on ultrasound in the transverse orientation at the level of the thyroid cartilage during inspiration:
<table>
<tr><th></th><th>Right vocal cord</th><th>Left vocal cord</th></tr>
<tr><td>A</td><td>Abducted</td><td>Abducted</td></tr>
<tr><td>B</td><td>Abducted</td><td>Adducted</td></tr>
<tr><td>C</td><td>Adducted</td><td>Abducted</td></tr>
<tr><td>D</td><td>Adducted</td><td>Adducted</td></tr>
</table></td><td>Answer: C. The recurrent laryngeal nerve (RLN) branches from the vagus nerve and supplies all the intrinsic muscles of the larynx, except the cricothyroid muscles. Complete paralysis of the RLN results in a partially adducted vocal cord, while partial paralysis results in a fully adducted vocal cord</td></tr>
<tr><td>9. A victim of a road traffic accident where the vehicle caught fire was brought into the emergency department with severe burns to his face, although his neck is relatively unscathed. The potential airway issues include:
A. Lower airway edema
B. Potential cervical spine instability
C. Upper airway injury
D. All of the above</td><td>Answer: D. This unfortunate patient will have all the attendant issues of trauma and smoke inhalation, not to mention burns and injuries to his face and upper airway</td></tr>
<tr><td>10. Advantages of a cricothyroidotomy over a tracheostomy in an emergency front of neck access include:
A. Relatively avascular structure
B. More superficial and palpable cricothyroid membrane compared to the deeper tracheal rings
C. Shorter insertion time required
D. All of the above</td><td>Answer: D. In an emergency situation, a cricothyroidotomy offers the fastest and least complicated means of front of neck airway access. However, it is thought to be associated with an increased risk of subglottic stenosis, and hence creation of a formal tracheostomy is often performed within 72 h of an emergency cricothyroidotomy</td></tr>
<tr><td>11. Postsurgical tracheostomy creation, a ward nurse notices swelling around the tracheostomy site. Ultrasound evaluation reveals anechoic areas in the subcutaneous and peri-muscular planes
The cause of the swelling is likely to be:
A. Blood
B. Subcutaneous emphysema
C. Soft tissue swelling
D. An overly tight tracheostomy strap</td><td>Answer: A. Fluid, such as blood, appears anechoic on ultrasound and will cast posterior acoustic enhancement (bright area). Air will cause posterior shadowing (dark area). Ultrasound of the airway is a useful bedside examination that is portable, can be done rapidly and noninvasively, and gives immediate information which can be critical to preventing adverse patient outcomes</td></tr>
<tr><td>12. Structures that may overlie the cricothyroid membrane (CTM) DO NOT include:
A. The cricothyroid artery and vein (in the upper 1/3)
B. The pyramidal lobe of the thyroid gland
C. Recurrent laryngeal nerve
D. Lymph nodes</td><td>Answer: C. All the other structures may be found in variable positions overlying cricothyroid membrane and care should be taken in the event a cricothyroidotomy needs to be performed</td></tr>
</table>

Questions	Answers
13. Differences between the ultrasound appearance of the pediatric airway compared to that of an adult include all EXCEPT: A. A cartilaginous and hypoechoic hyoid bone B. Measurement of the tracheal diameter for endotracheal tube sizing at the level of the thyroid cartilage C. Thinner and less echogenic cricothyroid membrane D. An elliptical rather than circular subglottic airway	Answer: B. The narrowest part of the pediatric airway is at the level of the cricoid cartilage, and airway measurement should take place here. Ultrasound sizing of the airway is more accurate compared to age-based and height-based formulas in estimating ETT size (outer diameter) for pediatric patients [25, 26]
14. A 12-year-old child with cerebral palsy and severe scoliosis requires a spine operation to improve his respiratory function. He has very limited cervical extension. Which of the following ultrasound techniques may help in this situation? 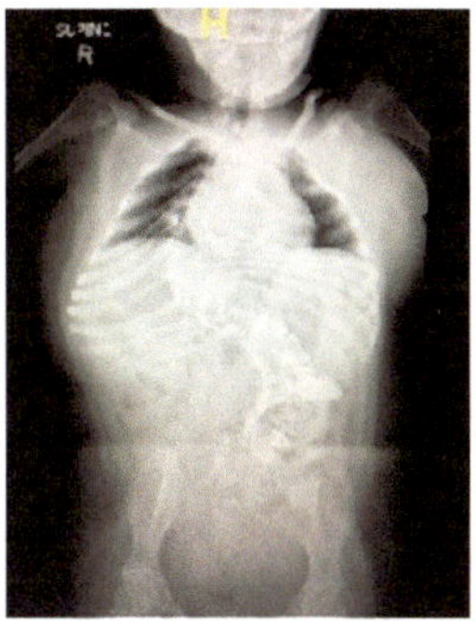 A. Assessment of the tracheal diameter for endotracheal tube (ETT) sizing at the level of the sternal notch B. Use of ultrasound to perform a superior laryngeal nerve block for an awake intubation C. Use of a curvilinear probe to assess the mentohyoid distance D. Use of a small "hockey stick probe" to identify the cricothyroid membrane	Answer: B. This patient is an airway challenge because of his limited range of motion. Ultrasound will be difficult because of his inability to extend his neck, and such patients are generally small for their age. Ultrasound is a reliable tool to predict ETT size for pediatric patients with thoracic or lumbar scoliosis. However, pediatric patients with cervical lateral bending will need an ETT smaller than the size predicted by ultrasonography [27]. Real-time imaging of the airway during intubation can also help to ensure that the ETT is placed at an appropriate depth, but this requires a second operator
15. Ultrasound features of an intubated airway include all except: A. Reverberation artifacts in the airway B. Double track lines in the sagittal plane C. Posterior shadow in the airway D. Comet-tail artifacts in the airway	Answer: A. The air column within the endotracheal tube causes a linear posterior shadow within the airway. Radial comet-tail artifacts may also be seen. Double track lines indicate the presence of a tube within the airway 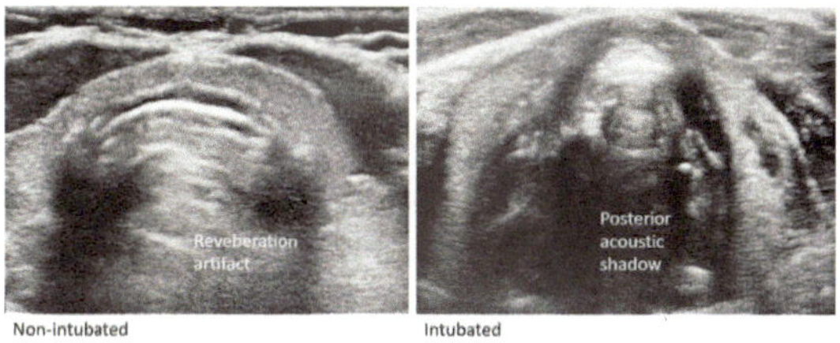

Questions	Answers
16. A 45-year-old patient attempted suicide by drinking a large volume of corrosive fluid and alcohol. He presents to the emergency department. He is extremely agitated, trashing, and has pulled out his intravenous cannulas. His breathing is stridorous and his pulse oximetry reading is 88%. What is the most reasonable plan of action? 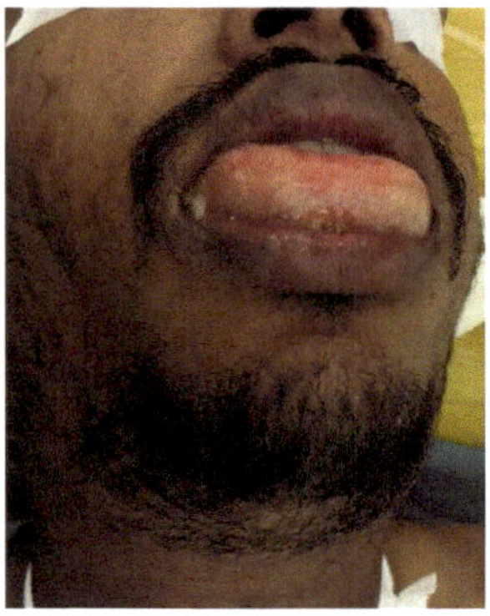 A. Avoid sedation, attempt awake bronchoscopic intubation B. Avoid sedation, perform percutaneous dilatational tracheostomy C. Sedate with IM or inhalational agents, perform cricothyroidotomy D. Sedate with IM or inhalational agents, paralyze patient, and attempt nasal or oral intubation	Answer C: The patient likely has upper airway edema and is agitated from a combination of intoxication and hypoxia. He is in respiratory distress and his airway needs to be secured. He is likely to be difficult to manage without sedation but should be kept spontaneously ventilating where possible. He will not be able to cooperate with an awake intubation Rapid focused ultrasound assessment of the airway should be done to identify the cricothyroid membrane as well as to evaluate airway edema and soft tissue swelling. Serial ultrasounds can also be used to monitor progress
17. Which of the following is true about ultrasound appearance of airway structures? A. Cartilage appears homogenously hypoechoic B. The cricothyroid membrane appears as a bright line because it is relatively solid compared to cartilage C. Reverberation artifacts appear as hyperechoic radial lines D. Air causes posterior acoustic enhancement	Answer: A The air-mucosa interface, such as that at the cricothyroid membrane, appears as a bright line because of the significant difference between soft tissue and air, resulting in a strong reflection of soundwaves Reverberation artifacts are generated due to the reflective properties of the air-mucosa interface and appear as regularly spaced parallel hyperechoic lines deep to the air-mucosa interface Air columns, such as that within an endotracheal tube, will cast an acoustic shadow, obscuring structures deep into it

Questions	Answers
18. A patient presents with the following lesion on CT scan and is being brought to the operating theatre for intubation and emergency surgery 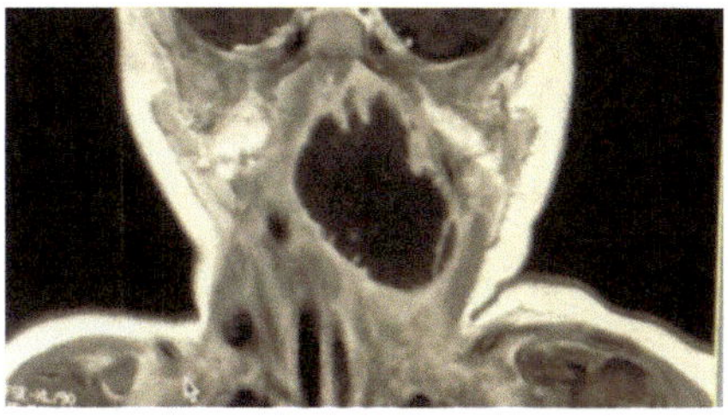 During a pre-intubation ultrasound scan of the patient's airway, which area do you expect to see the lesion in? 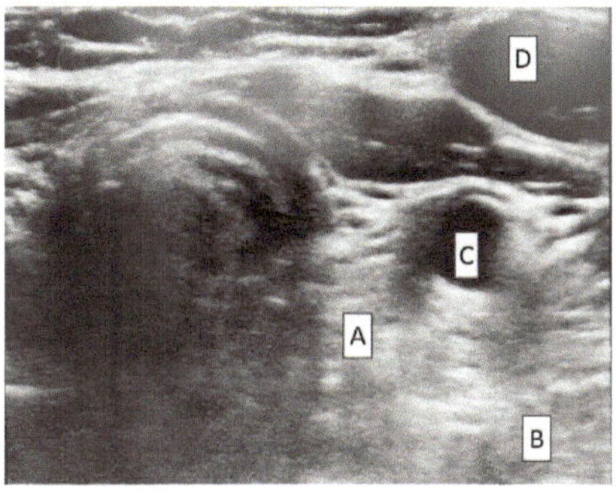	Answer: A. This patient has a large retropharyngeal abscess. Airway anatomy may be distorted, and ultrasound can help especially with ensuring accurate endotracheal tube sizing, as well as with the identification of critical airway structures
19. The best level to measure the airway diameter to select a left-sided double lumen endotracheal tube size is at the: A. Hyoid B. Thyroid cartilage C. Suprasternal notch D. Cricoid cartilage	Answer: C. The suprasternal notch provides an easily visualized and measured point of the airway for the purposes of sizing of a double lumen endotracheal tube, according to its outer diameter
20. Which of the following ultrasound features may predict a difficult airway? A. Skin to tracheal distance of 23 mm at the suprasternal notch B. Tongue width of 27 mm C. Skin to epiglottis distance of 22 mm D. Mentohyoid distance of 42 mm	Answer: D. The skin to tracheal distance at the suprasternal notch is not proven to be a marker of airway difficulty, although a larger distance would probably correspond to a prominent chest which may interfere with the handle of a standard laryngoscope It is important to remember that no single parameter can predict airway difficulty well. Multiple ultrasound airway parameters, together with clinical assessment, can help to increase the rate of identification of difficult airways and enable management by informing the clinician of the level at which they are most likely to encounter difficulty

<table>
<tr><th>Clinical exam scenarios</th><th>Answers</th></tr>
<tr>
<td>
A young man was brought into ED after a bar fight. He is intoxicated and unable to give a consistent history, but you note some mild bruising and swelling over his neck. He has no other injuries
His vital signs are as follows:
Blood pressure: 114/74 mmHg
Heart rate: 90 beats/min
Pulse oximetry: 94% on room air
Physical examination: No noisy breathing/stridor, not cyanotic, not in respiratory distress
1. What are your airway concerns for this patient?
2. Ultrasound reveals the following. There are no other abnormalities. What is the likely diagnosis?
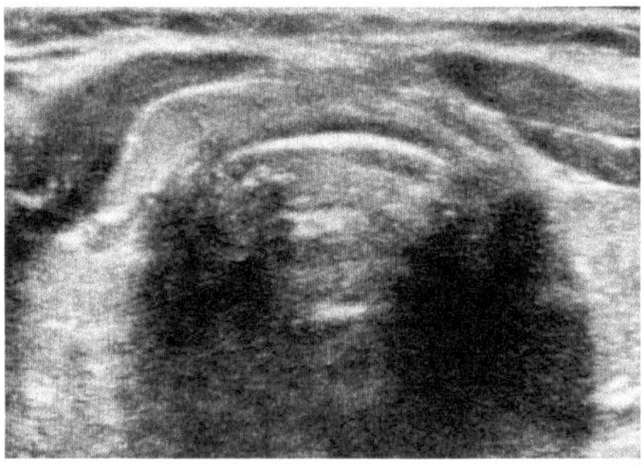
3. How would you manage this patient?
</td>
<td>
1. What are your airway concerns for this patient?
• Cervical spine injury
• Airway patency and continuity
• Soft tissue swelling
2. Likely diagnosis?
• Cricoid cartilage injury, indicated by the loss of continuity and depression of the cricoid cartilage
• There may be accompanying soft tissue swelling and edema
• Likely cause in this patient is blunt laryngeal trauma
3. Management?
Laryngeal trauma can be categorized as penetrating or blunt laryngeal trauma. Management can be guided by the Schaefer Classification System of Severity of Laryngeal Injuries in the table below [28, 29]
<table>
<tr><th>Severity</th><th>Management</th></tr>
<tr><td>Group 1: Minor endolaryngeal hematomas or lacerations without detectable fractures</td><td>Conservative; Consider medical adjunctive management such as steroids, antibiotics, anti-reflux medication, humidification, and voice rest</td></tr>
<tr><td>Group 2: More severe edema, hematoma, minor mucosal disruption without exposed cartilage, or nondisplaced fractures</td><td>Conservative initially but with serial examination as injuries may progress over time. Medical adjuncts as for Group 1</td></tr>
<tr><td>Group 3: Massive edema, large mucosal lacerations, exposed cartilage, displaced fractures, or vocal cord immobility</td><td>Direct laryngoscopy or esophagoscopy should be performed in the operating room. Tracheostomy, surgical exploration, and repair are often required</td></tr>
<tr><td>Group 4: Same as group 3, but more severe, with disruption of anterior larynx, unstable fractures, two or more fractures lines, or severe mucosal injuries</td><td>Direct laryngoscopy and esophagoscopy must be performed emergently. Tracheostomy mandated and surgical repair may involve stent placement</td></tr>
<tr><td>Group 5: Complete laryngotracheal separation</td><td>Patient will present with severe respiratory distress, necessitating urgent airway evaluation and management. Altered anatomy may make airway management difficult. Close communication and joint management between the surgical and anesthetic teams are critical</td></tr>
<tr><td colspan="2">Schaefer Classification System of Severity of Laryngeal Injuries and Suggested Management</td></tr>
</table>
</td>
</tr>
</table>

Clinical exam scenarios	Answers
An unknown elderly male was knocked down by a motorcycle while crossing the road. He sustained lower limb fractures and focused assessment with sonography in trauma (FAST) shows free fluid in his abdomen. He is hypotensive and tachycardic, and pulse oximetry is 86% on bag-mask ventilation with 100% oxygen. He is noted to have a tracheostomy, which was dislodged in the accident, as well as bilateral neck scars. Medical records are unavailable as he was not carrying any identity documents 1. What are your treatment priorities in this patient? 2. Bag-mask ventilation does not seem to be improving the patient's oxygenation, and he has become unconscious. Attempts at recanalization of the tracheostomy have failed, and the clinical team decides to intubate orally. Suspecting a difficult airway, an airway ultrasound is performed and reveal the following What is the implication of this ultrasound finding? 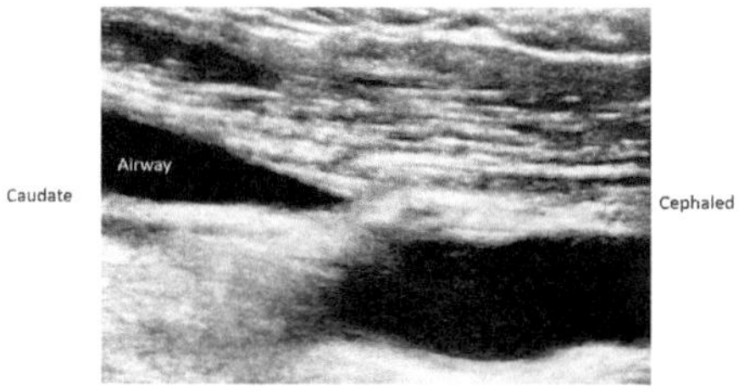 3. What is the most reasonable plan of management to secure the patient's airway?	**1. What are your treatment priorities in this patient?** This patient has sustained polytrauma, and it is imperative to rapidly secure his airway, oxygenate him and improve his hemodynamics with fluid, blood, and pressor support **2. Ultrasound of airway—findings and implications** The airway of this patient appears to terminate at the mid-tracheal level. This implies that the patient likely had a total laryngectomy and that the upper airway is not continuous with the lower airway. Hence, oral intubation will not be possible **3. Plan of management** Careful but rapid exploration of the tracheostomy site can be performed. A bougie or flexible suction catheter may be gently passed into the tracheotomy track. Real-time ultrasound monitoring can help to ascertain intratracheal placement and avoid creating a false passage. A tracheostomy tube or armored endotracheal tube can then be railroaded into the trachea, and ultrasound is used to confirm placement, as well as the depth of insertion
A patient was intubated 6 days ago for airway protection after an episode of torrential epistaxis, which has now resolved. The patient is a 40 kg elderly female of small build. A size 7.5 ETT was used. She is now ready to be extubated, but the clinical team is encountering resistance when attempts are made to withdraw the ETT. The patient is otherwise well and breathing spontaneously on FiO_2 0.28. They request for the anesthetic team's assistance in attempting extubation in the operating theatre 1. How would you assess the patient's fitness for extubation? 2. What are the risk factors for developing subglottic stenosis? 3. What ultrasound airway parameters are useful in the evaluation of this patient for extubation?	**1. How would you assess the patient's fitness for extubation?** Acronym: MOVEC • Mental status—GCS >8 (with some rare exceptions) • Oxygenation—The patient should be able to maintain adequate oxygenation with low levels of support. The PaO_2/FiO_2 ratio should be more than 150, and $FiO_2 < 0.4$ • Ventilation—Positive End Expiratory Pressure should be <10 cmH_2O, and minute ventilation requirements <15 L/min • Expectoration—Secretions should not be excessive or cause mucous plugging • Cardiovascular—instability should not be present **2. What are the risk factors for developing acquired subglottic stenosis?** • Paediatric—Prolonged intubation, low birth weight [30] • Adults—High body mass index, diabetes [31], prolonged intubation **3. What ultrasound parameters are useful in evaluation of this patient?** • Air column width during cuff deflation at the level of the cricothyroid membrane is a predictor of post-extubation stridor (PES) [32] • Evaluation of vocal cord function and airway edema • Ultrasound of the lung and diaphragm can also help to predict readiness for extubation

<table>
<tr><th>Clinical exam scenarios</th><th>Answers</th></tr>
<tr><td>

A 6-year-old child presents to the emergency department with a sorethroat, drooling, and stridor. He is distressed and anxious

1. How would you assess patency of this child's airway?
2. How can ultrasound of the airway help?
3. What are the differential diagnoses?
4. Ultrasound of the airway in the sagittal section using a curvilinear probe at the submental level shows the following appearance. What is the most likely diagnosis?

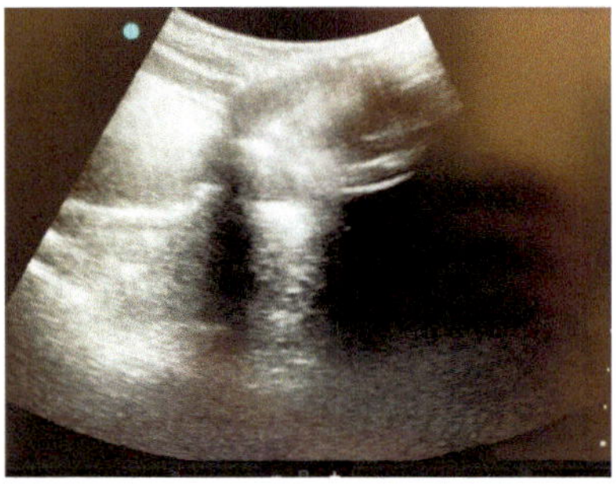

</td><td>

1. **How would you assess patency of this child's airway?**
   - Rapid assessment of patient's airway, breathing, and circulation
   - Airway—accessory muscle use, tracheal tug, stridor
   - Breathing—respiratory rate, breathing effort, and ability to move air in and out of lungs
   - Circulation—presence of cyanosis, hypoxia, heart rate, consciousness
2. **How can ultrasound of the airway help?**
   - Assess patency of airway
   - Identify cricothyroid membrane in the event emergency front of neck access is needed
   - Right-sizing of an endotracheal tube or tracheostomy tube
   - Evaluate potential causes for patient's symptoms
   - Noninvasive, bedside test that can be done with parental presence to encourage child's cooperation
3. **Differential diagnoses?**
   - Infective—epiglottitis, viral croup, bacterial tracheitis
   - Allergy—anaphylaxis, angioedema
   - Foreign body inhalation
   - Trauma
   - Inhalation of corrosive or irritative gas
4. **Ultrasound appearance of epiglottitis**
   - Using a curvilinear probe in the longitudinal orientation and at the level of the hyoid bone, the epiglottis appears as the head of the "alphabet P," and the acoustic shadow cast by the hyoid bone forms the stem of the letter P. A swollen and oedematous epiglottis is indicative of epiglottis [33]
   - Evaluation can also be made in the transverse orientation, just below the hyoid, seeing the hypoechoic cartilaginous epiglottis in the middle of the tongue [34]

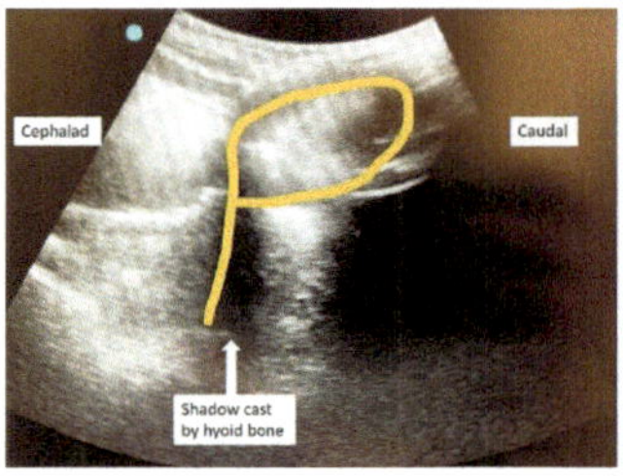

</td></tr>
</table>

<table>
<tr><th>Clinical exam scenarios</th><th>Answers</th></tr>
<tr><td>A 35-year-old male patient presents to the emergency department with a penetrating neck wound across his neck. The patient is sitting upright. Supplemental oxygen is being administered via a non-rebreather mask, and oxygen saturation is 85–88%. His blood pressure is 95/50 mmHg and heart rate is 102 beats per minute. The subcutaneous tissue below the mandible and oropharynx is grossly traumatized and bleeding heavily. The patient is conscious and able to breath, but there is a bubbling sound in his neck area with each breath
1. What are your initial goals of airway management in this patient?
2. How would you secure this patient's airway?
3. How would you utilize ultrasound in this scenario?
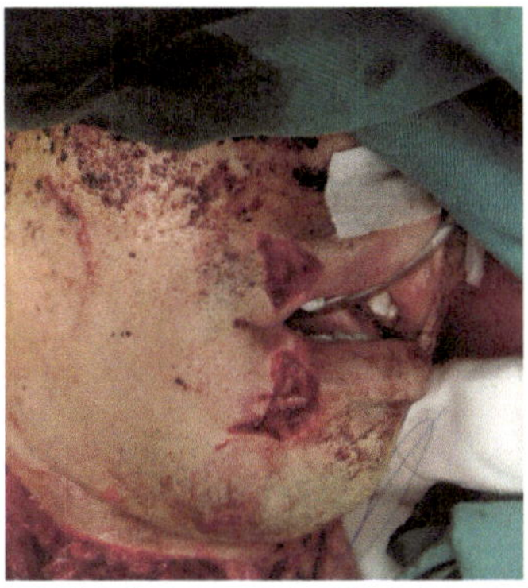</td>
<td>1. Initial goals of management
• Airway—maintain airway patency
• Breathing—maintain spontaneous ventilation and supplemental oxygen
• Circulation—ensure good vascular access and administer fluids, blood, and vasopressors as needed
• Disability—assess for other injuries
2. How would you secure this patient's airway?
This is an airway fraught with difficulties. There is likely trauma to the trachea itself, along with blood that will obscure visualization and soft tissue swelling which will worsen
The airway needs to be secured together with surgical expertise, and the management plan would need to be formulated according to the suspected level of injury. The patient may need to be sedated for this, but spontaneous ventilation should be maintained as far as possible. Avoid a cannot intubate, cannot ventilate situation
3. Use of ultrasound
Combination of airway and lung ultrasound can help to evaluate the success of endotracheal tube (ETT) insertion, whether by the oral, nasal, or front of neck access route. Tracheal ultrasound (either in real time or immediately after intubation) can exclude the presence of the ETT in the esophagus and possibly visualize the ETT in the trachea. Confirm the presence of lung sliding on the left, the absence of which may indicate right endobronchial intubation. Finally, confirm the presence of lung sliding on the right [35]</td></tr>
<tr><td>A 48-year-old patient, with a body mass index of 51 kg/m^2 requires intubation with a double lumen endotracheal tube for surgical removal of a right lung mass. She has limited neck extension, a small mouth opening, and has hypertension and diabetes. She is unsure if she has symptoms of obstructive sleep apnea
1. What are the ultrasound features that may suggest that the patient has obstructive sleep apnoea?
2. What may help make to optimize the performance of an airway ultrasound examination in this patient?
3. If double lumen tube intubation is not possible, what are the alternatives to achieve lung isolation?
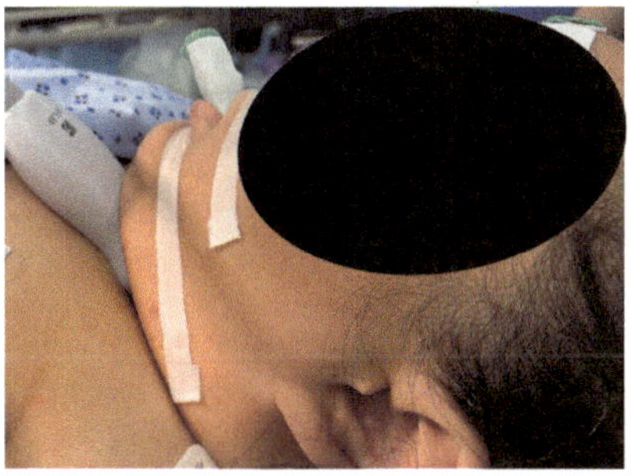</td>
<td>1. What are the ultrasound features that may suggest that the patient has obstructive sleep apnea (OSA)?
• Tongue width (between the lingual arteries) > 28 mm
• Retro-lingual space <37 mm and retropalatal space <30 mm
• Distance between the lateral edge of the pharynx and carotid artery, usually 30–50 mm. A greater distance correlates with greater severity of OSA [4, 24, 36]
2. Optimizing airway ultrasound examination
Ultrasound in morbidly obese patients may be challenging, especially with limited neck extension. Placing the patient's upper body in a ramped position may help to increase access to the patient's neck, as well as improve ventilation for the intubation process. Sufficient ultrasound gel is also essentialThe cricothyroid membrane (CTM) is often impalpable in morbidly obese patients. Ultrasound localization of the CTM can be performed faster than palpation. Tube sizing and real-time monitoring of intubation help to avoid airway injury [37]
3. If double lumen tube intubation is not possible, what are the alternatives to achieve lung isolation?
Insertion of a single lumen ETT, followed by the use of a bronchial blocker is one method. Alternatively, the single lumen ETT can be advanced to the left bronchus as an intentional endobronchial intubation</td></tr>
</table>

References

1. Gottlieb M, Holladay D, Burns KM, Nakitende D, Bailitz J. Ultrasound for airway management: An evidence-based review for the emergency clinician. Am J Emerg Med. 2020;38(5):1007–13.
2. Cherian A, Kundra P. Ultrasound imaging of the airway and its applications. Airway. 2018;1(1):17–24.
3. Adi O, Kok MS, Abdull Wahab SF. Focused airway ultrasound: an armamentarium in future airway management. J Emerg Crit Care Med. 2019;3:31.
4. Zetlaoui PJ. Ultrasonography for airway management. Anaesth Crit Care Pain Med. 2021;40(2):100821.
5. Jang YE, Kim EH, Song IK, Lee JH, Ryu HG, Kim HS, et al. Prediction of the mid-tracheal level using surface anatomical landmarks in adults: clinical implication of endotracheal tube insertion depth. Medicine (Baltimore). 2017;96(12):e6319.
6. Thomas VK, Paul C, Rajeev PC, Palatty BU. Reliability of ultrasonography in confirming endotracheal tube placement in an emergency setting. Indian J Crit Care Med. 2017;21(5):257–61.
7. Kuriyama A, Jackson JL, Kamei J. Performance of the cuff leak test in adults in predicting post-extubation airway complications: a systematic review and meta-analysis. Crit Care. 2020;24(1):640.
8. Schnell D, Planquette B, Berger A, Merceron S, Mayaux J, Strasbach L, et al. Cuff leak test for the diagnosis of post-extubation stridor: a multicenter evaluation study. J Intensive Care Med. 2019;34(5):391–6.
9. Venkategowda PM, Mahendrakar K, Rao SM, Mutkule DP, Shirodkar CG, Yogesh H. Laryngeal air column width ratio in predicting post extubation stridor. Indian J Crit Care Med. 2015;19(3):170–3.
10. Ding L-W, Wang H-C, Wu H-D, Chang C-J, Yang P-C. Laryngeal ultrasound: a useful method in predicting post-extubation stridor. A pilot study. Eur Respir J. 2006;27(2):384–9.
11. Sustić A, Miletić D, Protić A, Ivancić A, Cicvarić T. Can ultrasound be useful for predicting the size of a left double-lumen bronchial tube? Tracheal width as measured by ultrasonography versus computed tomography. J Clin Anesth. 2008;20(4):247–52.
12. Liao YC, Wu WC, Hsieh MH, Chang CC, Tsai HC. Ultrasound-guided superior laryngeal nerve block assists in anesthesia for bronchoscopic surgical procedure: a case report of anesthesia for rigid bronchoscopy. Medicine (Baltimore). 2020;99(27):e20916.
13. Sawka A, Tang R, Vaghadia H. Sonographically guided superior laryngeal nerve block during awake fiberoptic intubation. A A Case Rep. 2015;4(8):107–10.
14. Kristensen MS, Teoh WH. Ultrasound identification of the cricothyroid membrane: the new standard in preparing for front-of-neck airway access. Br J Anaesth. 2021;126(1):22–7.
15. Kristensen MS, Teoh WH, Rudolph SS, Tvede MF, Hesselfeldt R, Børglum J, et al. Structured approach to ultrasound-guided identification of the cricothyroid membrane: a randomized comparison with the palpation method in the morbidly obese. Br J Anaesth. 2015;114(6):1003–4.
16. Osman A, Sum KM. Role of upper airway ultrasound in airway management. J Intensive Care. 2016;4(1):52.
17. Kristensen MS, Teoh WH, Graumann O, Laursen CB. Ultrasonography for clinical decision-making and intervention in airway management: from the mouth to the lungs and pleurae. Insights Imaging. 2014;5(2):253–79.
18. Srinivasarangan M, Akkamahadevi P, Balkal VC, Javali RH. Diagnostic accuracy of ultrasound measurements of anterior neck soft tissue in determining a difficult airway. J Emerg Trauma Shock. 2021;14(1):33–7.
19. Abraham S, Himarani J, Mary Nancy S, Shanmugasundaram S, Krishnakumar Raja VB. Ultrasound as an assessment method in predicting difficult intubation: a prospective clinical study. J Maxillofac Oral Surg. 2018;17(4):563–9.
20. Komatsu R, Sengupta P, Wadhwa A, Akça O, Sessler DI, Ezri T, et al. Ultrasound quantification of anterior soft tissue thickness fails to predict difficult laryngoscopy in obese patients. Anaesth Intensive Care. 2007;35(1):32–7.
21. Ezri T, Gewürtz G, Sessler DI, Medalion B, Szmuk P, Hagberg C, et al. Prediction of difficult laryngoscopy in obese patients by ultrasound quantification of anterior neck soft tissue. Anaesthesia. 2003;58(11):1111–4.
22. Daniel SJ, Bertolizio G, McHugh T. Airway ultrasound: point of care in children-The time is now. Paediatr Anaesth. 2020;30(3):347–52.
23. You-Ten KE, Siddiqui N, Teoh WH, Kristensen MS. Point-of-care ultrasound (POCUS) of the upper airway. Can J Anaesth. 2018;65(4):473–84.
24. Singh M, Tuteja A, Wong DT, Goel A, Trivedi A, Tomlinson G, et al. Point-of-care ultrasound for obstructive sleep apnea screening: are we there yet? A systematic review and meta-analysis. Anesth Analg. 2019;129(6):1673–91.
25. Stafrace S, Engelhardt T, Teoh WH, Kristensen MS. Essential ultrasound techniques of the pediatric airway. Paediatr Anaesth. 2016;26(2):122–31.
26. Ahn JH, Park JH, Kim MS, Kang HC, Kim IS. Point of care airway ultrasound to select tracheal tube and determine insertion depth in cleft repair surgery. Sci Rep. 2021;11(1):4743.
27. Hao J, Zhang J, Dong B, Luo Z. The accuracy of ultrasound to predict endotracheal tube size for pediatric patients with congenital scoliosis. BMC Anesthesiol. 2020;20(1):183.
28. Adi O, Sum KM, Ahmad AH, Wahab MA, Neri L, Panebianco N. Novel role of focused airway ultrasound in early airway assessment of suspected laryngeal trauma. Ultrasound J. 2020;12(1):37.
29. Omakobia E, Micallef A. Approach to the patient with external laryngeal trauma: the schaefer classification. Otolaryngology. 2016;6(230):2.

30. Dankle SK, Schuller DE, McClead RE. Risk factors for neonatal acquired subglottic stenosis. Ann Otol Rhinol Laryngol. 1986;95(6 Pt 1):626–30.
31. Nicolli EA, Carey RM, Farquhar D, Haft S, Alfonso KP, Mirza N. Risk factors for adult acquired subglottic stenosis. J Laryngol Otol. 2017;131(3):264–7.
32. El Amrousy D, Elkashlan M, Elshmaa N, Ragab A. Ultrasound-guided laryngeal air column width difference as a new predictor for postextubation stridor in children. Crit Care Med. 2018;46(6):e496–501.
33. Hung TY, Li S, Chen PS, Wu LT, Yang YJ, Tseng LM, et al. Bedside ultrasonography as a safe and effective tool to diagnose acute epiglottitis. Am J Emerg Med. 2011;29(3):359.e1–3.
34. Ko DR, Chung YE, Park I, Lee HJ, Park JW, You JS, et al. Use of bedside sonography for diagnosing acute epiglottitis in the emergency department: a preliminary study. J Ultrasound Med. 2012;31(1):19–22.
35. Senussi MH, Kantamneni PC, Latifi M, Omranian AP, Krveshi L, Barakat AF, et al. Protocolized tracheal and thoracic ultrasound for confirmation of endotracheal intubation and positioning: a multicenter observational study. Crit Care Explor. 2020;2(9):e0225.
36. Isaiah A, Mezrich R, Wolf J. Ultrasonographic detection of airway obstruction in a model of obstructive sleep apnea. Ultrasound Int Open. 2017;3(1):E34–e42.
37. De Jong A, Molinari N, Pouzeratte Y, Verzilli D, Chanques G, Jung B, et al. Difficult intubation in obese patients: incidence, risk factors, and complications in the operating theatre and in intensive care units. Br J Anaesth. 2015;114(2):297–306.

4 Point-of-Care Ultrasound of the Lungs

Archit Sharma and Sudhakar Subramani

4.1 Introduction

Over the last two decades, ultrasound has emerged as a new imaging technique for the thorax, even though the possibility of exploring the lung by using ultrasound dates back to the 1960s [1]. Lung parenchyma is one of the challenging structures to evaluate using ultrasound, primarily due to high air/tissue ratio. However, in the early 1990s, with the advent of descriptors like lung sliding, and B-lines, it became possible to evaluate lung in a systematic way. With a growing interest in the technique, many other features of lung ultrasound, such as artifactual images of normal aeration (i.e., A-lines), and the real images mirroring pathologic conditions (e.g., consolidations, pleural effusion) have been described in the comprehensive examination. Many societies have formulated a structured way of performing lung ultrasound (LUS) and proposed it as an effective and accurate goal-directed diagnostic tool that can be applied in real time for the bedside assessment of patients with respiratory disorders [2].

LUS has been shown to outperform physical examination and chest radiography for both diagnosis and monitoring of many pulmonary and pleural conditions, especially in acute care settings such as an emergency department and intensive care units [2, 3]. In addition, suboptimal radiography may mask or mimic clinically significant abnormalities and at the same time, differentiation of pleural and parenchymal structures can be challenging in these acute settings. Moreover, chest ultrasound is increasingly used to guide various interventional procedures such as placement of intercostal drains. Subsequently, the role of LUS expanded to many non-acute care settings and widely used in the assessment of patients with chronic diseases with lung involvement, such as chronic heart failure, chronic kidney diseases, and autoimmune diseases [4]. LUS has been established as one of the key diagnostic tools in the neonatal and pediatric critical care setting as well [5]. In this chapter, the authors have focused on a detailed description of the physics and physiology of LUS, how to perform LUS, description of sonographic appearances of normal lung and in various pathological conditions, utilization in many clinical settings, limitations and pitfalls, and comparative outcomes with other commonly used diagnostic modalities.

Supplementary Information The online version contains supplementary material available at [https://doi.org/10.1007/978-981-16-7687-1_4].

A. Sharma
Divisions of Cardiothoracic Anesthesiology, Solid Organ Transplant and Critical Care, Department of Anesthesia, Iowa City, IA, USA
e-mail: Archit-Sharma@UIOWA.edu

S. Subramani (✉)
Department of Anesthesia, Division of Cardiothoracic Anesthesiology, Iowa City, IA, USA
e-mail: Sudhakar-subramani@uiowa.edu

A. Chakraborty, B. Ashokka (eds.), *A Practical Guide to Point of Care Ultrasound (POCUS)*,
https://doi.org/10.1007/978-981-16-7687-1_4

4.1.1 Ultrasound Properties of Lung

Acoustic impedance (Z), a measure of the resistance of particles in a medium to mechanical vibrations determines the appearance of LUS. If the density of the given medium and propagation velocity of US in the medium increases, the overall resistance to sound signal increases. In the thoracic region, there are mediums with different impedances that cause some of the sounds to be transmitted and some to be reflected as an echo. The amount of reflection is based on the differences in acoustic impedance: fluid appears as black due to constant Z resulting in no echo, and soft tissues have a minimal reflection. Majority of the reflection happens between soft tissue and air reflect 99.9% rendering this interface virtually impenetrable to the US. This leads to inability to visualize normal aerated lung beneath the pleura and only artifacts can be seen [6].

Overall, LUS images are based on the relative amounts of air and fluid in the lung. If the lung is highly fluid-filled, then it can be directly visualized, whereas in case of pneumothorax, due to air being present below the parietal pleura, one is unable to visualize the lung tissue directly. Although in the past significant attenuation of US signals had discouraged clinicians to utilize US for the assessment of lung, in the current day and age, a better understanding of physical properties and new and improved ultrasound probes have played a significant role in expanding the use of LUS.

4.1.2 Types of Ultrasound Transducers for LUS

Table 4.1 shows properties, usefulness, and limitations of three commonly used probes for LUS (Fig. 4.1).

Table 4.1 Comparison of three LU transducers

Curvilinear probe	Phased array probe	Linear probe
• Low frequency (3–5 MHz) • Higher penetration • Larger sector width • Not ideal for rapid movement structures • Large footprint need more angulation to avoid ribs • Lung sliding can be easily visualized • Effusions, consolidated lung, and the diaphragm well imaged	• Low frequency (3–4.5 MHz) • Greater penetration • Poor quality of image • Small footprint allows to avoid ribs	• Higher frequency (5–10 MHz) • Poor penetration • Narrow sector width • Not ideal for deeper structures • Great image quality for superficial structures • Large footprint needs significant angulation to avoid ribs • No ideal for rapid movement structures

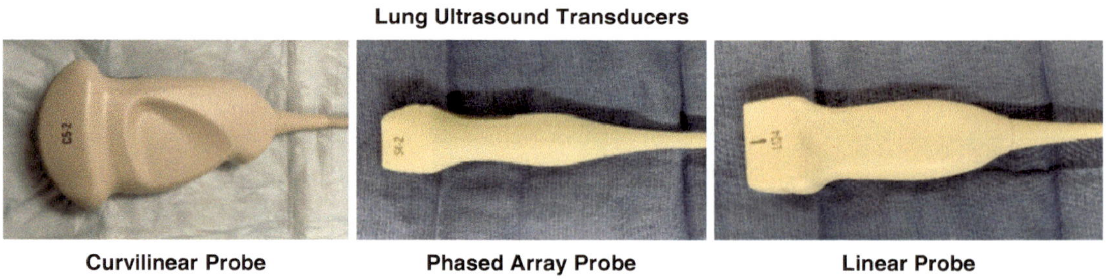

Fig. 4.1 Types of LU transducers

4.1.3 Performing LUS

Transthoracic chest US can be performed with one of the three probes, as described in Fig. 4.1. Initially, a curvilinear probe can be used for a quick survey of the chest wall, pleura, and lungs. Once an abnormality has been identified, a high-resolution linear probe can be used to provide a detailed depiction of any chest wall, pleural, or peripheral lung abnormality. In 2D images, the echogenicity of a lesion can be compared with that of the liver and characterized as hypoechoic, isoechoic, or hyperechoic. The color and quantitative Doppler can be used to identify vasculature. For improving the color Doppler imaging, the sensitivity should be set to a low-velocity scale (typically 0.25 m/s), along with a wall filter to minimize rejection of small frequency shifts and to avoid interference from respiratory or cardiac movements. It is also suggested to increase the color Doppler gain until a light, but uniform, background colored "snowstorm" is obtained. The Doppler angle should be less than 60° for accurate evaluation of vascular flow and needs to be repeated at least twice to ensure reproducibility of the spectral waveform. M-mode is used to demonstrate certain artifacts to diagnose lung/pleural abnormality.

Prior to image acquisition, the operator should ensure correct image orientation displayed on the screen such that the left side of the image should correspond with either the right side of the patient (if transverse) or cephalad (if longitudinal). A comprehensive examination can be performed in supine position especially in acute care settings or in sitting or decubitus positions. We will discuss a few of the protocols that have been described in the literature to examine the thorax [7]. Growing application of LUS in different settings has led to a difference in the approach and the nomenclature. A panel of experts from the First International Consensus Conference on Lung Ultrasound (ICC-LUS) have provided evidence-based recommendations on "point-of-care" LUS that predominantly focus on six major areas such as terminology, technology, technique, clinical outcomes, cost effectiveness, and future research [2].

One of the simplest and quick ways of evaluating lungs is a three-point (upper anterior, lower anterior, and postero-lateral) examination of each lung and is considered as a great starting point for a novice. To locate the three points, apply two hands side by side (without thumbs) over the anterior chest with your wrists in the anterior axillary line and your upper little finger resting along the clavicle. Your lower little finger will be aligned with the lower border of the lung (the phrenic line) (Fig. 4.2). Upper anterior point corresponds to the base of the middle and ring fingers on the upper hand and it lies over the upper lobe. Lower anterior point corresponds to the middle of the palm on the lower hand and it lies over the middle or lingular lobe. For postero-lateral point, move the probe laterally and posteriorly as far as possible behind the posterior axillary line from the lower anterior point and it lies over the lower lobe. In the three-point examination, all views are obtained in longitudinal orientation. Raising the arm above the patient's head increases the rib space distance and facilitates scanning with the patient in erect or recumbent positions. The posterior chest is best imaged with the patient sitting upright, while the anterior and lateral chest may be assessed in the lateral decubitus position. Maximum visualization of the lung and pleural space is achieved by scanning along the intercostal spaces. US should be performed during quiet respiration, to allow for assessment of normal lung movement, and in suspended respiration, when a lesion can be examined in detail with 2D or color Doppler (Fig. 4.2).

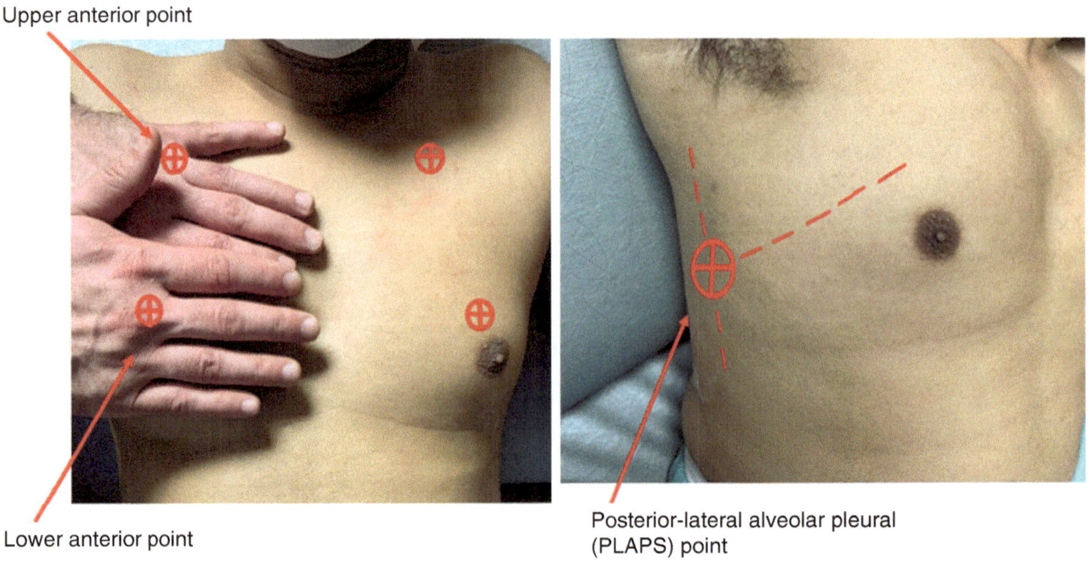

Fig. 4.2 Three point examination

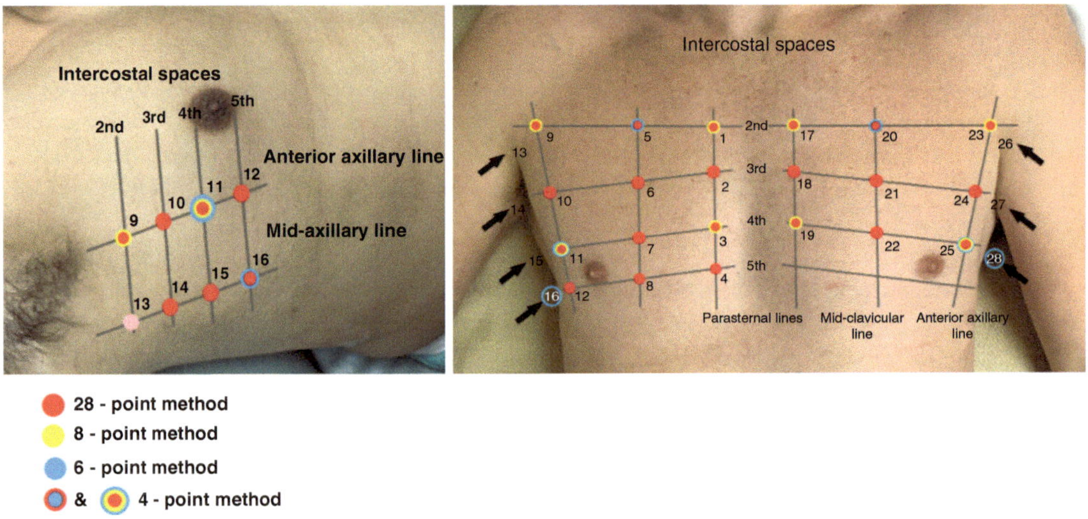

Fig. 4.3 Various scanning sites

4.1.4 Blue Protocol (Four-Point Method)

Blue protocol is based on a four-points assessment, which is basically upper and lower anterior points, on both sides of the chest wall. A positive point is defined as the presence of at least three B-lines. For positive examination, for certain acute respiratory disorders, at least three B-lines on each scanning site must be present [8].

Other least commonly used methods are six-point, eight-point, and 28 points. A six-point method consists of two blue points and an additional scanning site on the fifth intercostal space at mid-axillary line [9]. In the eight-point method, two anterior points between the sternum and the anterior axillary line, and two lateral points between the anterior and the posterior axillary line are the scanning sites [10]. In the 28-points method, scanning sites are at 16 points on the right side and 12 points on the left as shown in Fig. 4.3

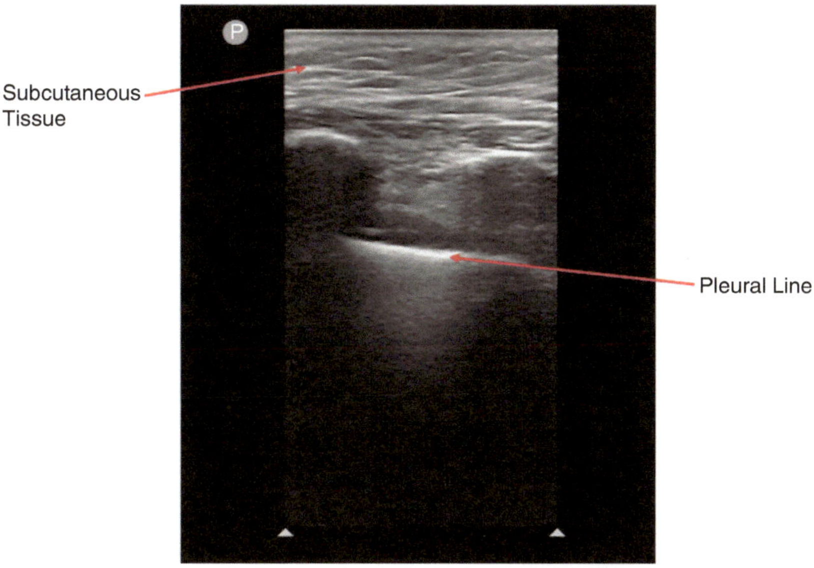

Fig. 4.4 LUS of normal lung

[11]. The supplementary videos 4.41–4.4 provide an example of scanning the chest wall from various positions. Video 4.1: Right upper anterior point using phased array probe, Video 4.2: Right lower anterior point using a transverse probe, Video 4.3: Right Posterior-lateral alveolar pleural point, Video 4.4: Right costophrenic view.

4.1.5 Ultrasound Image of Normal Lung

Visualization of the chest wall is achieved with the placement of the transducer in sagittal orientation in any intercostal space between second and seventh space. All signs in LUS arise from the pleural line, except for subcutaneous emphysema which will not display the pleural line due to the presence of air in the superficial tissue. The normal chest wall appears as a series of echogenic soft tissue layers, representing the layers of muscles and the fascia planes. The following structures and artifacts can be obtained from normal lung ultrasound from superficial to deep: (a) subcutaneous tissues and intercostal muscles; (b) upper and lower ribs with acoustic shadowing beneath the ribs due to near complete reflection of the ultrasound beam at bone (Fig. 4.4 acoustic shadowing), if you turn the transducer along long axis of ribs, the anterior cortex should appear as a continuous smooth echogenic line; (c) pleural line, caused by near-complete reflection of the ultrasound beam at the aerated lung and it appears as a hyperechoic homogeneous horizontal line between the pleura and aerated lung tissue, the visceral pleura usually appears thicker than the parietal pleura, the curvilinear probe unable to differentiate visceral and parietal pleura as it appears as echogenic bands measuring up to 2 mm thick; (d) multiple hyperechoic horizontal lines called A-lines appears below the pleural line, spaced at multiples of the distance between the probe and the pleural line, A-lines are due to reverberation artifacts generated from the strong reflection of the pleural line (Fig. 4.5).

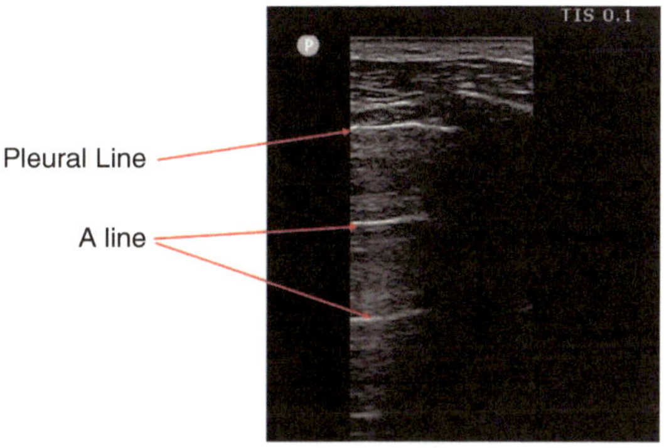

Fig. 4.5 LUS avoiding ribs shows multiple A-line

4.1.6 Lung Sliding and Lung Pulse

The lung sliding and lung pulse are the two dynamic findings found in a normal lung ultrasound. These two features are caused by the movement of the lung surface (visceral pleura) in relation to the innermost chest wall (parietal pleura). The lung sliding represents air movement during respiration and lung pulse indicates the transmission of cardiac contractions through the lung. Turning the probe transversely will abolish the rib shadows so more of the pleural line can be seen. The danger of this is that an inexperienced user may interpret a rib as the pleural line and incorrectly diagnose absent lung sliding. M-mode imaging will be helpful to exclude pneumothorax as it shows seashore sign, one of the characteristic features of lung sliding. The horizontal line represents subcutaneous tissue above the pleural line while the movement of lung sliding appears as sand in far field (Fig. 4.6).

4.1.7 Pneumothorax

The key LUS findings associated with pneumothorax are the absence of lung sliding, absent B-lines, lung pulse, and presence of the lung point. In supine patients, air, being nondependent tends to collect anteriorly. In order to exclude or to diagnose pneumothorax, it is recommended to place the probe on the highest point of the anterior chest to demonstrate lung sliding. Absence of lung sliding has a 95% sensitivity and 100% negative predictive value in predicting a pneumothorax [12]. M-mode imaging will be helpful in certain challenging patients to diagnose pneumothorax. It demonstrates only horizontal lines without sandy appearance, normal appears in near field termed as "stratosphere sign" or barcode sign (Fig. 4.7) However, one should be aware of other conditions causing absence lung sliding such as pleural effusion or if both pleurae fused together due to underlying pneumonia, pleurodesis, or ARDS. Moreover, the lung sliding

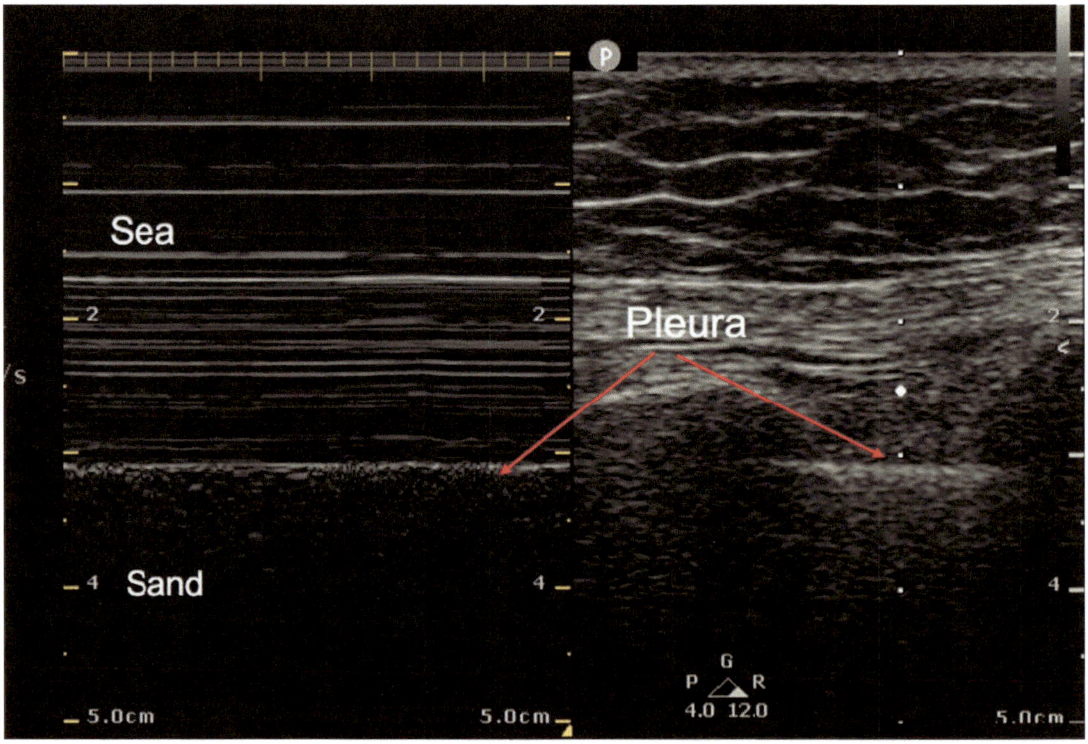

Fig. 4.6 Seashore sign

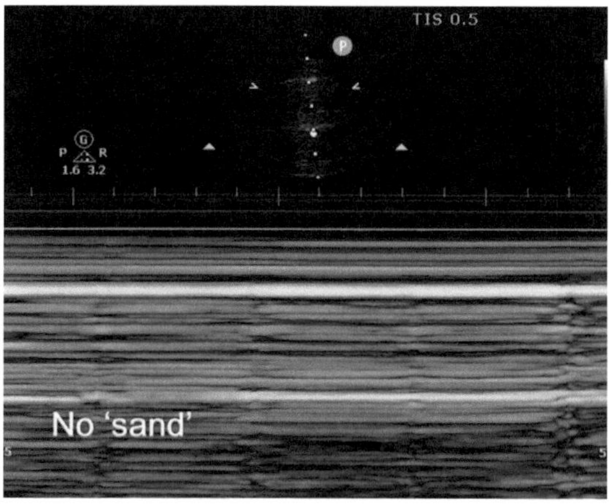

Fig. 4.7 Stratosphere or barcode sign

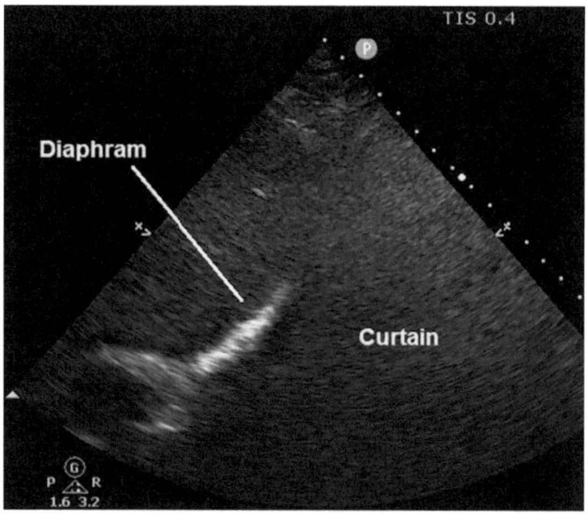

Fig. 4.8 Curtain sign from hydropneumothorax

will be reduced with low tidal volume ventilation or in hyperinflated lungs. Also, lung sliding will be absent if there is no respiration in one lung due to pneumonectomy or one lung intubation.

In some situations, if one is unable to demonstrate absence of lung sliding in suspected patients, demonstrating B-lines arising at visceral pleura-lung boundary, will be helpful to exclude pneumothorax. If there is no evidence of lung sliding and B-lines, then one should look for lung point, the point at which the two pleural layers rejoin one another [13]. It is also explained by the inspiratory increase of parietal contact of the collapsed lung. Lung point is noticed in the lateral aspect of chest wall and to demonstrate it, the ultrasound transducer needs to be moved laterally. Detection by LUS has a sensitivity is 66% for fully collapsed lungs and 79% for occult pneumothorax [14]. It is also helpful to indirectly judge the volume of air in the pleural cavity to determine appropriate intervention.

Finally, if the lung point cannot be demonstrated then the "lung pulse" should be sought. Cardiac pulsation will be transmitted to pleura by lung only if the pleural layers are still adjacent to one another causing a small amount of motion in 2D in relation with the heartbeat [15]. M-mode will be useful to demonstrate vertical lines running from the pleural line to the bottom of the image in time with cardiac pulsation called T lines. Hydropneumothorax can also be identified with LUS with the "curtain sign" describing reverberation artifacts originating from the air within the pleura that obscures the underlying effusion during inspiration (Fig. 4.8) [16]. The simplified algorithm for pneumothorax is shown in Fig. 4.9.

Use of a combination of absent lung sliding and the loss of B-lines has a reported sensitivity of 100%, specificity of 96.5%, and negative predictive value of 100% [17].

4.1.8 Limitations for Identification of Pneumothorax

Certain patient-specific factors such as obesity, edema, or heavy musculature may degrade image quality, making it hard to clearly demonstrate pleural line. The presence of subcutaneous emphysema or conditions causing pleural thickening or calcifications can block visualization of the pleural line [18]. In patients with ARDS, vigorous intercostal muscle contraction adjacent to the pleura results in movement of the adjacent parietal pleural surface. There will be potential operators to misdiagnose this abnormal movement as the presence of lung sliding. One should be aware of the differences between the movement of the pleural line by intercostal muscle contraction and from the shimmering movement of lung sliding [19].

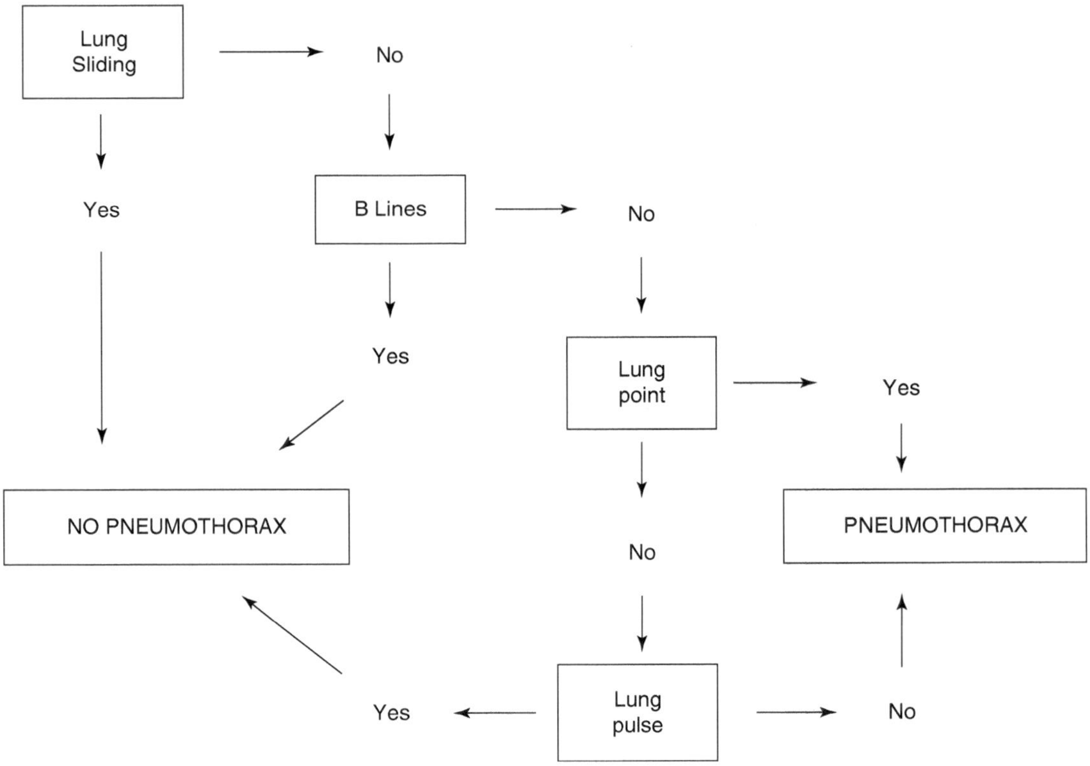

Fig. 4.9 Simplified algorithm for pneumothorax.

4.1.9 Pulmonary Edema and Interstitial Lung Disease

Until recently, it was thought that ultrasound of the lung tissue would be ineffective because the air in the lung parenchyma would cause too much acoustic impedance. However, this has been shown to not be the case; and specifically, when the air content decreases (as in pulmonary edema or any interstitial lung disease), an acoustic mismatch needed to reflect the ultrasound beam is created, and a signature ultrasound finding appears (B-lines). This reflection of the beam creates some comet-tail reverberation artifacts, called B-lines or ultrasound lung comets. A B-line is a discrete, laser-like, vertical, hyperechoic image that arises from the pleural line, extending to the bottom of the screen without fading, and moves synchronously with respiration. Multiple B-lines (>2) are the sonographic sign of interstitial lung disease and their number increases along with decreasing air content as shown in Fig. 1.10. When the air content is further decreased, such as in lung consolidations, the acoustic window on the lung becomes completely open and the lung may be directly visualized as a solid parenchyma, like the liver or the spleen. It has been reported that one can assess the space between B-lines to help determine further detail about the pathology of the airspace disease [20].

A positive region is defined by the presence of three or more B-lines in a longitudinal plane between two ribs. Multiple B-lines which are 7 mm apart characterize subpleural interlobular septal edema or thickening (Fig. 4.10). Closely spaced (≤3 mm) and coalescent B-lines suggest subpleural fluid-filled alveoli which correspond to ground glass opacities in CT. The term "B-pattern" should be used in the description of multiple B-lines in patients with interstitial syndrome [21]. In either case, the number and intensity of B-lines increase with the degree of loss of aeration. It is important to realize that absence of normal artifacts may also provide useful information. One such artifact is what are termed A-lines, which

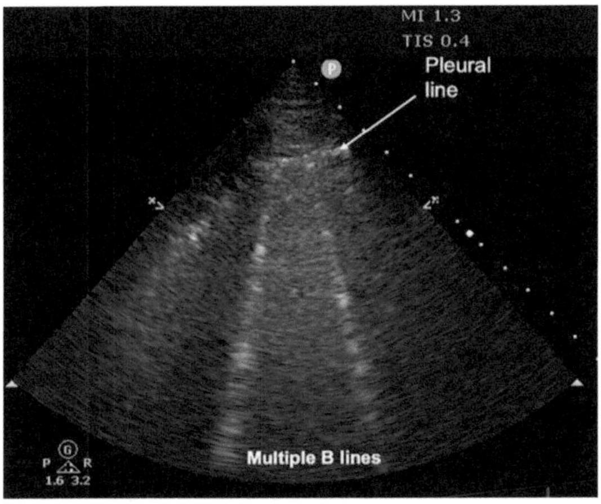

Fig. 4.10 B-lines in pulmonary edema and interstitial lung disease

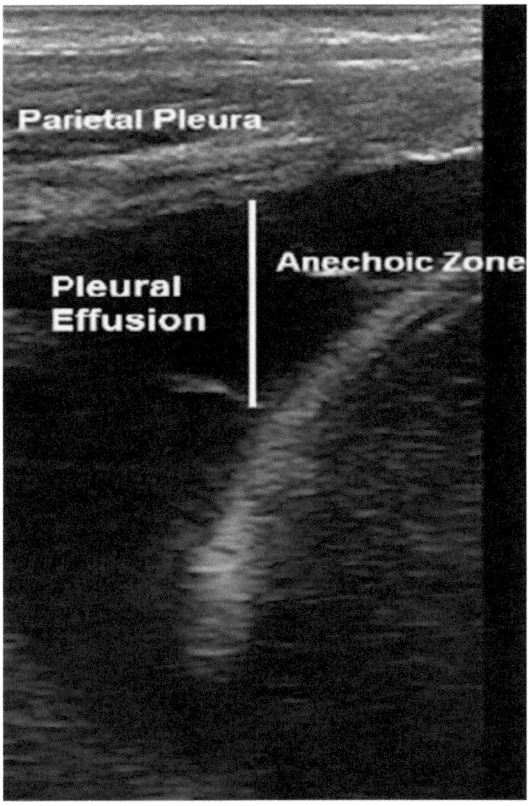

Fig. 4.11 Pleural effusion along with collapsed lung

represent the reverberation artifact of lung pleura. This artifact is a hyperechoic horizontal line that is parallel to the pleural line. The distance from A-line to pleural line is equal to the distance between skin and pleural line, and this may repeat further down the ultrasound image. The presence of A-lines is a sign of normal aeration but may also occur in the setting of pneumothorax. One must always assess for pleural sliding when A-lines are visualized. Also, since the presence of A-lines is a sign of normal aeration (assuming normal pleural sliding) one should not often see A-lines and B-lines in the same image.

4.1.10 Pleural Effusion

The appearance of effusion between parietal and visceral pleura in ultrasound images depends on its nature. Most transudates, as well as some exudates, appear as anechoic space (dark shadow) between pleura because at pleura-effusion boundary negligible echo is produced. This is well demonstrated in Fig. 4.11. The presence of internal echoes (grey smoky shadows) in this anechoic space is suggestive of exudate or hemorrhage which can be confirmed by thoracentesis. The visceral pleura-lung boundary appears as a hyperechoic line in a normally aerated lung.

In a free effusion and aerated lung, the variation in interpleural distance during respiratory cycle is easily visualized in M-mode as sinusoid movement of visceral pleura and called sinusoid sign, as is demonstrated in Fig. 4.12.

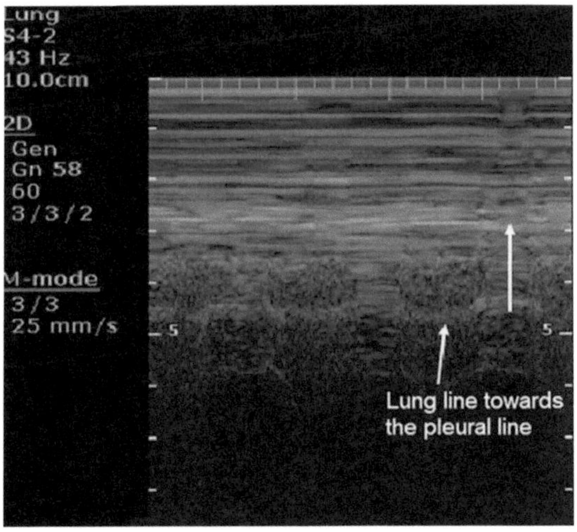

Fig. 4.12 Sinusoid sign caused by pleural movement

The posterior axillary line above the diaphragm is the optimal site for the detection of non-loculated pleural effusion [22]. Various ultrasound-guided approaches have been suggested for assessment of volume of pleural effusion. Interpleural distance of ≥50 mm between posterior chest wall and lung is predictive of pleural effusion ≥500 mL [23]. The LUS is superior to supine chest X-ray in the diagnosis of pleural effusion and distinguishing it from other causes of white opacities in chest X-ray. The LUS is as good as CT in the diagnosis of pleural effusion [2]. A hydropneumothorax can be identified by a dynamic air-fluid margin, with features of pneumothorax above air-fluid level.

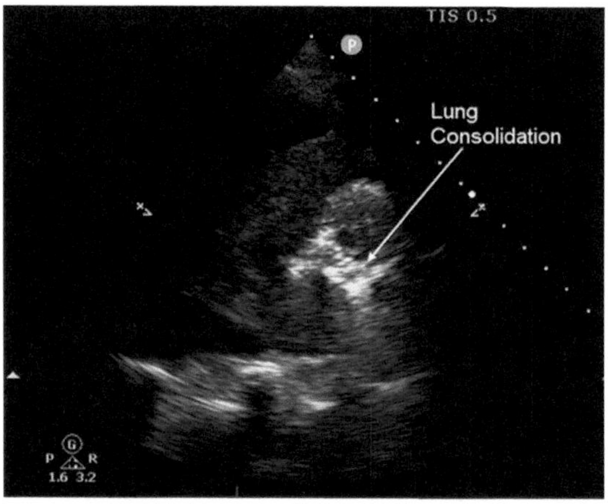

Fig. 4.13 Lung consolidation demarcated from normal lung tissue

4.1.11 Consolidation

The appearance of LUS depends on the relative aeration of alveoli. Pneumonia is an inflammatory, and infectious process involving the lungs. Typically, the alveoli in intensely inflamed areas fill with inflammatory fluid or pus, and this is known as consolidation. The changes may be widespread, patchy, or lobar. Ultrasound can detect the pulmonary changes associated with pneumonia as long as the process involves some of the pleural surface. Pneumonia progresses through stages, and the ultrasound changes vary depending on the degree and extent of consolidation. In the appropriate clinical setting, a localized patch of numerous B-lines, often with tiny areas of subpleural consolidation, suggests early pneumonia.

As the disease progresses, inflammatory and purulent fluid fills the alveoli and the lung appears solid, with a homogenous relatively fine echotexture similar to liver. The sonographic appearance of frank consolidation looks remarkably liver-like and is also termed *hepatization*. More commonly there are smaller areas of consolidation, as demonstrated in Fig. 4.13. Where these abut the pleural surface, they are linear, but their deeper borders usually demonstrate an irregular interface with underlying aerated lung. This irregular junction between consolidated and aerated lung is known as the "shred sign." Air within the consolidated area may remain in small aerated patches of lung, or more commonly air remains within small bronchi. The echogenic appearance of small air bubbles all lined up within a bronchus is known as the sonographic air bronchogram.

4.1.12 Atelectasis

Subpleural echo-poor region or tissue-like echotexture is seen in compression or obstructive atelectasis. This appearance is due to the absence of peripheral lung expansion. Compression atelectasis caused by massive pleural effusion is seen as floating wedge-shaped tissue-like structure, as is demonstrated in Fig. 4.14 [21]. The absence of dynamic air/fluid in this tissue like echotexture helps in differentiating it from pneumonia. Loss of aeration in lung at various stages due to gradually increasing pleural effusion can be seen as compression atelectasis develops. Compression or resorptive atelectasis shows early and late signs along with tissue-like echotexture. Early signs are abolished lung sliding with lung pulse, standstill cupola. Residual trapped air with static air bronchogram is a late sign. Air is completely absorbed subsequently.

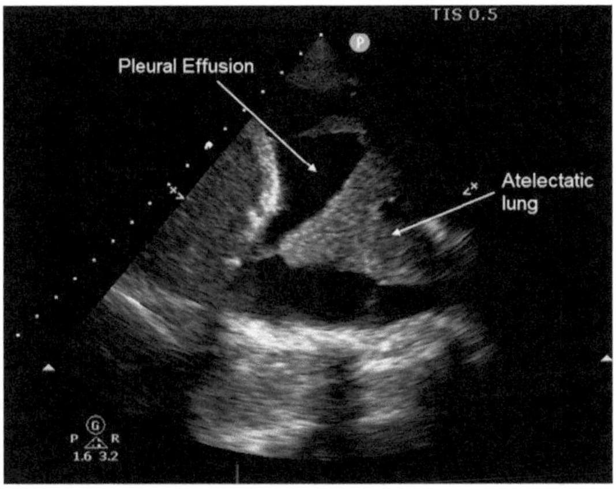

Fig. 4.14 Pleural effusion along with atelectatic lung floating in the pleural fluid

4.1.13 Asthma/Chronic Obstructive Pulmonary Disease

The presence of pleural line, lung sliding, A-Lines in 2D, and seashore sign in M-mode in both lungs as characteristic LUS picture of aerated lung have been mentioned above. In conditions like COPD, asthma and pulmonary embolism subpleural aeration are usually not affected. Lung sliding may be reduced by hyperinflation [24]. These conditions usually present with a similar LUS picture of aerated lung, as shown in Fig. 4.15. The BLUE protocol has described this LUS picture as A-profile and suggested a decision tree to differentiate these chronic conditions [25].

4.1.14 Pulmonary Embolism

In the case of a pulmonary embolism, usually an A-profile or A-pattern is seen in LUS. The BLUE protocol suggests searching for venous thrombosis if A-profile is present. If venous thrombosis is present, diagnosis of pulmonary embolism is considered in patients with acute respiratory failure. Peripheral pulmonary embolism is seen as multiple hypoechoic subpleural wedge-shaped tissue-like echotexture. There can be local or basal pleural effusion also [26].

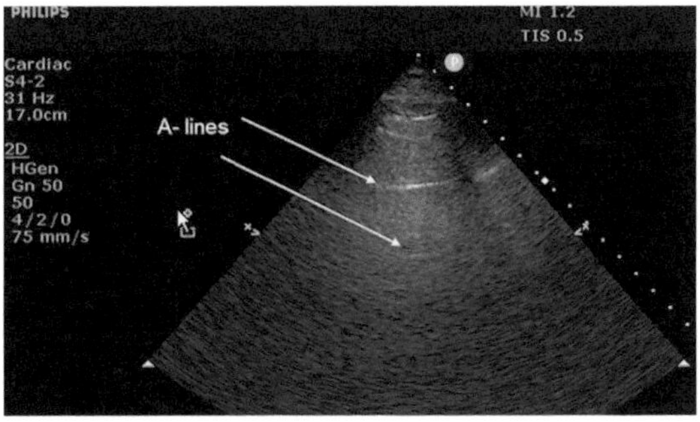

Fig. 4.15 Hyperinflated lung in a patient with COPD, with A-line appearance

The BLUE protocol has been proposed to help in the diagnosis of various lung conditions, as described before [26, 27]. Each region or zone is then sonographically characterized. Integration of various LUS findings in all regions/zones gives sonographic diagnosis. Finally, interpretation of sonographic diagnosis is done in context with history, clinical assessment, other investigations, and laboratory data. One algorithm is suggested in Fig. 4.16. Table 4.2 summarizes the major LUS findings in different pathological states.

4.1.15 Lung Ultrasound in COVID-19

POCUS has found its wide application in emergency and critical care medicine [2]. Many studies have shown that ultrasound imaging is more sensitive than chest X-ray examination in the diagnosis of ventilator-associated pneumonia [28] and community-acquired pneumonia (CAP) [29–31]. It can also make a sensitive diagnosis of viral pneumonia such as H1-N1 or H7-N9 earlier than chest X-ray examination [32] and thus has been recommended as an alternative screening method for such pneumonia in endemic areas [33, 34]. However, ultrasound identification between viral pneumonia and bacterial pneumonia remains a huge challenge. Use of LUS is feasible in the diagnosis of COVID-19, and the ultrasound images are mainly manifested as B-line artifacts, rocket

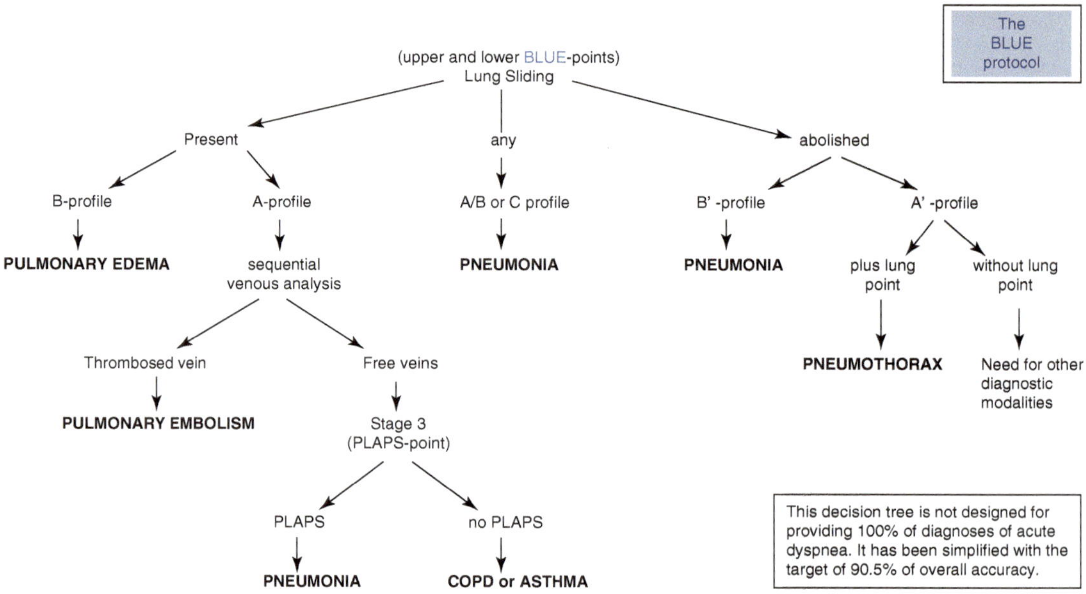

Fig. 4.16 The blue protocol

Table 4.2 Ultrasound findings of different pathologies

Lung pathology	USG features	Distribution
Normal lungs	Ribs and rib shadows: Present Hyperechoic pleural line: Present Lung sliding: Present A-profile A-lines: Present M-mode: Seashore sign present Isolated B-line may be seen	Both lungs In laterobasal areas
Subcutaneous emphysema asthma/COPD	Ribs and rib shadows: Absent E lines: Present A-profile ↓ Lung sliding, if hyperinflation is present	In affected areas In involved lung
Pulmonary embolism	A-profile Peripheral pulmonary embolism Subpleural wedge-shaped tissue like echo may be seen Focal/basal pleural effusion may be present	Both lungs Focal/multifocal inhomogeneous
Pneumothorax	Ribs and rib shadows: Present Hyperechoic pleural line: Present Lung sliding: Absent A-lines: Present B-lines: Absent characteristic Lung point: Present Lung pulse: Absent M-mode: Stratosphere sign present	In affected lung Focal
Pleural effusion	Ribs and rib shadows: Present Hyperechoic pleural line and lung sliding: Absent Anechoic (dark) space: Present (internal echoes present, if it is transudate) Hyperechoic lung line present if the underlying lung is aerated M-mode: Sinusoid sign, quad sign present, if underlying lung aerated	In affected hemithorax

Table 4.2 (continued)

Lung pathology	USG features	Distribution
Pulmonary edema	Ribs and rib shadows: Present Hyperechoic pleural line and lung sliding: Present Pleural line and subpleural abnormalities: Absent A-lines: Present B-lines: Significant and ≥2 bilateral regions +	Both lungs Homogeneous Dependent areas
ALI/ARDS	Ribs and rib shadows: Present Pleural line: Present Lung sliding: Present/may be ↓ Pleural and subpleural abnormalities: Present Anterior subpleural tissue like echo may be seen A-lines: Present B-lines: Significant but irregularly spaced	Both lungs Inhomogeneous Spared areas of normal Appearance seen
Pulmonary fibrosis	Ribs and rib shadows: Present Pleural line and lung sliding: Present Lung sliding: Normal/may be ↓ Pleural line and subpleural abnormalities: Present A-lines: Present B-lines: Significant and spaced	Affected lung may be bilateral or unilateral Focal/multifocal Inhomogeneous
Lung contusion	Ribs and rib shadows: Present Pleural line and lung sliding: Present Lung sliding: Normal/may be ↓ Pleural line and subpleural abnormalities: Present A-lines: Present B-lines: Significant and spaced/crowded	In affected lung May be bilateral or unilateral Focal/multifocal Inhomogeneous
Interstitial/ broncho-pneumonia	Ribs and rib shadows: Present Plural line and lung sliding: Present Lung sliding: Normal/may be ↓ Pleural line and subpleural abnormalities: Present A-lines: Present B-lines: Significant and spaced/crowded	In affected lung May be bilateral or unilateral Focal/multifocal Inhomogeneous
Pneumonia consolidation	Ribs and rib shadows: Present Pleural line and lung sliding: Absent Tissue like echotexture of consolidated lung Dynamic air/fluid bronchogram: Present Shred sign: Present	In affected lung May be unilateral or bilateral Focal/multifocal Inhomogeneous
Atelectasis	Ribs and rib shadows: Present Pleural line and lung sliding: Absent Tissue like echotexture of atelectatic lung Dynamic air/fluid bronchogram: Absent Shred sign: Absent Attendant signs of atelectasis: Present Evolving atelectasis Image characteristics depend on aeration	In affected lung

COPD chronic obstructive pulmonary disease, *USG* use of ultrasonography
* Correlate USG image with history, clinical examination, and clinical presentation

sign, and partially or completely diffused B-line. Small consolidation and abnormal pleural lines are detected in some cases. Ultrasound images of CAP were often manifested as large and circumscribed consolidation accompanied by bronchial gas phase or liquid phase, and pleural effusion was more common in CAP patients while their lung lesions were, to some extent, limitedly distributed compared with those of COVID-19 patients. Consolidations are more extensive in bacterial pneumonia because a large number of fibrinogens permeated out from blood vessel to alveoli as the permeability of the blood vessel increases. A limited number of studies [35] showed that the pathologic features of COVID-19 were mainly manifested by diffused interstitial inflammation alveolar damage, including apoptosis and shedding of alveolar epithelial cells, formation of pulmonary hyaline membrane, obviously widened lobar space, and infiltration of inflammatory cells composed of lymphocytes and monocytes.

The similar pathologic features among COVID-19, SARS, and Middle East Respiratory Syndrome [36, 37] were the pathologic basis for the formation of lung ultrasound signs among patients with such diseases. The unique ultrasound signs of interstitial pneumonia included the disappearance of pleural line and the overlapping of B-line, as well as white lung, waterfall sign, and small consolidations in patients with severe interstitial pneumonia. Combined with other studies, this study indicated that different viral pneumonias had similar sonographic features, and there was still no evidence of obvious identification characteristics among them. However, compared with pulmonary edema and interstitial lung fibrosis, diffuse B-line patterns were more commonly detected in COVID-19 patients. The reasons might be that the more severe pulmonary inflammation and more abundant mucus were conducive to the formation and fusion of B-line in such patients [38, 39].

Unexpectedly, large consolidation was rarely seen in COVID-19, and either bronchial fluid phase or gas phase was rarely seen in the consolidation, whereas nearly all the pleural abnormalities were detected in this study. The main

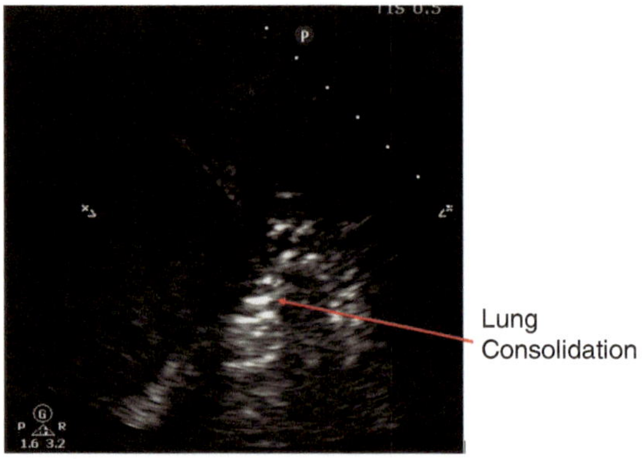

Fig. 4.17 Bilateral ground glass opacifications in a COVID-19 patient

sonographic features of COVID-19 were as follows: (i) thickening, blurred and irregular, and fragmented pleural line; (ii) dispersed B-line and rocket sign, partially diffused B-line, completely diffused B-line for white lung or waterfall sign, pulmonary consolidations or subpleural focal lesions, generally less than 1.0 cm and shown as a C-line sign, were often seen among severe COVID-19 patients, while large pulmonary consolidation was uncommon. Fig. 4.17 demonstrates the characteristics of the lung in a COVID-positive patient.

4.1.16 Role of LUS in Thoracic Interventions/Procedures

Ultrasound can be used as a guide during thoracentesis procedures or for the placement of chest tubes in patients with pleural effusions (inflammatory, infectious, neoplastic) or inflammatory infiltrates involving the lung parenchyma or chest wall. Imaging can also be used to collect samples of expanding bone lesions of the ribs, which are a frequent site of distant metastases and involvement from disease arising in other contiguous structures. For complicated, antibiotic-resistant effusions which can form fibrous septa, ultrasound can also be used as a guide for intracavitary administration of fibrinolytic agents, which lyse adhesions and septa, improving the chances for effective drainage. Ultrasound-guided biopsy is indicated for Pancoast tumors, whose pleural and extrapleural extension can be evaluated in part by sonography. The use of color Doppler is fundamental for evaluating the vessels of this region.

The complications commonly associated with interventional procedures involving the chest, regardless of the type of guidance used, are pneumo- and hemothorax, hemoptysis, vasovagal reactions, and if a malignant lesion is being biopsied, neoplastic seeding along the needle tract. When interventional procedures are performed under ultrasound guidance, the rate of complications is around 1% [40], which is lower than the rates reported for CT-guided procedures [41].

4.1.17 Advantages of LUS

All intensivists prefer the least invasive tool, all else being equal. Ultrasound is an answer to the long-standing dilemma: "Radiography or CT in the ICU?" Radiography is a familiar tool that lacks sensitivity [42]: about 60–70% [43]. CT has high accuracy but severe drawbacks: cost, transportation of critically ill patients, delay between CT and the resulting therapy, renal issues, anaphylactic shock, and mainly high irradiation [44]. Ultrasound has quite similar performances to CT [12, 45] being on occasion superior: better detection of pleural septations, necrotic areas, real-time measurement allowing assessment of dynamic signs: lung sliding, air bronchogram [46], and diaphragm [47]. Ultrasound should be considered as reasonable, bedside "gold standard." For all assessed disorders, it provides quantitative data. Pleural effusions can be quantified [48]. Lung consolidation can be monitored, which is useful for those who want to increase end-expiratory pressure [49]. The volume and progression of a pneumothorax are monitored using the lung point location [50]. Lung ultrasound will favor programs allowing decrease in bedside radiographs and CTs in the next decades.

4.1.18 Limitations

Dressings and subcutaneous emphysema create limitations to performing a good ultrasound exam. Exceptional cases provide difficult interpretation, even for experts. Is lung ultrasound easy? Some experiences show high interobserver agreement [8]. A burgeoning literature, up to a consensus conference, seems to confirm this accessibility [2]. A scientific assessment of the learning curve remains to be done, not in volunteers (creating a selection bias), but in unselected physicians. Care should be taken to confide training to experts choosing simplicity, although one can practice lung ultrasound with any machine, any probe, and any teaching approach.

In conclusion, the scope of LUS in emergency and critical care settings has expanded extensively. This imaging modality is easily available at bedside, real time, and free of radiation hazards in comparison to conventional imaging modalities of lung, in critically ill patients. It can be used easily at the bedside to assess initial lung morphology in severely hypoxemic patients and can be easily repeated, allowing the effects of therapy to be monitored. Its use in the diagnosis of lung diseases is real but with some practical limitations. Importance of history taking and clinical examination cannot be undermined, and one should not jump to the conclusion using just the LUS findings.

Self-Assessment Questions: Select the Best Answer

1. The maximum reflection of ultrasound signals during thoracic ultrasound happens at
   A. Skin and subcutaneous
   B. Subcutaneous and muscle layer
   C. Soft tissue and pleura
   D. Pleura and lung parenchyma
2. Following are the features of using a linear ultrasound probe in LUS except
   A. Deeper penetration
   B. Has narrow sector width
   C. Large footprint
   D. Not recommended for rapidly moving structures

3. For better image quality using color Doppler all are recommended except
   A. Using wall filter for rapidly moving structures
   B. High scale velocity
   C. Adjust color gain to get "snowstorm" appearance
   D. Doppler angle must be less than 60°
4. The structure highlighted in the following image represents

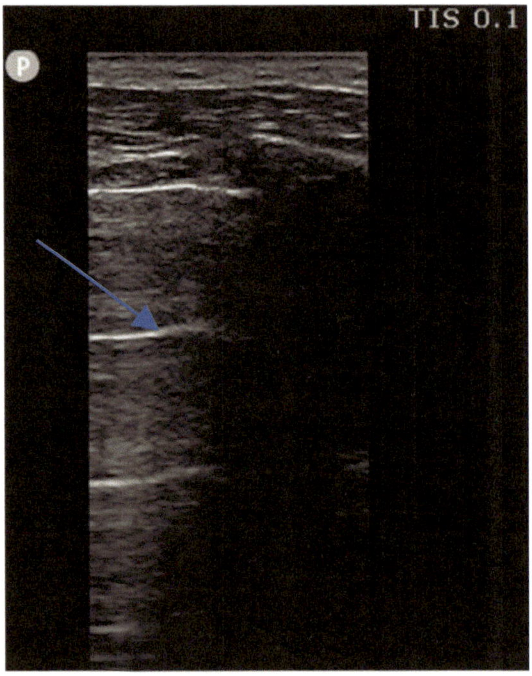

   A. Pleural line
   B. B-line
   C. A-line
   D. Z-line
5. The most appropriate technique to avoid acoustic shadowing from ribs is
   A. Using curvilinear probe
   B. Scanning in sagittal plane
   C. Phased array probe parallel to rib
   D. Using linear probe
6. A-lines are one of the common artifacts observed in LUS. The true statement about A-line is
   A. Reflection from bony surface
   B. Refraction from pleural surface
   C. Reverberation from pleural line
   D. Refraction from fascial plane
7. Following are advantages of using curvilinear probe in LUS except
   A. Smaller footprint
   B. Higher penetration
   C. Ideal for assessment of diaphragm
   D. Lower frequency
8. Blue protocol is one of the commonly employed methods for comprehensive assessment of lung using ultrasound. A positive blue point represents
   A. Presence of two B-lines
   B. Presence of one B-line
   C. Presence of three B-lines
   D. Presence of four B-lines
9. Absence of lung sliding is one of the essential features of LUS to diagnose pneumothorax. Presence of the following respiratory condition will cause false lung sliding due to vigorous intercostal muscle contraction
   A. Emphysema
   B. Chronic bronchitis
   C. Acute respiratory distress syndrome
   D. Bronchial asthma
10. The highlighted structure/artifact in the following ultrasound image represents

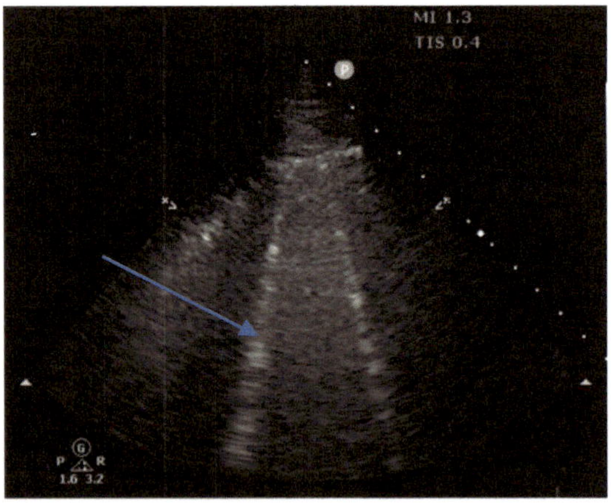

   A. A-line
   B. Pleural line
   C. T-line
   D. B-line
11. You have high peak ventilation pressures after intubating a patient with advanced COPD. You find bilateral anterior B-lines but cannot find lung sliding over the right ante-

rior thorax. What is the most likely cause of high peak pressures?
   A. Pleural effusion
   B. Pulmonary edema
   C. Pneumothorax
   D. Pericardial tamponade

12. You are taking care of a trauma patient who is admitted after a collision between the car that he was an unrestrained driver in ran into a tree. The patient has multiple rib fractures and has a high oxygen requirement of 70% oxygen on a noninvasive BiPAP machine to maintain oxygenation. He is also complaining of dyspnea and chest fullness. You perform a lung ultrasound, and the attached picture is displayed. What is the most likely reason for his respiratory condition?

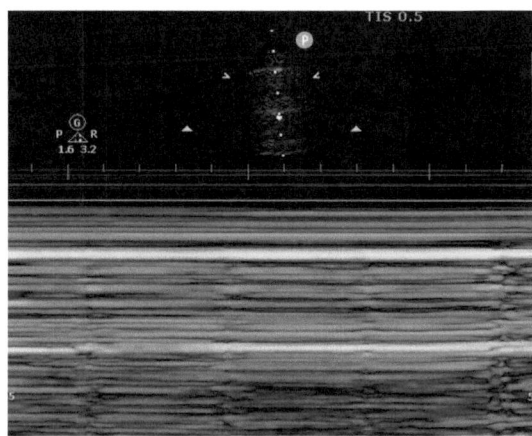

   A. Pleural effusion
   B. Pulmonary contusions
   C. Pericardial effusion
   D. Pneumothorax

13. A 50-year-old patient presents with a week-long history of dyspnea. Fever, and cough. His blood pressure is 90/50 and he is requiring four liters of oxygen to maintain his saturation. The attached picture represents the ultrasound exam with the probe held in place at the base of the lung. What is the most likely diagnosis?

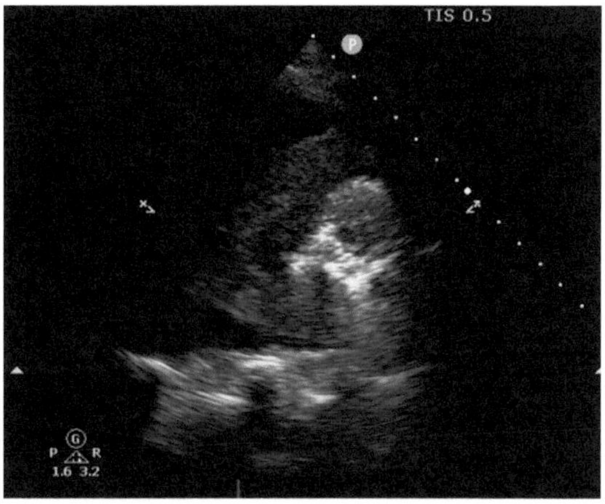

   A. COPD
   B. Pneumonia
   C. Pericardial effusion
   D. Pneumothorax

14. A 75-year-old woman, with chronic myeloid leukemia presents with dyspnea and fever. She presented to her doctor a week ago with fever and cough, for which she was treated with azithromycin. She was feeling better for a while but has been declining for the past couple of days. Please interpret her lung ultrasound findings

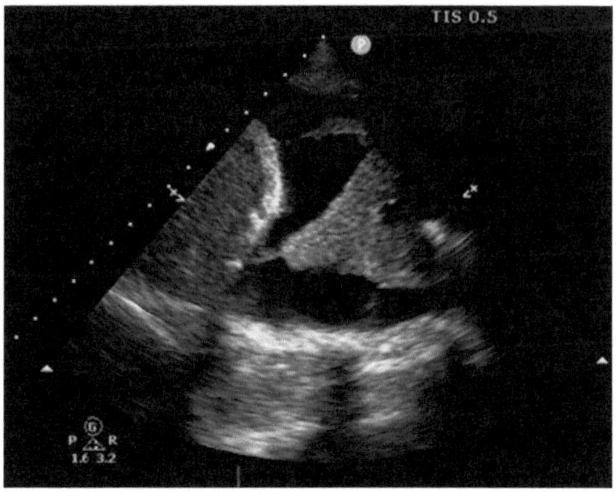

   A. Pleural effusion
   B. Pneumonia
   C. Pericardial effusion
   D. Pneumothorax

15. You are called on the floor to evaluate a 90-year-old man with diastolic dysfunction. His diuretics have been held for the past week due to renal dysfunction (currently his creatinine has plateaued at 4.2 mg/dL). He has been placed on BiPAP but continues having substantial work of breathing. The following images are obtained from his right thorax. What is the most likely cause of his pulmonary dysfunction, based on the ultrasound findings

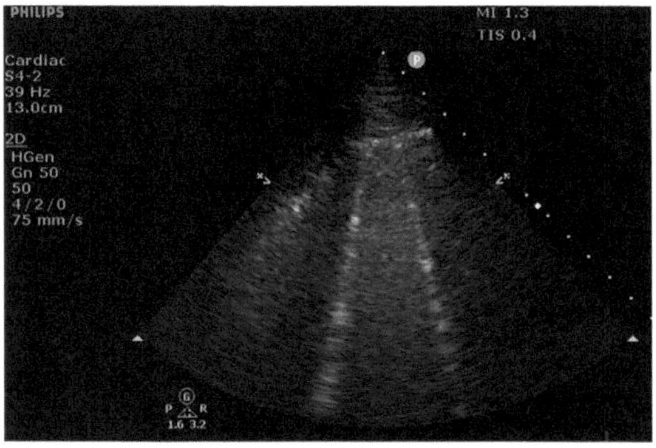

A. Pleural effusion
B. Pneumonia
C. Pericardial effusion
D. Pulmonary edema

16. A 29-year-old male, weighing 134 kg is brought to the emergency department after a motor vehicle accident. He has lost a lot of blood and is hypotensive and anemic with a Hb of 6.2. An emergent central line is placed in his right internal jugular and is challenging to place, given his body habitus. The patient becomes hemodynamically unstable after line placement and there is some concern that he might have developed an iatrogenic pneumothorax due to accidental puncture during line placement. A lung ultrasound over the right upper chest shows the following picture

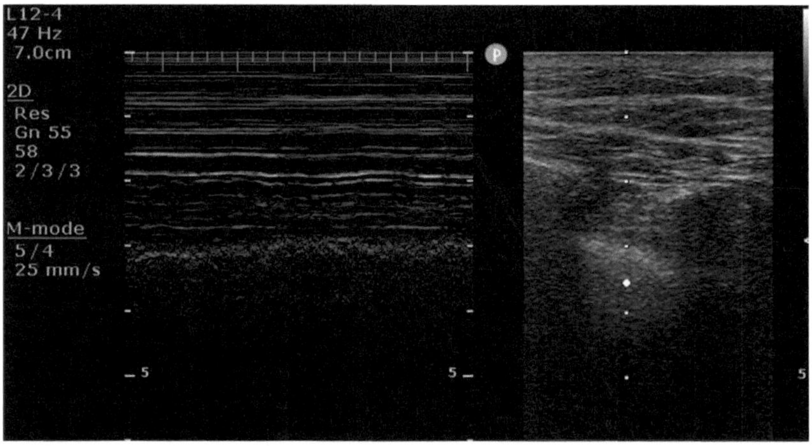

What is the most accurate statement?
A. Patient does not have pneumothorax
B. Patient does not have pneumothorax, at that point. A more comprehensive lung exam is required
C. Patient needs an emergent chest tube
D. Patient has a hemothorax that needs to be drained

17. Which one of the following statements about B-lines is TRUE?
A. B-lines are reverberation artifacts arising from volumetric variations between aerated and fluid-filled parts of the lung tissue
B. B-lines are evenly spaced horizontal lines at integer multiples of the distance from the skin to the pleural line
C. B-lines indicate well-aerated lung
D. B-lines are diagnostic with for pneumothorax

18. Absence of pleural lung sliding can occur in all of the following situations except
A. Pneumothorax
B. Apnea

C. Bronchial intubation
D. Bronchial obstruction
E. Pleural adhesion
F. All of the above

19. A 64-year-old female, with a history of HTN, HLD, and COPD has an onset of shortness of breath and sudden chest pain for the past few hours, after a coughing spell. The physician evaluates the heart and lungs with ultrasound. When looking at the lungs, the physician notices multiple horizontal lines between two hypoechoic columns as well as a lung point however he does not see any lung sliding. What is the most likely diagnosis?
A. Pleural effusion
B. Pneumonia
C. Pericardial effusion
D. Pneumothorax

20. A 82-year-old male with a past history of CAD, systolic heart failure with EF of 30%, COPD, and a 3-year history of progressively worsening dyspnea on exertion finally presents to his PCP for workup. The doctor notices distended jugular veins and upon auscultation hears an S3 and a holosystolic murmur over the apex. The physician performs a chest ultrasound exam and sees the following. Based on this exam, which of the following is true?

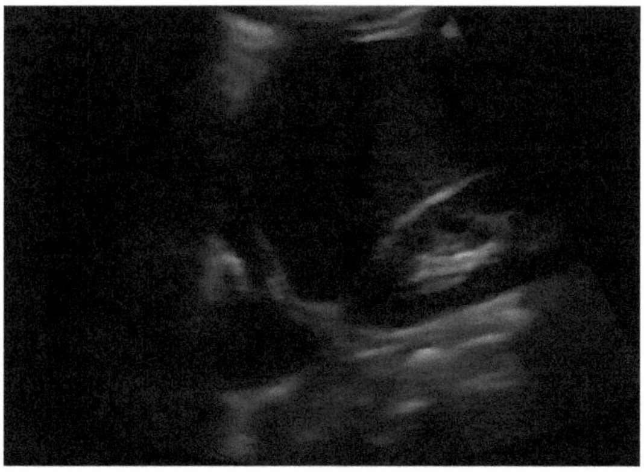

A. Patient has a pleural effusion
B. Patient has fluid in the hepatorenal recess
C. Patient has free fluid surrounding the bladder
D. Patient is completely healthy

References

1. Ross AM, Genton E, Holmes JH. Ultrasonic examination of the lung. J Lab Clin Med. 1968;72(4):556–64.
2. Volpicelli G, Elbarbary M, Blaivas M, Lichtenstein DA, Mathis G, Kirkpatrick AW, International Liaison Committee on Lung Ultrasound (ILC-LUS) for International Consensus Conference on Lung Ultrasound (ICC-LUS), et al. International evidence-based recommendations for point-of-care lung ultrasound. Intensive Care Med. 2012;38(4):577–91.
3. Mojoli F, Bouhemad B, Mongodi S, Lichtenstein D. Lung ultrasound for critically ill patients. Am J Respir Crit Care Med. 2019;199(6):701–14.
4. Gargani L, Volpicelli G. How I do it: lung ultrasound. Cardiovasc Ultrasound. 2014 Jul;4(12):25. https://doi.org/10.1186/1476-7120-12-25.
5. Singh Y, Tissot C, Fraga MV, Yousef N, Cortes RG, Lopez J, et al. International evidence-based guidelines on point of care ultrasound (POCUS) for critically ill neonates and children issued by the POCUS Working Group of the European Society of Paediatric and Neonatal Intensive Care (ESPNIC). Crit Care. 2020;24(1):65.
6. Aldrich JE. Basic physics of ultrasound imaging. Crit Care Med. 2007;35(Suppl):S131–7.
7. Buessler A, Chouihed T, Duarte K, Bassand A, Huot-Marchand M, Gottwalles Y, et al. Accuracy of several lung ultrasound methods for the diagnosis of acute heart failure in the ED: a multicenter prospective study. Chest. 2020;157(1):99–110.
8. Lichtenstein D, Goldstein I, Mourgeon E, Cluzel P, Grenier P, Rouby JJ. Comparative diagnostic performances of auscultation, chest radiography, and lung ultrasonography in acute respiratory distress syndrome. Anesthesiology. 2004;100(1):9–15.
9. Pivetta E, Goffi A, Lupia E, Tizzani M, Porrino G, Ferreri E, SIMEU Group for Lung Ultrasound in the Emergency Department in Piedmont, et al. Lung ultrasound-implemented diagnosis of acute decompensated heart failure in the ED: a SIMEU multicenter study. Chest. 2015;148(1):202–10.
10. Volpicelli G, Mussa A, Garofalo G, Cardinale L, Casoli G, Perotto F, et al. Bedside lung ultrasound in the assessment of alveolar-interstitial syndrome. Am J Emerg Med. 2006;24(6):689–96.
11. Jambrik Z, Monti S, Coppola V, Agricola E, Mottola G, Miniati M, Picano E. Usefulness of ultrasound lung comets as a nonradiologic sign of extravascular lung water. Am J Cardiol. 2004;93(10):1265–70.
12. Lichtenstein DA, Menu Y. A bedside ultrasound sign ruling out pneumothorax in the critically ill. Lung sliding. Chest. 1995;108(5):1345–8.
13. Lichtenstein D, Mezière G, Biderman P, Gepner A. The lung point: an ultrasound sign specific to pneumothorax. Intensive Care Med. 2000;4:1434–40.
14. Lichtenstein D, Mezière G, Lascols N, Biderman P, Courret JP, Gepner A, Tenoudji-Cohen M. Ultrasound diagnosis of occult pneumothorax. Crit Care Med. 2005;4:1231–8.

15. Lichtenstein D, Lascols N, Prin S, Mezière G. The lung pulse: an early ultrasound sign of complete atelectasis. Intensive Care Med. 2003;4:2187–92.
16. Targhetta R, Bourgeois JM, Chavagneux R, Marty-Double C, Balmes P. Ultrasonographic approach to diagnosing hydropneumothorax. Chest. 1992;101:931–4.
17. Koh DM, Burke S, Davies N, Padley SP. Transthoracic US of the chest: clinical uses and applications. Radiographics. 2002;22(1):e1.
18. Volpicelli G. Sonographic diagnosis of pneumothorax. Intensive Care Med. 2011 Feb;37(2):224–32.
19. Alrajhi K, Woo MY, Vaillancourt C. Test characteristics of ultrasonography for the detection of pneumothorax: a systematic review and meta-analysis. Chest. 2012;141(3):703.
20. Copetti R, Soldati G, Copetti P. Chest sonography: a useful tool to differentiate acute cardiogenic pulmonary edema from acute respiratory distress syndrome. Cardiovasc Ultrasound. 2008;6:16.
21. Bouhemad B, Zhang M, Lu Q, Rouby JJ. Clinical review: bedside lung ultrasound in critical care practice. Crit Care. 2007;11:205.
22. Pneumatikos I, Bouros D. Pleural effusions in critically ill patients. Respiration. 2008;76:241–8.
23. Roch A, Bojan M, Michelet P, Romain F, Bregeon F, Papazian L, et al. Usefulness of ultrasonography in predicting pleural effusions>500 mL in patients receiving mechanical ventilation. Chest. 2005;127:224–32.
24. Via G, Storti E, Gulati G, Neri L, Mojoli F, Braschi A. Lung ultrasound in the ICU: from diagnostic instrument to respiratory monitoring tool. Minerva Anestesiol. 2012;78:1282–96.
25. Lichtenstein DA, Mezière GA. Relevance of lung ultrasound in the diagnosis of acute respiratory failure: the BLUE protocol. Chest. 2008;134:117–25.
26. Reissig A, Kroegel C. Transthoracic ultrasound of lung and pleura in the diagnosis of pulmonary embolism: a novel non-invasive bedside approach. Respiration. 2003;70:441–52.
27. Wang XT, Liu DW, Zhang HM, He HW, Liu Y, Chai WZ, et al. The value of bedside lung ultrasound in emergency-plus protocol for the assessment of lung consolidation and atelectasis in critical patients. Zhonghua Nei Ke Za Zhi. 2012;51:948–51.
28. Mongodi S, Via G, Girard M, Rouquette I, Misset B, Braschi A, Mojoli F, Bouhemad B. Lung ultrasound for early diagnosis of ventilator-associated pneumonia. Chest. 2016;149:969–80.
29. Ho MC, Ker CR, Hsu JH, Wu JR, Dai ZK, Chen IC. Usefulness of lung ultrasound in the diagnosis of community-acquired pneumonia in children. Pediatr Neonatol. 2015;56:40–5.
30. Alzahrani SA, Al-Salamah MA, Al-Madani W, Elbarbary MA. Systematic review and meta-analysis for the use of ultrasound versus radiology in diagnosing of pneumonia. Crit Ultrasound J. 2017;9:6.
31. Reissig A, Copetti R, Mathis G, Mempel C, Schuler A, Zechner P, et al. Lung ultrasound in the diagnosis and follow-up of community-acquired pneumonia: a prospective, multicenter, diagnostic accuracy study. Chest. 2012;142:965–72.
32. Testa A, Soldati G, Copetti R, Giannuzzi R, Portale G, Gentiloni-Silveri N. Early recognition of the 2009 pandemic influenza a (H1 N1) pneumonia by chest ultrasound. Crit Care. 2012;16:R30.
33. Lissaman C, Kanjanauptom P, Ong C, Tessaro M, Long E, O'Brien A. Prospective observational study of point-of-care ultrasound for diagnosing pneumonia. Arch Dis Child. 2019;104:12–8.
34. Tsai NW, Ngai CW, Mok KL, Tsung JW. Lung ultrasound imaging in avian influenza a (H7 N9) respiratory failure. Crit Ultrasound J. 2014;6:6.
35. Tsung JW, Kessler DO, Shah VP. Prospective application of clinician-performed lung ultrasonography during the 2009 H1 N1 influenza a pandemic: distinguishing viral from bacterial pneumonia. Crit Ultrasound J. 2012;4:16.
36. Shen MS, Yin T, Ji XL. Pathological diagnosis and differential diagnosis of severe acute respiratory syndrome. J Clin Exp Pathol. 2003;19:387–9.
37. Xu Z, Shi L, Wang Y, Zhang J, Huang L, Zhang C, et al. Pathological findings of COVID-19 associated with acute respiratory distress syndrome. Lancet Respir Med. 2020;8:420–2.
38. Zhu ZX, Lian XH, Zeng YM, Wu WJ, Xu ZR, Chen YJ, et al. Point-of-care ultrasound- a new option for early quantitative assessment of pulmonary edema. Ultrasound Med Biol. 2020;46:1–10.
39. Zeng LQ, Lyu GR, Lian XH, Zhu ZX, Chen YJ, Xu ZR, Guo YN. Study on the correlation between B line in ultrasound and severity of pulmonary edema. Chinese J Ultrasound Med. 2019;35:272–4.
40. Yang PC. Ultrasound-guided transthoracic biopsy of the chest. Radiol Clin N Am. 2000;38(2):323–43.
41. Sheth S, Hamper UM, Stanley DB, Wheeler JH, Smith PA. US guidance for thoracic biopsy: a valuable alternative to CT. Radiology. 1999;210:721–6.
42. Hendrikse K, Gramata J, ten Hove W, Rommes J, Schultz M, Spronk P. Low value of routine chest radiographs in a mixed medical-surgical ICU. Chest. 2007;4:823–8.
43. McGonigal MD, Schwab CW, Kauder DR, Miller WT, Grumbach K. Supplemented emergent chest CT in the management of blunt torso trauma. J Trauma. 1990;4:1431–5. https://doi.org/10.1097/00005373-199012000-00001.
44. Lauer MS. Elements of danger - the case of medical imaging. N Engl J Med. 2009;4:841–3. https://doi.org/10.1056/NEJMp0904735.

45. Lichtenstein D, Hulot JS, Rabiller A, Tostivint I, Mezière G. Feasibility and safety of ultrasound-aided thoracentesis in mechanically ventilated patients. Intensive Care Med. 1999;4:955–8.
46. Lichtenstein D, Mezière G, Seitz J. The dynamic air bronchogram. An ultrasound sign of alveolar consolidation ruling out atelectasis. Chest. 2009;4:1421–5.
47. Lerolle N, Guérot E, Dimassi S, Zegdi R, Faisy C, Fagon JY, Diehl JL. Ultrasonographic diagnosis criterion for severe diaphragmatic dysfunction after cardiac surgery. Chest. 2009;4:401–7.
48. Vignon P, Chastagner C, Berkane V, Chardac E, Francois B, Normand S, et al. Quantitative assessment of pleural effusion in critically ill patients by means of ultrasonography. Crit Care Med. 2005;4:1757–63.
49. Bouhemad B, Brisson H, Le-Guen M, Arbelot C, Lu Q, Rouby JJ. Ultrasound assessment of positive end-expiratory pressure-induced lung recruitment. Am J Respir Crit Care Med. 2011;4:341–7.
50. Oveland NP, Lossius HM, Wemmelund K, Stokkeland PJ, Knudsen L, Sloth E. Using thoracic ultrasonography to accurately assess pneumothorax progression during positive pressure ventilation. A comparison with CT scanning. Chest. 2013;4(2):415–22.

Point-of-Care Ultrasound of the Heart: Transthoracic Echocardiogram

5

Rohit Vijay Agrawal, Sudipta Mukherjee, Chang Chuan Melvin Lee, Arunangshu Chakraborty, and Manojit Lodha

5.1 Echocardiography

5.1.1 Background

Point-of-care ultrasonography (PoCUS) is increasingly employed in a variety of clinical settings—particularly in emergency departments and critical care units. A part of PoCUS is point-of-care echocardiography which may be employed to provide rapid diagnosis for respiratory and circulatory failure or the etiology of cardiac arrest, answer specific clinical questions, and facilitate goal-directed care, such as fluid management or inotropic support. Point-of-care echocardiography is increasingly employed by nontraditional practitioners of echocardiography, and a limited structural assessment of the heart and inferior vena cava (IVC) can be performed by acute medicine practitioners such as emergency physicians, intensivists, and anesthesiologists.

An evolving patient care landscape, coupled with increased availability of ultrasound has made bedside echocardiography an important tool in patient assessment. The role of point-of-care testing improves efficiency and can improve patient outcomes [1]. The role of point-of-care echocardiography is to answer specific clinical questions in a dichotomous manner in order to facilitate early diagnosis and guide therapy. Point-of-care echocardiography is typically one part of a PoCUS protocol, and the findings should be considered together with the rest of the ultrasound examination, such as lung and vascular ultrasound. The findings obtained from point-of-care echocardiography also have to be interpreted in conjunction with bedside clinical examination findings and laboratory data.

While the conduct of a comprehensive diagnostic echocardiogram is well beyond the scope of this book, this chapter aims to serve as a primer for anesthetic and critical care trainees to understand essential sonographic principles underlying echocardiography, and point-of-care assessment of cardiac function to identify life-threatening pathology and basic assessment of cardiac function to augment the bedside cardiac examination and make better-informed decisions for patient care.

R. V. Agrawal
National University Health System, Singapore, Singapore

Surgical Intensive Care Unit, National University Health System, Singapore, Singapore

S. Mukherjee
Tata Medical Center, Kolkata, West Bengal, India

C. C. M. Lee (✉)
National University Health System, Singapore, Singapore

A. Chakraborty
Department of Anaesthesia, Critical Care and Pain, Tata Medical Center, Newtown, Kolkata, West Bengal, India

M. Lodha
Tata Medical Center, Kolkata, West Bengal, India

Vivekananda Institute of Medical Sciences, Kolkata, West Bengal, India

A. Chakraborty, B. Ashokka (eds.), *A Practical Guide to Point of Care Ultrasound (POCUS)*,
https://doi.org/10.1007/978-981-16-7687-1_5

It is also important to understand the limitations of point-of-care echocardiography. Unlike a comprehensive echocardiographic study, the point-of-care echocardiography does not acquire images from all possible windows and views, it is mainly a qualitative assessment, just sufficient to answer the specific clinical query by detecting pathological states relevant to the clinical setting. Furthermore, the impact of inter-individual variation cannot be discounted as the study is interpreted by providers with a wide range of expertise and skill levels. Lastly, the study shows a single snapshot in the course of a patient's care and repeated reassessment to evaluate the effectiveness of treatment or clinical trajectory may be required. At present, most hemodynamic calculations, such as stroke volume and ejection fraction, require manual operator measurement or assessment, and thus if continuous cardiovascular and hemodynamic assessment is required, it is not the optimal tool for monitoring.

5.1.1.1 Sonography Principles and Instrumentation

The fundamentals of knobology and ultrasound physics have been covered elsewhere in this book, and this section will briefly cover 3 areas which are particularly relevant to bedside echocardiography.

Phased array transducers. Echocardiography probes, unlike most other PoCUS methods, utilizes phased array transducers with adjustable focus and steering. These transducers have multiple piezoelectric elements which are electronically separate [2]. In newer pocket-sized handheld devices, the piezoelectric elements are replaced by a novel ultrasound-on-chip technology which generates a voltage through a membrane that generates ultrasound waves [3]. Individual elements are fired sequentially to steer the ultrasound beam by creating a radially propagating scan line. This allows a probe with a small footprint to allow imaging of a wider field of view which is essential in cardiac imaging. The small square footprint also helps to be accommodated within intercostal space and to avoid obstruction by the ribs. In order to produce three-dimensional echocardiography, specialized matrix array transducers are required, but these are beyond the scope of this book.

Transducer orientation. All transducers have a marker on one side of the probe which corresponds with the orientation marker on the image produced on the ultrasound screen [4]. This is relevant as the transducer orientation marker is important in view acquisition during echocardiography. In addition, the operator may notice that, by convention, the transducer orientation marker on the ultrasound screen is on the left of the image, while this is reversed for echocardiography (i.e., on the right of the screen).

Spectral Doppler. Spectral Doppler imaging is important in echocardiography, as it allows for the measurement of blood flow velocity to calculate pressure gradients and flow. Two forms of spectral doppler exist—pulsed wave Doppler (PW) which uses short bursts of ultrasound, or range gating to measure velocities in a specific area or depth (sample volume). However, at high velocities above the Nyquist limit range ambiguity, or aliasing occurs, precluding measurement by PW, which is the main disadvantage of PW. The Nyquist limit, defined as (Nyquist limit = pulse repetition frequency/2), is the maximum velocity that can be measured by PW. This can be increased by adjusting the baseline shift and scale. Continuous wave Doppler (CW) in contrast, utilizes continuously emitting and receiving crystals to measure velocities across the entire scan line. Generally speaking, CW displays the highest velocity along the scan line. While this allows it to have no maximum velocity, the signal is not gated, and localization of the signal is not possible.

5.1.1.2 Normal Transthoracic Echocardiography (TTE)

The American Society of Echocardiography (ASE) divides transthoracic echocardiography (TTE) into different categories—the ultrasound-assisted physician examination, cardiac PoCUS, critical care echocardiography, limited echocardiography, and comprehensive echocardiography [5]. The focused TTE is incorporated as part of several protocols such as the Rapid Ultrasound for Shock and Hypotension (RUSH) and

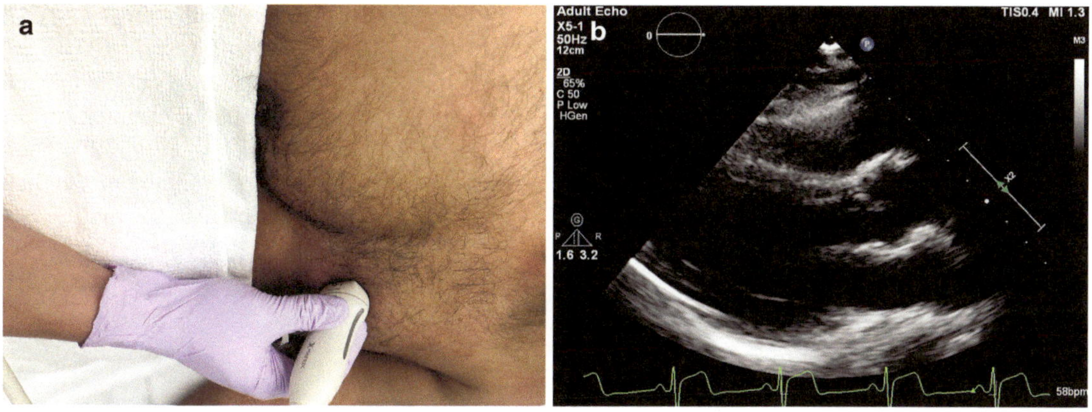

Fig. 5.1 (**a**) Probe positioning for the parasternal long-axis view, with the transducer orientation marker pointing towards the patient's left shoulder. (**b**) The parasternal long-axis view, with the left ventricle shown posterior (lower half of the image) to the right ventricle, and the mitral and aortic valves can be seen towards the right of the image

Sonography in Hypotension and Cardiac Arrest (SHoC) protocols [6–9]. While each protocol has its own philosophy and utilizes a different permutation of views, they share the same basic views covered below.

Parasternal long-axis view (PLAX). Cardiac imaging traditionally commences with the parasternal windows. Although some echocardiography laboratories perform echocardiography with the patient in the left lateral decubitus position, this is not practical in most scenarios, especially in critically ill patients, where PoCUS is often performed. Nonetheless, a semi-rotated position towards the left, by placing a pillow under the patient's right back and hip, may help improve image acquisition. The initial probe position is just to the left of the sternum, in the third or fourth intercostal space (Fig. 5.1a). Acquisition of the PLAX view is obtained with the alignment of the transducer orientation marker pointing towards the patient's right shoulder. In this view (Fig. 5.1b), the right ventricle is seen anteriorly, and the left ventricle and atrium inferiorly. The mitral and aortic valves should be clearly visualized towards the right of the image, and M-Mode echocardiography directed towards the anterior mitral leaflet from this view can be used to acquire the E-Point Septal Separation (EPSS)—a semiquantitative measure of left ventricular systolic function covered later in this chapter

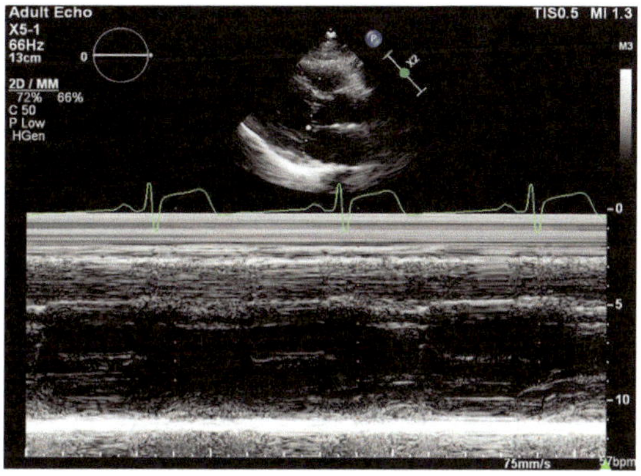

Fig. 5.2 M-Mode echocardiography demonstrating the E-Point Septal Separation (EPSS) acquired from the parasternal long-axis view

(Fig. 5.2) [10, 11]. The anteroseptal and inferolateral walls of the left ventricle are visualized in this view, although the cardiac apex is usually poorly visualized. Tilting the probe towards the patient's right hip allows visualization of the right ventricular inflow view in which the tricuspid valve and its leaflets can be visualized. From this view, Doppler interrogation of the tricuspid valve can be performed.

Parasternal short-axis view (PSAX). Rotation of the probe 90° clockwise from the PLAX view is probably the most efficient way of obtaining the PSAX view. The transducer orientation marker should now point towards the patient's left shoulder. The PSAX view demonstrates different structures at different levels, of which there are five different scan planes. Generally, most PoCUS providers will focus on the mid-ventricular SAX view (Fig. 5.3a, b) where LV is seen in cross-section with the 2 papillary muscles. This view is attractive to PoCUS providers as it allows visual estimation of left ventricular systolic function, myocardial thickening, and movement of all six wall segments at this level, as well as LV filling. From this view, M-Mode sonography can be aligned perpendicu-

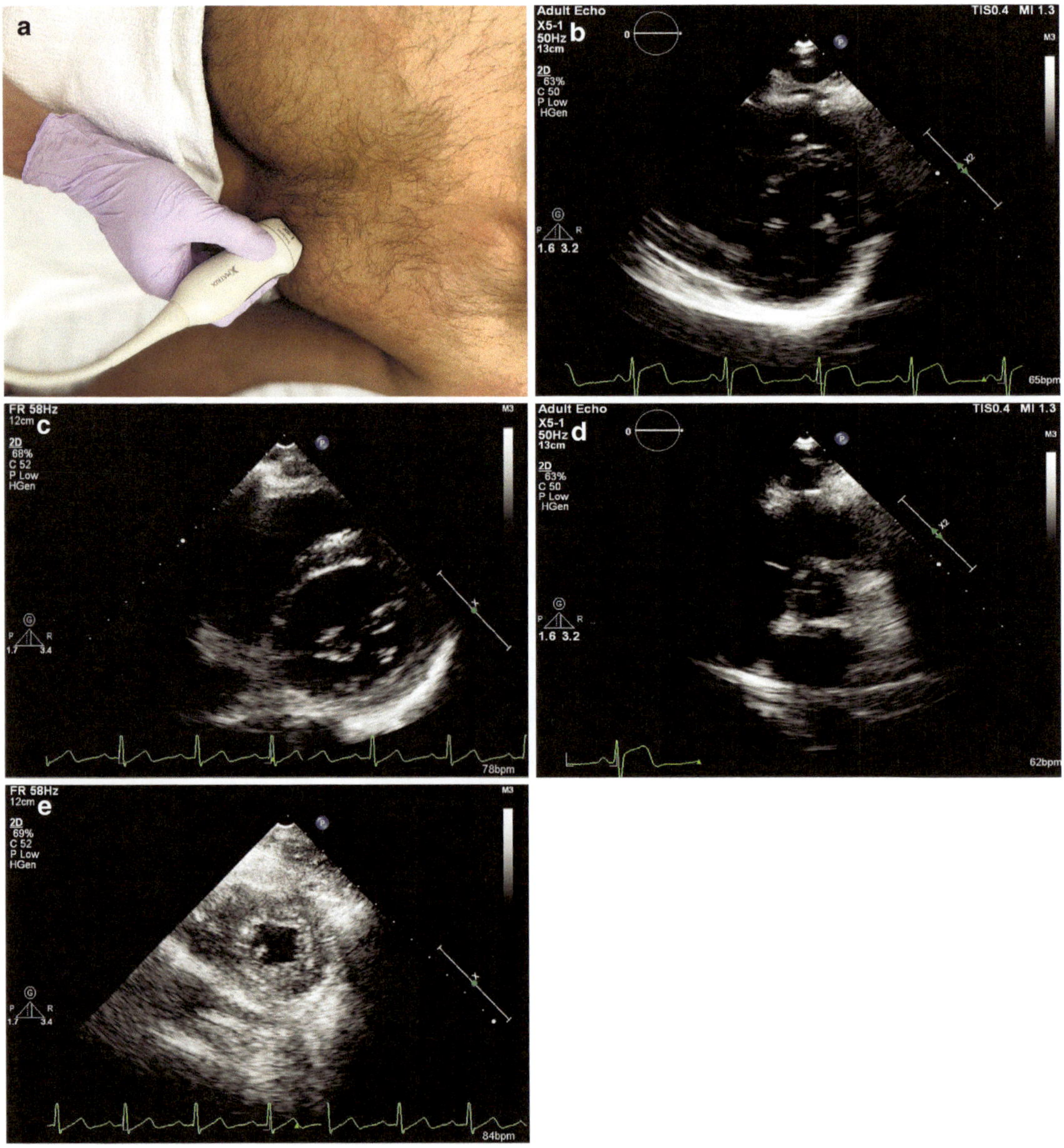

Fig. 5.3 (**a**) Probe positioning for the parasternal short-axis view, with the transducer orientation marker pointing towards the patient's left shoulder. (**b**) The parasternal mid-ventricular short-axis view, with the left ventricle shown in cross-section with the two papillary muscles. (**c**) The parasternal short-axis view at the basal level, demonstrating the "fish mouth" appearance of the mitral valve. (**d**) The aortic valve short-axis view. (**e**) The parasternal short-axis view at the level of the cardiac apex

lar to the inferior wall passing through the center of the LV cavity allow assessment of LV end-diastolic and end-systolic diameter, which can also be used to calculate fractional shortening and estimate ejection fraction based on geometric formulae such as Teicholz's formula or the modified Quinone's equation [12–14]. This is covered further later in this chapter.

From the mid-ventricular view, the probe can be angled cephalad towards the base of the heart and first produces the "fish mouth" appearance of the mitral valve (Fig. 5.3c). The anterior and posterior mitral valve leaflets can be visualized in this view, with the anterior leaflet of the mitral valve towards the top of the screen (anteriorly) and the posterior leaflet below. The anterior and posterior mitral valve leaflets are each divided into three scallops (A1–A3 and P1–P3). A1 and P1 are on the right of the image and the A3 and P3 scallops are on the left. This view is of limited clinical utility in the context of PoCUS.

The probe is further directed cephalad to obtain the aortic valve short-axis view (Fig. 5.3d), in which the three cusps of the aortic valve appear symmetrical. The tricuspid valve can be seen to the left of this image, and the pulmonary valve anterior to the aortic valve. The anatomy of the aortic valve can be assessed in this view, as well as the presence of any tricuspid regurgitation. Doppler interrogation of the tricuspid valve can be performed in this view. Further cephalad direction of the probe from the aortic valve short-axis view brings the main pulmonary artery into view, although this is of limited clinical utility, except in the rare case of a massive acute pulmonary embolism, in which a thrombus may be visible in the main pulmonary artery.

Caudal direction of the probe allows assessment of the cardiac apex (Fig. 5.3e) for wall motion abnormalities and ballooning, of which the latter may indicate Takotsubo cardiomyopathy. Otherwise, this view does not yield much clinical information for PoCUS providers.

Apical 4-chamber view (A4C). The A4C is obtained at the cardiac apex—which can vary significantly between individuals. This view is usually obtained by starting just inferolaterally to the left nipple or left breast, with the transducer orientation marker pointing towards the patient's left shoulder (Fig. 5.4a). The probe is directed towards the patient's right shoulder and then moved laterally until the cardiac apex is visualized in the middle of the upper part of the screen. The probe should then be tilted until the interventricular septum runs down the middle of the image. This view shows all 4 cardiac chambers and allows the operator to estimate the relative sizes of the right- and left-sided chambers, and visualize both atrioventricular valves (Fig. 5.4b). Application of color flow Doppler allows the detection of mitral and/or tricuspid regurgitation, or turbulent flow suggestive of stenosis. Furthermore, this view allows for good alignment for continuous wave Doppler interrogation of a tricuspid regurgitation jet for estimation of right ventricular systolic pressure. Both left and right ventricular systolic function can be estimated or measured in this view. Tricuspid annulus peak systolic excursion (TAPSE) (Fig. 5.4c), a surrogate measure of right ventricular systolic function, can be measured in this view by aligning M-Mode ultrasound to the lateral tricuspid annulus. In this view, the anterolateral and inferoseptal walls of the left ventricle can be seen. The presence of any pericardial collection can also be seen from this view.

A cephalad and leftward redirection of the probe from the A4C view produces the apical 5-chamber view which allows for visualization of the left ventricular outflow tract and aortic valve, from which Doppler measurements can be performed.

The A4C view is important as it forms the basis from which additional views such as the apical 2-chamber, apical 3-chamber, and apical 5-chambers views can be obtained, although these are generally not part of PoCUS protocol, but necessary for advanced measurements and assessment of global left ventricular function.

Apical 2-chamber (A2C). A 90° counterclockwise rotation of the probe from the A4C view generates the A2C view (pic), which allows assessment of the anterior and posterior walls of the left ventricle for wall motion abnormalities, as well as left ventricular function. Furthermore, biplane measurements of left ventricular systolic function, such as Simpson's biplane, require tracing end-diastolic and end-systolic endocardial borders of

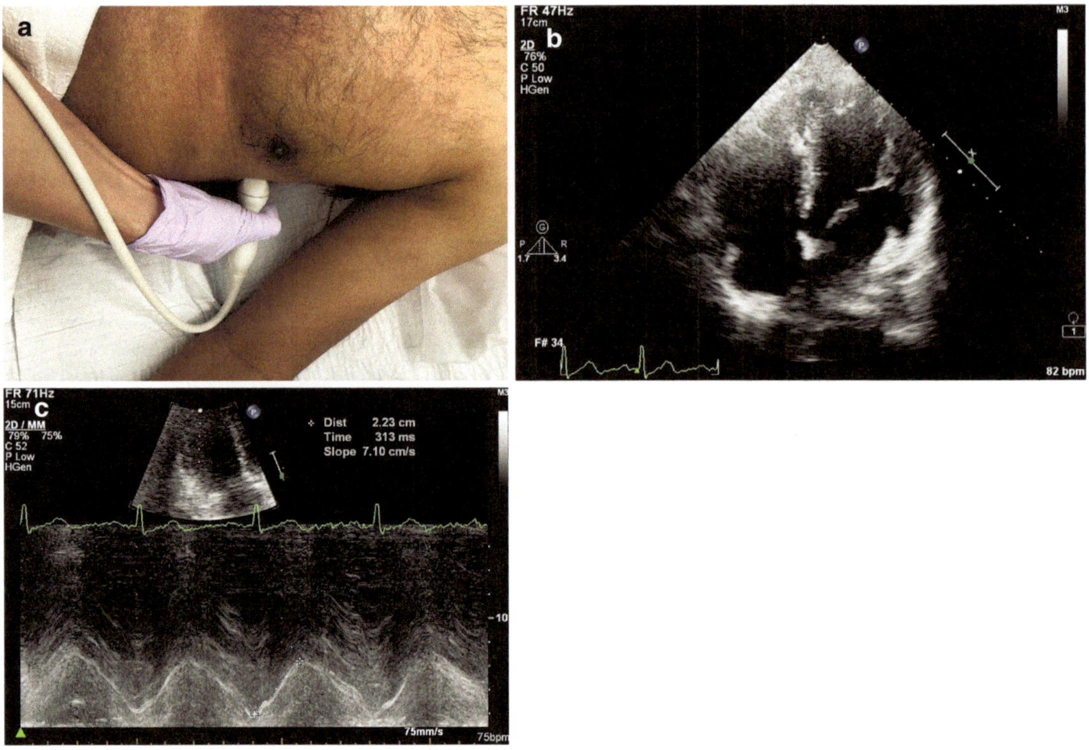

Fig. 5.4 (**a**) Probe positioning for the apical 4-chamber view, with the transducer orientation marker pointing towards the patient's left. (**b**) The apical 4-chamber view with the right ventricle on the left of the screen. (**c**) The tricuspid valve peak systolic excursion (TAPSE), measured by M-Mode echocardiography aligned to the lateral tricuspid annulus

the left ventricle in orthogonal views; thus, measurements performed in the A4C view will need to be complemented by measurements in the A2C view. Further counterclockwise rotation of the probe from the A2C position generates the apical 3-chamber (A3C) or apical long-axis view, analogous to the PLAX view. In this view, the anteroseptal and inferolateral walls of the left ventricle, as well as the left ventricular outflow tract and aortic valve can be visualized, and unlike the parasternal long axis, allows for alignment of a Doppler beam for pulsed wave and continuous-wave measurements of flow across the left ventricular outflow tract and aortic valve. Unlike the PLAX view, the A3C view usually allows for visualization of the apex of the left ventricle.

Subcostal window. The subcostal window can be accessed by placing the transducer in the subxiphoid space (Fig. 5.5a) with patient in supine position and legs bent at the knees to relax abdominal muscles. Subcostal window is particularly important in those patients where apical and parasternal windows are difficult to obtain, like the patients on ventilator and COPD patients. From this window, a 4-chamber view can be obtained to visualize any pericardial collections and allow gross estimation of chamber sizes, ventricular filling, and systolic function (Fig. 5.5b). Alignment also usually does not allow for adequate alignment for quantitative techniques which use pulsed wave or continuous wave Doppler. The apex is also typically not well visualized, only the septal and lateral walls of the left ventricle, precluding assessment of regional wall motion abnormalities, and limiting the utility of this view to visual estimates of function. Nonetheless, application of color flow Doppler in this view can still allow for visualization of gross

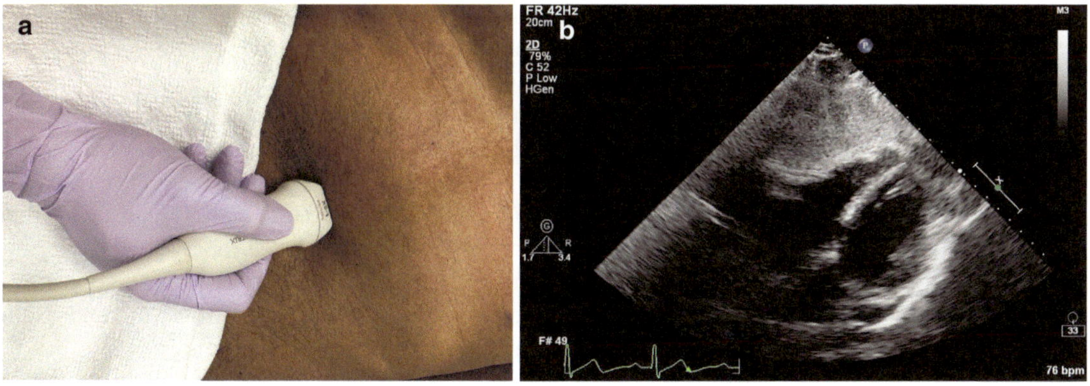

Fig. 5.5 (**a**) Probe positioning for the subcostal view, with the transducer orientation marker pointing to the patient's left. (**b**) The subcostal 4-chamber view. The right ventricle and atrium and anterior (upper half of the screen), and the left ventricle and atrium seem posterior. The liver and inferior vena cava can be seen on the left of the screen

valvular pathology such as regurgitation, as well as flow across the interatrial or interventricular septum. As it is comparatively easier to obtain a subcostal window compared to the parasternal or apical windows, especially in ventilated patients, modifications of other views are sometimes obtained from this window. Rotation of the probe counterclockwise produces a subcostal short-axis view that cuts through the mid-papillary region of the left ventricle that can allow for assessment of volume status. A modified short-axis view of the aortic valve can also be obtained from the subcostal window.

Inferior vena cava (IVC) view. This is a modification of the subcostal window. A cephalad orientation of the transducer from subcostal long-axis view will create IVC view (Fig. 5.6). The orientation marker is directed towards the head of the patient (cephalad). It will identify the IVC draining into the right atrium. Approximately 3 cm from the junction of inferior vena cava (IVC) and right atrium, the hepatic vein can be visualized to drain into IVC. This anatomical landmark is important as all the measurements of IVC in terms of volume status is supposed to be done just proximal to drainage point of hepatic vein and is standardized at this level. Measurements of IVC diameter can be performed with M-Mode echocardiography (Fig. 5.7). The abdominal aorta that is situated next to the IVC, needs to be differentiated from, and can be easily done so by its pulsations relative to the QRS complex of the ECG, or the patient's pulse based on the arterial waveform or plethysmography. Furthermore, the abdominal aorta has a thicker wall, with less respiratory variability and does not drain into the right atrium; this can be further confirmed by color flow or spectral Doppler interrogation.

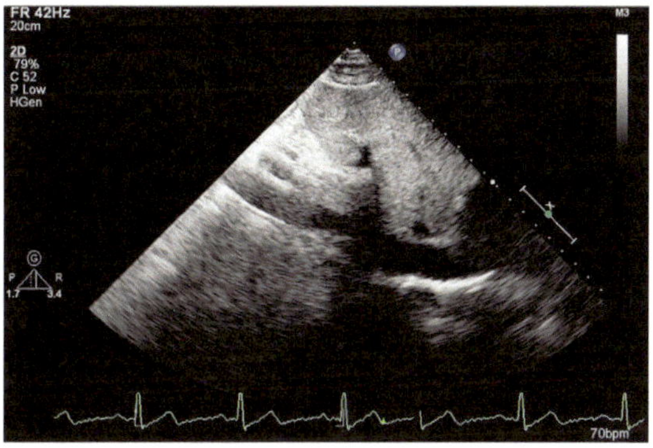

Fig. 5.6 The subcostal inferior vena cava view

Suprasternal window. The suprasternal view is usually not performed as part of PoCUS. It is acquired with the probe in the suprasternal notch and the transducer orientation marker pointing cephalad in a 12 o'clock position. In this view, the ascending aorta, aortic arch, and part of the proximal descending thoracic aorta can be clearly

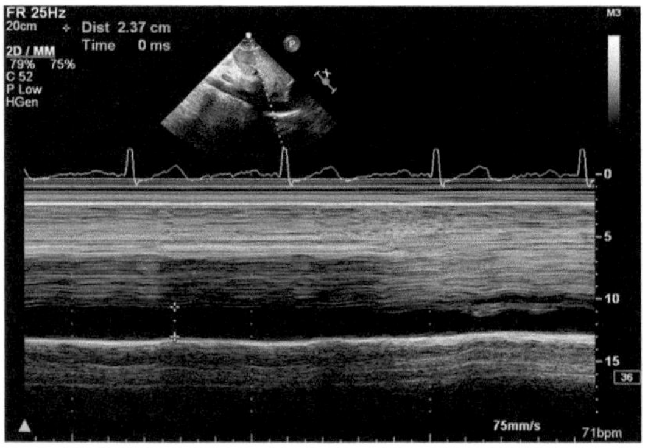

Fig. 5.7 Measurements of inferior vena cava diameter using M-Mode echocardiography

visualized, as well as the right pulmonary artery inferior to the aortic arch, and the aortic arch branches—the innominate artery, left common carotid artery, and left subclavian artery. This view allows for the identification of a proximal aortic aneurysm or dissection.

5.1.1.3 Normal Transesophageal Echocardiography (TOE)

There is increasing interest in the use of transesophageal echocardiography (TOE) in both acute care and perioperative medicine, due to its ability to circumvent poor transthoracic windows from positive pressure ventilation, chest wall injuries, and dressings, and provide good visualization of cardiac structures [15, 16].

Unlike transthoracic echocardiography, the TOE probe consists of a single ultrasound array that can be rotated around the long axis of the beam from 0 to 180°. The probe is inserted to various depths, and a multiplane angle is applied to rotate the beam in order to view cardiac structures across different scan planes [17].

Due to its small risk of serious complications, formal training in probe handling and manipulation is currently required by many centers. The indications for TOE are diverse. These range from hemodynamic monitoring, such as in basic perioperative TOE, to structural heart assessment of pathologies (such as valvular abnormalities) not achievable by TTE, to specific procedural indications such as during open-heart surgery, and catheter-based cardiac interventions. The *American Society of Echocardiography* has put forward a consensus statement detailing the 11 basic views required for a basic perioperative TOE examination, which are listed below (Table 5.1) with their approximate acquisition angles [18]. The basic perioperative TOE examination is a noncomprehensive examination aimed at assessing hemodynamic function, and exclusion of life-threatening pathology.

5.1.1.4 Left Ventricular Systolic Function Assessment

Left ventricular systolic function should be assessed in the presence of undifferentiated shock as it has important implications for treatment. Patients with left ventricular systolic dysfunction and a dilated left ventricle may benefit from inotropic support, rather than further fluid resuscitation. Furthermore, the presence of left ventricular systolic dysfunction is of prognostic value, and its presence portends worse outcomes.

The assessment of left ventricular systolic function is commonly assessed in the PLAX, PSAX, and A4C views. In patients with poor transthoracic windows (chronic obstructive pulmonary disease, left-sided pneumothorax, left-sided thoracic surgery, etc.), the subcostal 4-chamber view may also provide useful information. Visual estimates of ejection fraction are most commonly performed as part of PoCUS as traditional methods of quantifying ejection fraction, such as Simpson's biplane or fractional area change are time-consuming, require training, and a subject of interobserver variability. Furthermore, studies have demonstrated the feasibility and accuracy of qualitative visual estimates of ejection fraction in the management of the critically ill [19].

Quantitative measures of left ventricular systolic function can be obtained from PoCUS. Fractional shortening (FS) of the left ventricle can be measured in the PLAX or PSAX views via M-Mode echocardiography which

Table 5.1 The 11 basic views which constitute a basic perioperative transesophageal echocardiographic examination

View	Approximate depth and angle	Structures visualized and acquisition from previous view (if any maneuvers required)
ME 4-chamber view	ME, 30–40 cm 0–10°	Both atria and ventricles, atrioventricular valves (mitral and tricuspid) interatrial septum, and interventricular septum Inferoseptal and anterolateral walls of the LV Right-sided chambers are seen on the right side of the image
ME 2-chamber view	ME, 30–40 cm 00–100°	Left atrium and ventricle, left atrial appendage, and mitral valve Anterior and posterior walls of the LV are seen
ME long-axis view	ME, 40–50 cm 120–140°	Left atrium and ventricle, mitral valve, aortic valve, and left ventricular outflow tract Aortic root and proximal ascending aorta Anteroseptal and inferolateral walls of the LV Right ventricle and right ventricular outflow tract in the far field of the image
ME ascending aortic long-axis view	ME, 30–40 cm 90–110°	Transducer withdrawn slightly from the ME long-axis view The mid-ascending portion of the aorta and right pulmonary artery is seen
ME ascending aortic short-axis view	ME, 30–40 cm 20°	The mid-ascending portion of the aorta and main pulmonary artery and its bifurcation, as well as the superior vena cava. The left pulmonary artery is not well visualized
ME aortic valve short-axis view	ME, 30–40 cm 0–30°	Probe advanced from the ME ascending aortic short-axis view Aortic valve, interatrial septum, left main coronary artery, both atria, pulmonary valve, and the right ventricular outflow tract can be seen
ME RV inflow-outflow view	Me, 30–40 cm 60–80°	Aortic valve, interatrial septum, both atria, pulmonary and tricuspid valves, and the right ventricular outflow tract are visualized
ME bicaval view	ME, 30–40 cm 90–110°	Left and right atria, interatrial septum, superior and inferior vena cavae on the right and left of the screen, respectively. The tricuspid valve may be seen in the far field with increasing angles
TG mid-papillary short-axis view	TG, 40–45 cm 0–20°	Probe advanced from the mid-oesophageal views The LV, papillary muscles, and all six walls at the mid-ventricular level. Part of the RV may be seen
Descending aortic short-axis view	ME to TG, 30–40 cm 0°	The probe is withdrawn to a ME to TG level The descending thoracic aorta and left hemithorax is seen
Descending aortic long-axis view	ME to TG, 30—40 cm 90°	The descending thoracic aorta and left hemithorax is seen

Abbreviations: *ME* midesophageal, *RV* right ventricle, *TG transgastric, LV* left ventricle

allows the calculation of LV end-diastolic and end-systolic dimensions (Fig. 5.8). Its normal value is >30%. Usually, ejection fraction (EF) is considered to be double of FS. Fractional shortening is a unidimensional assessment and is not clinically appropriate in the presence of regional wall motion abnormalities or septal dyskinesia. Fractional area change (FAC) can be measured in the PSAX view (mid-papillary segment). This is a two-dimensional assessment of left ventricular area change during end-systole and end-diastole, the end-systolic area (ESA) and end-diastolic area (EDA), respectively. Normally it is 35–65%, and is calculated by FAC = (EDA − ESA) × 100/EDA. Ejection fraction, the difference between end-diastolic volume and end-systolic volume of the left ventricle can be calculated by geometric formulae (Table 5.2), such as the Teicholz's equation or the modified Quinone's equation (from M-Mode echocardiography) or the modified Simpson's biplane method of disks (from tracing endocardial borders). Both Teicholz's formula and the modified Quinone's equation have their limitations as linear measurements which make assumptions regarding the shape of the left ventricle and thus may be inaccurate in situations where there is asymmetrical left ventricular contraction such as ischemic heart disease. An alternative is to use Simpson's biplane method of disks, which requires tracing of LV endocardial borders in orthogonal views (i.e., 4-chamber and 2-chamber views) in both end-diastole and end-systole. This method divides the LV cavity into an a priori defined number of disks (usually 20), and the volume of each disk is calculated based on the tracing of the LV cavity [12–14, 20, 21].

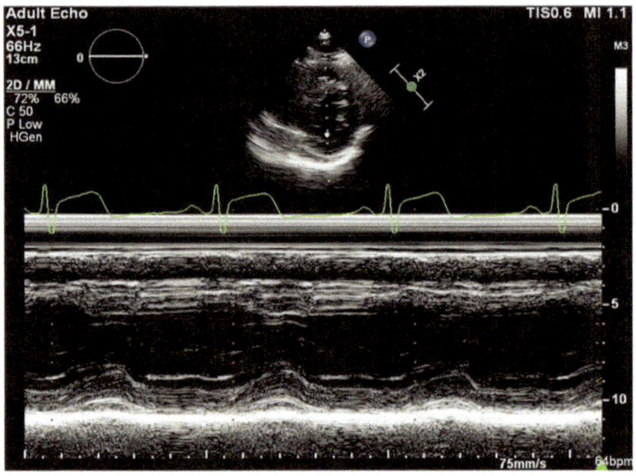

Fig. 5.8 M-Mode echocardiography demonstrating the left ventricular cavity. From this view, left ventricular end-diastolic and end-systolic dimensions can be measured, and calculations of fractional shortening or ejection fraction performed

Another semiquantitative measure of left ventricular systolic function easily obtained by echocardiography is the E-point septal separation (EPSS) which is the minimum distance between the tip of the anterior mitral valve leaflet endocardial border of the interventricular septum. The normal value of the EPSS is <7 mm, which corresponds with a normal ejection fraction [10, 11]. Based on magnetic resonance imaging studies, ejection fraction may be estimated from EPSS using the equation ejection fraction = 75.5 − (2.5 × EPSS).

Apart from the estimate of ejection fraction, the operator should also consider wall motion

Table 5.2 Teicholz's formula and the modified Quinone's equation [12–15]

Formula	Description
Teicholz's formula:	
Vol = $7D^3/(2.4 + D)$, where D is the LV diameter (mm) LVEF = (EDV − ESV)/EDV	Calculates LV volume using only LV diameter (D), and thus its accuracy is based on geometric assumptions regarding the shape of the LV Measurements are performed in end-diastole and end-systole in order to calculate the EDV and ESV, respectively
Modified Quinone's equation:	
$\%\Delta D^2 = (LVEDD^2 - LVESD^2)/LVEDD^2$ $LVEF = (\%\Delta D^2) + [(1 - \%\Delta D^2)(\%\Delta L)]$ Where LVEDD is the averaged LV end-diastolic dimension (mm), and LVESD is the averaged LV end-systolic dimension (mm) %ΔL: Correction for apical contraction +15% Normal apex +5% Hypokinetic apex +0% Akinetic apex −5% Slightly dyskinetic apex −15% Frankly dyskinetic apex	Calculates LVEF without planimetry by performing 8 averaged measurements of the LV internal diameter at different levels in the parasternal long-axis, apical 4 chamber, and long-axis views at end-diastole (LVEDD) and end-systole (LVESD). The formula further corrects for apical contraction visualized in the long axis (%ΔL) as with Teicholz's formula, the modified Quinone's equation is a linear measurement based on geometric assumptions, which may be inaccurate in the context of LV distortion (e.g., asymmetrical wall motion abnormalities, focal aneurysms)

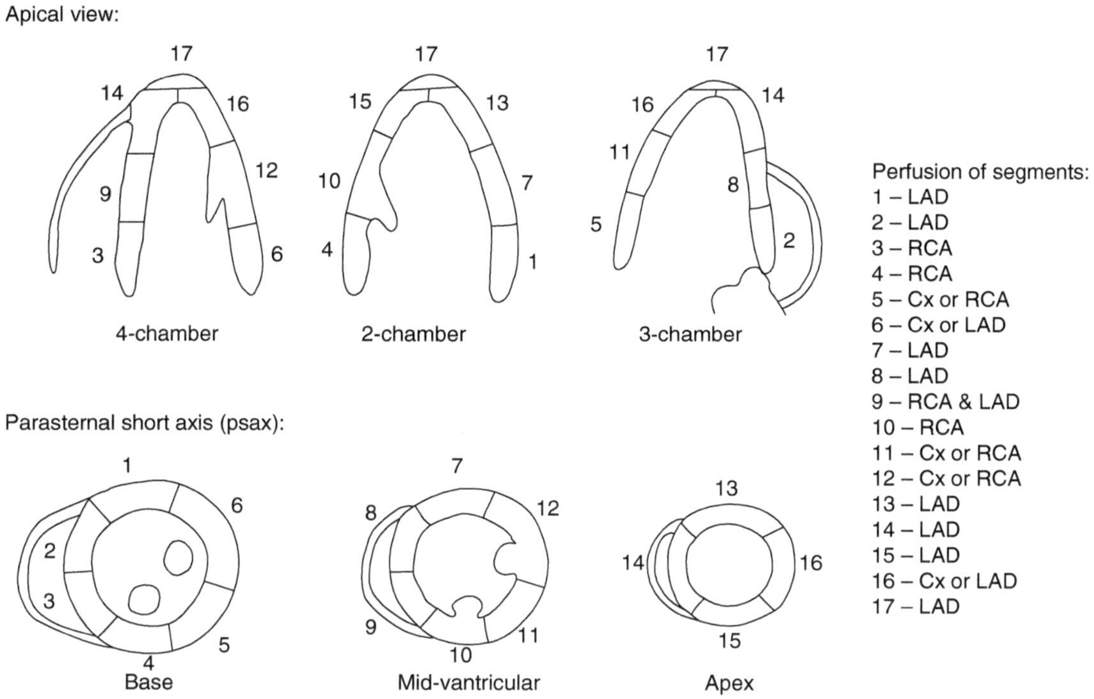

Fig. 5.9 The 17-segment model and its correspondence to perfusion by coronary arteries depicts the fundamental methodological approach. *Ortiz-Pérez JT, Rodríguez J, Meyers SN,* et al. *Correspondence between the 17-segment model and coronary arterial anatomy using contrast-enhanced cardiac magnetic resonance imaging. Cardiovasc Imaging. 2008; 1:282–93* [23]

abnormalities. The wall segments of the left ventricle should exhibit symmetrical systolic excursion towards the center of the cavity, and the myocardium should increase in thickness by >30% during systole. These findings are easily assessed from the PSAX view, as all six segments are visible. Evaluation for the presence of regional wall motion abnormalities (RWMA) is important for the diagnosis of acute coronary syndrome. Rise in cardiac biomarkers is delayed and time is the key in critically ill patients. Furthermore cardiac biomarkers, such as Troponin I can be elevated from other causes such as acute kidney injury, pulmonary embolism, and sepsis which need to be distinguished from acute coronary syndrome. ECG changes can also be a delayed finding, that makes echocardiography important for early evaluation of acute coronary syndrome. The presence of RWMAs may necessitate early coronary angiography and intervention. In critically ill patients stress cardiomyopathy can be similar to the presentation as ACS with similar ECG changes and rise in cardiac markers, but the characteristic ECHO finding of apical ballooning is distinctive. Regional wall motion abnormalities may be briefly evaluated with the PSAX view at the apical, mid-ventricular, and basal levels. However, a comprehensive evaluation also requires assessment with the A4C, A2C, A3C, and PLAX views. Depending on the occluded vessel (left anterior descending, right coronary, or left circumflex artery), different areas of the left ventricular wall may show hypokinesia, dyskinesia, or akinesia (Fig. 5.9; Table 5.2) [22, 23].

5.1.1.5 Left Ventricular Diastolic Function

When considering left ventricular function, far more attention is paid to systolic function compared to diastolic function. In diastolic dysfunction, there is impaired relaxation and noncompliance of the left ventricle (lusitropy). The long-standing consequence is an elevated left ventricular filling pressure, left atrial pressure, and left atrial dilatation. Measurement of diastolic dysfunction can be easily performed by using pulsed wave Doppler to measure mitral inflow velocities. The sample volume is placed at the coaptation point on an A4C view. This generates an E wave which corresponds to opening of the mitral valve and filling of the LV from the left atrium down a pressure gradient [24]. Diastasis then occurs as the left ventricular and atrial pressures equilibrate. Atrial systole then generates the A wave due to reacceleration of transmitral flow [24]. Identification of the E and A waves can be done by either observing the relative position to an ECG trace on the sonography platform (if applied) or the systolic wave on pulsed wave Doppler. The A wave occurs after the P wave on the ECG and precedes the systolic wave on pulsed wave Doppler. Measurement of time interval from the peak of the E wave to its extrapolated return to baseline is known as the deceleration time and is representative of the time required for left ventricular and atrial pressures to equalize [24].

In normal diastole, the mitral E wave is usually slightly higher than the A wave with a resultant ratio of the E and A waves exceeding 1.0 (E/A 1–1.5). A normal deceleration time of 180–220 ms is seen [24–27].

In grade I diastolic dysfunction or impaired relaxation, the active process of ventricular relaxation is slowed, with a reduction in the E velocity. This results in atrial systole contributing more to ventricular filling and a consequently larger A wave. The E/A ratio is reversed and E is < A (E/A < 0.75). The deceleration time is prolonged (>240 ms) congruent with the impaired lusitropy [24–27].

In grade II diastolic dysfunction, pseudonormalization is seen as a result of elevated left atrial pressures. The increased left atrial pressure results in a pressure gradient that reestablishes flow once the mitral valve opens and the E wave is larger due to this increased blood flow. This restores a "normal" E/A ratio of >1.0 [24–27]. Grade II diastolic dysfunction should be suspected in patients with unexplained dilated LA and can be unmasked by valsalva maneuver or during tissue Doppler interrogation.

Further diastolic dysfunction results in restrictive ventricular filling. Due to the elevated left atrial pressures filling a stiff, noncompliant ventricle, a high inflow velocity is seen with diastasis achieved rapidly. Atrial contraction contributes little to ventricular filling against the elevated left ventricular pressures. The E wave is usually twice the peak velocity of the A wave (E/A > 2) and the deceleration time is short (<140 ms), reflecting the rapid pressure equilibrium and diastasis [24–27] (Table 5.3).

Grade IV Diastolic dysfunction is restrictive cardiomyopathy, which is sonologically the same

Table 5.3 Grading of diastolic dysfunction

	Normal	Mild (Grade I)	Moderate (Grade II)	Severe (Grade III)
Pathophysiology		↓ Relaxation	↓ Relaxation and ↑ LVEDP	↓ Compliance ↑↑ LVEDP
E/A ratio	1–2	<0.8	0.8–2.0	≥2.0
Valsalva ΔE/A		<0.5	≥0.5	≥0.5
DT (ms)	150–200	>200	150–200	<150
e′ velocity (cm/s)	≥10	<8	<8	<5
E/e′ ratio	≤8	≤8	9–14	≥15
IVRT (ms)	50–100	≥100	60–100	≤60
PV_S/PV_D	=1	S > D	S < D	S < <D
PV_S (ms)	<0.35	>0.35	≥0.35	≥0.35
B_{dur}–A_{dur} (ms)	<20	<20	≥30	≥30
LA volume	<34 ml/m^2	Mildly enlarged	Moderately enlarged	Severely enlarged
Clinical presentation		Mild diastolic dysfunction or impaired relaxation phase	Pseudonormalization, Increased stiffness of the LV, elevated LAP	Restrictive filling (reversible) High LAP, noncompliant LV. May be reversible with reduction of preload (e.g., diuretics, Valsalva)

as Grade III, the only difference being it is not reversible with Valsalva maneuver.

5.1.1.6 Right Ventricular Function Assessment

Generally, the left ventricle (LV) receives much more attention during echocardiographic evaluation, particularly the systolic function of the LV. However, the importance of the right ventricle (RV) and its assessment has garnered increased recognition. Right ventricular dysfunction has important physiologic and prognostic implications [28]. Conditions that may result in RV dysfunction include primary RV failure (e.g., myocardial infarction, severe sepsis) or increased RV afterload (e.g., Pulmonary hypertension, pulmonary embolism, acute respiratory distress syndrome). Assessment of RV size can guide fluid resuscitation, and is important, as further fluid loading in the context of RV dysfunction can further worsen RV function, create interventricular septal bowing that compromises LV filling, and worsen hemodynamics.

Furthermore, certain causes of RV dysfunction necessitate specific therapy. Pulmonary emboli may require anticoagulation or thrombolysis, and massive saddle embolism with severe obstructive shock may require surgical embolectomy. In patients with pulmonary hypertension, specific physiological and pharmacological strategies may be required in addition to treating the underlying etiology—these may include inhaled nitric oxide (iNO), inodilator administration (e.g., Milrinone, Dobutamine), or pulmonary vasodilator therapy.

Fractional area change (FAC) is a commonly employed measure of RV systolic function. End-diastolic area (EDA) and end-systolic area (ESA) can be measured by tracing the endocardial borders of the right ventricle, allowing calculation of FAC by the formula FAC = (EDA − ESA) × 100/EDA. Values of FAC correlate well with RV ejection fraction obtained by cardiac magnetic resonance imaging (CMR) measurements, which are regarded as the gold standard in the quantification of RV systolic function. Fractional area change values of <35% indicate RV systolic dysfunction [29, 30].

However, tracing of endocardial borders may not be practical at the bedside with portable sonography platforms. During systole, the right ventricular free wall contracts towards the apex.

Contractility of the right ventricular free wall contributes minimally (15%) to the cardiac output. It is the vertical annular movement that is the most important contributor of RV systolic function. Tricuspid Annular Plane Systolic Excursion (TAPSE) can be measured by M-Mode echocardiography with the cursor aligned to the base of the lateral tricuspid valve annulus. Normal TAPSE value is 16 mm or more. A TAPSE value less than that indicates RV systolic dysfunction [29, 30].

5.1.1.7 Pulmonary Artery Pressures

Systolic, mean, and end-diastolic pulmonary artery pressures can be estimated by echocardiography.

Right ventricular systolic pressure (RVSP) is used as a surrogate measure of pulmonary artery systolic pressure (PASP). This is calculated by sum of the estimated or measured right atrial pressure (RAP) and peak gradient (PPG) of the tricuspid regurgitation (TR) jet, expressed as RVSP = TR PPG + RAP. The peak TR gradient is obtained by aligning a continuous wave (CW) Doppler beam to the TR jet to measure the peak velocity (TR V_{max}) and hence gradient by Bernoulli's equation, across the tricuspid valve. Thus, RVSP = $4(\text{TR } V_{max})^2$ + RAP [31]. Similarly, mean Pulmonary artery = Mean TR gradient (obtained by tracing the TR jet in CW) + RAP. If there is insufficient TR to obtain a complete CW Doppler envelope, RVSP(and hence PASP) and mean PAP cannot be estimated.

Diastolic PA pressure can be estimated by measuring the end-diastolic velocity of PR (Vpr). Diastolic PAP = $4(\text{Vpr})^2$ + RAP.

In the absence of adequate TR to estimate RVSP, the acceleration time across the pulmonary valve can help predict the likelihood of pulmonary hypertension, and estimate mean pulmonary artery systolic pressure (MPAP) by Mahan's equation. A short pulmonary acceleration time (<92 ms) is suggestive of elevated MPAP.

5.1.1.8 Volume Assessment

Volume status assessment is important to guide fluid therapy. Knowing when to intensify fluid administration is important. However, volume loading is detrimental in patients with myocardial dysfunction, or those who are already clinically overloaded. Although simple clinical examination techniques such as the straight leg raise exist, these alone may not provide sufficient information. Surrogate measures of fluid status such as central venous pressure or pulmonary capillary wedge pressure (PCWP) are invasive, and may not be accurate. Furthermore, derived measures of arterial waveform analysis such as stroke volume variation can only be interpreted accurately in certain physiological states.

Left ventricular assessment. Hypovolaemia may be indicated by a small, under-filled left ventricular cavity. This can be visible on the parasternal long- and short-axis views, as well as the apical and subcostal 4 chamber views. On the parasternal short axis, kissing papillary muscles may be seen.

Right ventricular assessment. During the bedside echocardiographic examination, the size of the right ventricle should be noted, particularly the approximate ratio of the right ventricle diameter to that of the left ventricle (RV:LV ratio). The RV:LV ratio should be less than 1:1, that is, the RV should not be the same size or larger than the left ventricle [32, 33]. A dilated right ventricle should prompt caution with further fluid loading. However, the critically ill may have a dilated right ventricle for other reasons, such as positive pressure mechanical ventilation leading to an increased right ventricular afterload, or pulmonary embolism. The latter may result in a distinctive echocardiographic finding of regional right ventricular dysfunction known as McConnell's sign, in which there is akinesia of the mid-free wall but normal motion at the apex [34].

Inferior vena cava assessment. Both the inferior (IVC) and superior vena cavae (SVC) are sensitive to fluid changes. They are collapsible, and their diameters undergo cyclical changes during both spontaneous respiration and positive pressure mechanical ventilation. During spontaneous respiration, the vessels collapse on inspiration and expand on expiration; and the minimum ($IVCD_{min}$) and maximum ($IVCD_{max}$) diameters can be easily measured by M-Mode ultrasound or direct 2D measurements [35]. The IVC can be imaged in the subxiphoid (or subcostal) long-axis view. Measurements are typically performed 2 cm inferior to the junction of the IVC and the hepatic veins, although the IVC may collapse nonuniformly [36]. In spontaneously breathing patients, the IVC collapsibility index is used and calculated by: IVC collapsibility index = $[(IVCD_{max} - IVCD_{min})/IVCD_{max}]$. An IVC collapsibility index of >50% is associated with reduced RAP and hypovolaemia [37]. In mechanically ventilated patients however the positive intrathoracic pressure transmitted during inspiration leads to reduced venous return and increased IVC diameter during this phase of the respiratory cycle, and thus IVC distensibility is used instead of collapsibility. The IVC distensibility index is calculated by the same formula, $[(IVCD_{max} - IVCD_{min})/IVCD_{max}]$. A distensibility index of cut-off of >18% has been proposed to indicate fluid responsiveness [38].

The diameter of the IVC has also been proposed as an indicator of fluid overload. However, the utility of this has a few caveats. Firstly, the diameter of the IVC varies with position and may be dilated in healthy individuals, such as athletes [39, 40]. Nonetheless, a diameter > 2.5 cm may be considered dilated, and suggestive of elevated right atrial pressure [29, 40–42].

More about IVC assessment can be found in Chap. 6: Vascular POCUS.

Superior vena cava assessment. Superior vena cava distensibility has been proposed as a measure of fluid responsiveness as the superior vena cava (SVC) is subject to the same cyclical changes in intrathoracic pressure as the IVC [43, 44]. In their study, Vieillard-Baron et al. proposed a cut-off of 36% to indicate fluid responsiveness [43]. However, SVC variability is usually studied by transesophageal echocardiography as views of the SVC are difficult to acquire using transthoracic echocardiography, and even when obtainable usually does not provide good alignment for M-Mode measurements.

Doppler assessment. Stroke volume variation may be used to predict fluid responsiveness. In one of its more primitive forms, this is visualized as variation or "swing" in the peak of an arterial waveform that varies with the respiratory cycle. Stroke volume can be quantified using pulsed wave Doppler, with the sample volume placed in the left ventricular outflow tract (LVOT) on the apical 5-chamber or apical long-axis views. Respiratory variation should ideally be measured over a single respiratory cycle. Although stroke volume (SV) is calculated using the product of the LVOT area and time-velocity integral (VTI) of a pulsed wave Doppler measurement within the LVOT (i.e., $SV = LVOT_{area} \times VTI_{LVOT}$), the former does not change, and for the purposes of PoCUS, measurement of VTI is adequate. In some cases, simple visualization of the peak velocity variation across the LVOT will suffice. In mechanically ventilated patients, a 12–20% variation in VTI or peak aortic flow predicts fluid responsiveness [44, 45]. However, the stroke volume variation has a few caveats, which also apply to non-echocardiographic methods of quantification (e.g., pulse waveform analysis). Among these include the need for mechanical ventilation, a fixed tidal volume of 8 $mL.kg^{-1}$, and sinus rhythm [44–48]. In addition to static measurements of LVOT VTI variability, a passive leg raise can be performed, and the pre-leg raise and post-leg raise VTI values are compared. The leg raise is akin to subjecting the patient to a volume load, by returning the pooled venous blood in the lower limb to the right ventricle. A change of >12% is suggestive of fluid responsiveness [49, 50].

5.1.1.9 Cardiac Output

Cardiac output can be calculated noninvasively by echocardiography and has been shown to correlate well with that obtained by thermodilution techniques [51]. SV can be obtained by the formula $SV = LVOT_{area} \times VTI_{LVOT}$, described in the previous section. The apical 5 chamber and 3 chamber views can be used to measure LVOT VTI using pulsed wave doppler. Care has to be taken not to use continuous wave doppler as this modality measures the highest velocity along the scan line, which will occur at the aortic valve (and not the LVOT) thus leading to overestimation of SV. Once SV is calculated, a simple product against heart rate will yield the estimated cardiac output.

References

1. The College of Emergency Medicine. Crowding in the emergency department. Revised ed. London: The College of Emergency Medicine; 2014.
2. Lawrence JP. Physics and instrumentation of ultrasound. Crit Care Med. 2007;35(8 Suppl):S314–22.
3. Baribeau Y, Sharkey A, Chaudhary O, et al. Handheld point-of-care ultrasound probes: the new generation of POCUS. J Cardiothorac Vasc Anesth. 2020;34(11):3139–45.
4. Moore CL. Chapter 3. Ultrasound orientation. In: Carmody KA, Moore CL, Feller-Kopman D. eds. Handbook of critical care and emergency ultrasound. McGraw Hill; https://accessanesthesiology-mhmedical-com.ezproxy.anzca.edu.au/content.aspx?bookid=517&sectionid=41066789. Accessed 25 June 2021
5. Kirkpatrick JN, Grimm R, Johri AM, Kimura BJ, et al. Recommendations for echocardiography laboratories participating in cardiac point of care cardiac ultrasound (POCUS) and critical care echocardiography training: report from the American Society of Echocardiography. J Am Soc Echocardiogr. 2020;33(4):409–422.e4.
6. Stickles SP, Carpenter CR, Gekle R, Kraus CK, et al. The diagnostic accuracy of a point-of-care ultrasound protocol for shock etiology: a systematic review and meta-analysis. CJEM. 2019;21(3):406–17.
7. Seif D, Perera P, Mailhot T, Riley D, Mandavia D. Bedside ultrasound in resuscitation and the rapid ultrasound in shock protocol. Crit Care Res Pract. 2012;2012:503254.
8. Milne J, Atkinson P, Lewis D, et al. Sonography in hypotension and cardiac arrest (SHoC): rates of abnormal findings in undifferentiated hypotension and during cardiac arrest as a basis for consensus on a hierarchical point of care ultrasound protocol. Cureus. 2016;8(4):e564.
9. Vaishnav M, Sedgwick J. Point-of-care echocardiography – a road to future or a step backwards. Australas J Ultrasound Med. 2019;22:26–31.
10. McKaigney CJ, Krantz MJ, La Rocque CL, Hurst ND, Buchanan MS, Kendall JL. E-point septal separation: a bedside tool for emergency physician assessment of left ventricular ejection fraction. Am J Emerg Med. 2014;32(6):493–7.
11. Silverstein JR, Laffely NH, Rifkin RD. Quantitative estimation of left ventricular ejection fraction from mitral valve E-point to septal separation and compari-

son to magnetic resonance imaging. Am J Cardiol. 2006;97(1):137–40.
12. Wandt B, Bojö L, Tolagen K, Wranne B. Echocardiographic assessment of ejection fraction in left ventricular hypertrophy. Heart. 1999;82(2):192–8.
13. Picard MH, Popp RL, Weyman AE. Assessment of left ventricular function by echocardiography: a technique in evolution. J Am Soc Echocardiogr. 2008;21(1):14–21.
14. St John Sutton MG, Plappert T, Rahmouni H. Assessment of left ventricular systolic function by echocardiography. Heart Fail Clin. 2009;5(2):177–90.
15. Roscoe A, Strang T. Echocardiography in intensive care. Contin Educ in Anaesth Crit Care Pain. 2008;8(2):46–9.
16. Mayo PH, Narasimhan M, Koenig S. Critical care transesophageal echocardiography. Chest. 2015;148(5):1323–32.
17. Seward JB, Khandheria BK, Freeman WK, Oh JK, Enriquez-Sarano M, Miller FA, Edwards WD, Tajik AJ. Multiplane transesophageal echocardiography: image orientation, examination technique, anatomic correlations, and clinical applications. Mayo Clin Proc. 1993;68(6):523–51.
18. Reeves ST, Finley AC, Skubas NJ, Swaminathan M, Whitley WS, Glas KE, Hahn RT, Shanewise JS, Adams MS, Shernan SK. Council on Perioperative Echocardiography of the American Society of Echocardiography; Society of Cardiovascular Anesthesiologists. Basic perioperative transesophageal echocardiography examination: a consensus statement of the American Society of Echocardiography and the Society of Cardiovascular Anesthesiologists. J Am Soc Echocardiogr. 2013;26(5):443–56.
19. Hope MD, de la Pena E, Yang PC, Liang DH, McConnell MV, Rosenthal DN. A visual approach for the accurate determination of echocardiographic left ventricular ejection fraction by medical students. J Am Soc Echocardiogr. 2003;16(8):824–31.
20. Foley TA, Mankad SV, Anavekar NS, Bonnichsen CR, Morris MF, Miller TD, et al. Measuring left ventricular ejection fraction-techniques and potential pitfalls. European Cardiology. 2012;8(2):108–14.
21. Li J, Zhang L, Wang Y, Zuo H, Huang R, Yang X, Han Y, He Y, Song X. Agreement in left ventricular function measured by echocardiography and cardiac magnetic resonance in patients with chronic coronary Total occlusion. Front Cardiovasc Med. 2021;8:675087.
22. Iwaszczuk P, Kołodziejczyk B, Kruczek T, et al. Ischemic versus non-ischemic (neurogenic) myocardial contractility impairment in acute coronary syndromes: prevalence and impact on left ventricular systolic function recovery. Med Sci Monit. 2018;24:3693–701.
23. Ortiz-Pérez JT, Rodríguez J, Meyers SN, et al. Correspondence between the 17-segment model and coronary arterial anatomy using contrast-enhanced cardiac magnetic resonance imaging. Cardiovasc Imaging. 2008;1:282–93.
24. Nishimura RA, Borlaug BA. Diastology for the clinician. J Cardiol. 2019;73(6):445–52.
25. Nagueh SF, Smiseth OA, Appleton CP, Byrd BF 3rd, Dokainish H, Edvardsen T, Flachskampf FA, Gillebert TC, Klein AL, Lancellotti P, Marino P, Oh JK, Popescu BA, Waggoner AD. Recommendations for the evaluation of left ventricular diastolic function by echocardiography: an update from the American Society of Echocardiography and the European Association of Cardiovascular Imaging. J Am Soc Echocardiogr. 2016;29(4):277–314.
26. Silbiger JJ. Pathophysiology and echocardiographic diagnosis of left ventricular diastolic dysfunction. J Am Soc Echocardiogr. 2019;32(2):216–232.e2.
27. Schumacher A, Khojeini E, Larson D. ECHO parameters of diastolic dysfunction. Perfusion. 2008;23(5):291–6.
28. Anavekar NS, Skali H, Bourgoun M, Ghali JK, Kober L, Maggioni AP, McMurray JJ, Velazquez E, Califf R, Pfeffer MA, Solomon SD. Usefulness of right ventricular fractional area change to predict death, heart failure, and stroke following myocardial infarction (from the VALIANT ECHO study). Am J Cardiol. 2008;101(5):607–12.
29. Rudski LG, Lai WW, Afilalo J, Hua L, Handschumacher MD, Chandrasekaran K, Solomon SD, Louie EK, Schiller NB. Guidelines for the echocardiographic assessment of the right heart in adults: a report from the American Society of Echocardiography endorsed by the European Association of Echocardiography, a registered branch of the European Society of Cardiology, and the Canadian Society of Echocardiography. J Am Soc Echocardiogr. 2010;23(7):685–713. quiz 786-8
30. Dutta T, Aronow WS. Echocardiographic evaluation of the right ventricle: clinical implications. Clin Cardiol. 2017;40(8):542–8.
31. Armstrong DW, Tsimiklis G, Matangi MF. Factors influencing the echocardiographic estimate of right ventricular systolic pressure in normal patients and clinically relevant ranges according to age. Can J Cardiol. 2010;26(2):e35–9.
32. Frémont B, Pacouret G, Jacobi D, Puglisi R, Charbonnier B, de Labriolle A. Prognostic value of echocardiographic right/left ventricular end-diastolic diameter ratio in patients with acute pulmonary embolism: results from a monocenter registry of 1,416 patients. Chest. 2008;133(2):358–62.
33. Hendriks SV, Klok FA, den Exter PL, Eijsvogel M, Faber LM, Hofstee HMA, Iglesias Del Sol A, Kroft LJM, Mairuhu ATA, Huisman MV. Right ventricle-to-left ventricle diameter ratio measurement seems to have no role in low-risk patients with pulmonary embolism treated at home triaged by Hestia criteria. Am J Respir Crit Care Med. 2020;202(1):138–41.
34. Oh SB, Bang SJ, Kim MJ. McConnell's sign; a distinctive echocardiographic finding for diagnosing acute pulmonary embolism in emergency department. Crit Ultrasound J. 2015;7(Suppl 1):A20. https://doi.org/10.1186/2036-7902-7-S1-A20.

35. Yildizdas D, Aslan N. Ultrasonographic inferior vena cava collapsibility and distensibility indices for detecting the volume status of critically ill pediatric patients. J Ultrason. 2020;20(82):e205–9.
36. Blehar DJ, Resop D, Chin B, Dayno M, Gaspari R. Inferior vena cava displacement during respirophasic ultrasound imaging. Crit Ultrasound J. 2012;4(1):18.
37. Kircher BJ, Himelman RB, Schiller NB. Noninvasive estimation of right atrial pressure from the inspiratory collapse of the inferior vena cava. Am J Cardiol. 1990;66(4):493–6.
38. Barbier C, Loubières Y, Schmit C, Hayon J, Ricôme JL, Jardin F, Vieillard-Baron A. Respiratory changes in inferior vena cava diameter are helpful in predicting fluid responsiveness in ventilated septic patients. Intensive Care Med. 2004;30(9):1740–6.
39. Mookadam F, Warsame TA, Yang HS, Emani UR, Appleton CP, Raslan SF. Effect of positional changes on inferior vena cava size. Eur J Echocardiogr. 2011;12(4):322–5.
40. Goldhammer E, Mesnick N, Abinader EG, Sagiv M. Dilated inferior vena cava: a common echocardiographic finding in highly trained elite athletes. J Am Soc Echocardiogr. 1999;12(11):988–93.
41. Gadi SR, Ruth BK, Johnson A, Mazimba S, Kwon Y. Isolated marked inferior vena cava dilatation: unusual presentation or underrecognized common phenomenon? Case Rep Cardiol. 2018;2018:8396523.
42. Pellicori P, Carubelli V, Zhang J, Castiello T, Sherwi N, Clark AL, Cleland JG. IVC diameter in patients with chronic heart failure: relationships and prognostic significance. JACC Cardiovasc Imaging. 2013;6(1):16–28.
43. Vieillard-Baron A, Chergui K, Rabiller A, Peyrouset O, Page B, Beauchet A, Jardin F. Superior vena caval collapsibility as a gauge of volume status in ventilated septic patients. Intensive Care Med. 2004 Sep;30(9):1734–9.
44. Miller A, Mandeville J. Predicting and measuring fluid responsiveness with echocardiography. Echo Res Pract. 2016;3(2):G1–G12.
45. Charron C, Fessenmeyer C, Cosson C, Mazoit JX, Hebert JL, Benhamou D, Edouard AR. The influence of tidal volume on the dynamic variables of fluid responsiveness in critically ill patients. Anesth Analg. 2006;102:1511–1517.Vie.
46. Feissel M, Michard F, Mangin I, Ruyer O, Faller JP, Teboul JL. Respiratory changes in aortic blood velocity as an indicator of fluid responsiveness in ventilated patients with septic shock. Chest. 2001;119:867–73.
47. Heenen S, De Backer D, Vincent JL. How can the response to volume expansion in patients with spontaneous respiratory movements be predicted? Crit Care. 2006;10:R102.
48. De Backer D, Heenen S, Piagnerelli M, Koch M, Vincent JL. Pulse pressure variations to predict fluid responsiveness: influence of tidal volume. Intensive Care Med. 2005;31:517–23.
49. Bou Chebl R, Wuhantu J, Kiblawi S, Carnell J. Bedside echocardiography and passive leg raise as a measure of volume responsiveness in the emergency department. J Ultrasound Med. 2019;38(5):1319–26.
50. Maizel J, Airapetian N, Lorne E, Tribouilloy C, Massy Z, Slama M. Diagnosis of central hypovolemia by using passive leg raising. Intensive Care Med. 2007;33(7):1133–8.
51. Zhang Y, Wang Y, Shi J, Hua Z, Xu J. Cardiac output measurements via echocardiography versus thermodilution: a systematic review and meta-analysis. PLoS One. 2019;14(10):e0222105. https://doi.org/10.1371/journal.pone.0222105.

6 Vascular Ultrasound

Sudhakar Subramani, Satoshi Hanada, and Arunangshu Chakraborty

6.1 Introduction

Vascular ultrasound (VU) plays a significant role in visual depiction of arteries and veins. The procedure has, over the last two decades, undergone considerable upgrades in technology, approach, and utility to diagnose various vascular-related disorders in both major and minor vessels and determine management options for those conditions. In the case of arteries, VU gives information ranging from endothelial dysfunction over measuring the increase of intima media thickness to the detection of stenoses, occlusion, or aneurysm. VU helps to differentiate between primary vasculitis and arterial compression syndromes like entrapment syndrome of different arterial regions. It also plays an essential role in arterial cannulation of various vessels such as femoral, brachial, radial, and dorsalis pedis in a wide range of clinical settings. In the case of veins, VU is considered as the primary imaging modality to diagnose venous thrombosis, while follow-up controls help in the prediction of recurrent venous thrombosis. Ultrasound is a key tool to determine the cause and severity of chronic venous insufficiency and allows various therapeutic procedures for the treatment of varicose veins to be visually monitored. Like arterial cannulation, VU helps to cannulate major veins and the deeper veins in certain complex clinical settings. In this chapter, the authors give a broader view of the role of ultrasound in certain vascular structures.

The supplementary videos provided along with this chapter will help the beginners practice their skills at—Video 6.1: Assessment of IJ and Carotid artery, Video 6.2: Assessment of Subclavian vessels infraclavicular approach, Video 6.3: Assessment of IVC Trans abdominal coronal long axis, Video 6.4: Assessment of abdominal aorta, Video 6.5: Assessment of femoral vessels.

Supplementary Information The online version contains supplementary material available at [https://doi.org/10.1007/978-981-16-7687-1_6].

S. Subramani (✉) · S. Hanada
Department of Anesthesia, University of Iowa, Iowa City, IA, USA
e-mail: Sudhakar-subramani@uiowa.edu

A. Chakraborty
Department of Anaesthesia, Critical Care and Pain, Tata Medical Center, Newtown, Kolkata, West Bengal, India

6.2 Carotid Artery

6.2.1 Anatomy of Carotid Artery

The carotid arteries are the primary vessels that supply blood to the brain and the facial area. The right common carotid artery (RCCA) originates in the neck from the brachiocephalic artery while the left common carotid artery (LCCA) arises in the thoracic region from the arch of the aorta [1]

A. Chakraborty, B. Ashokka (eds.), *A Practical Guide to Point of Care Ultrasound (POCUS)*,
https://doi.org/10.1007/978-981-16-7687-1_6

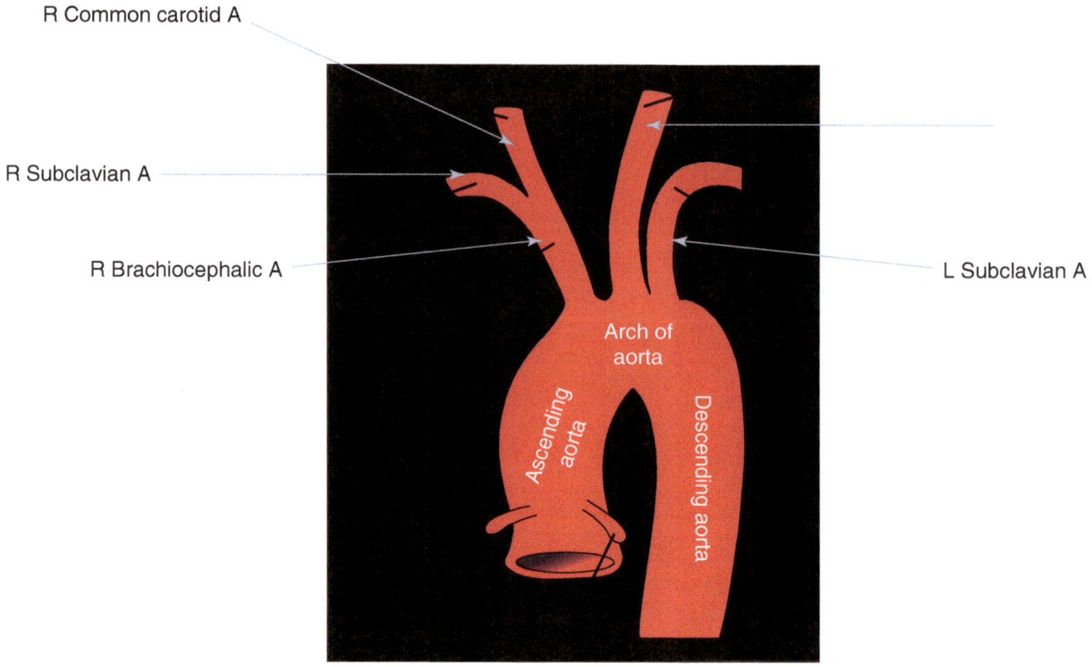

Fig. 6.1 Origin of left and right carotid arteries

(Fig. 6.1). The common carotid artery typically bifurcates at the upper border of the thyroid cartilage at the level of carotid sinus into the internal carotid artery (ICA) predominantly supplies the brain, and the external carotid artery (ECA) supplies the neck and face (Fig. 6.2). However, several studies have shown a variant in which the common carotid artery bifurcates more distally [2]. Generally, carotid bifurcation is the site of clinically meaningful atherosclerosis, and a more distal bifurcation may impact the ability to proceed with standard surgical or interventional approaches. Evaluating carotid artery anatomy is essential prior to cannulation or any interventional procedures.

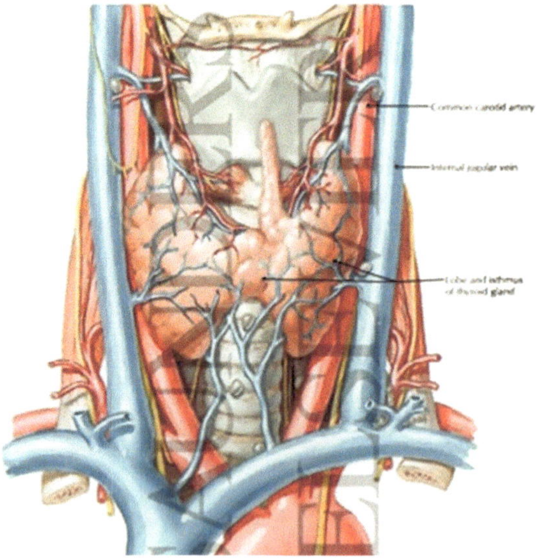

Fig. 6.2 Course of common carotid artery and IJV

6.2.2 Ultrasound Assessment of Carotid Artery

Ultrasound of carotid artery (CA) remains a longstanding and reliable tool in the current armamentarium of diagnostic modalities used to assess vascular morbidity, especially in an early stage. Both grayscale (two-dimensional—2D) and Doppler US can be used for the evaluation of extracranial segments of the CA, with the complexity of these two methods commonly being referred to as duplex ultrasound (DUS). The 2D US helps predominantly for the assessment of morphology including size, variations in carotid bifurcation, anomaly, and of vascular wall atherosclerotic changes (Figs. 6.3a, b and 6.4 normal carotid artery sax and lax). From the peri-operative and critical care aspects, knowing variations in CA is essential to minimize inadvertent arterial cannulation while placing a central venous cannula in the internal jugular vein (Fig. 6.5 variations in carotid artery). Although the 2D US could differentiate between calcified and noncalcified portions of the plaque, the advancement of technology using three-dimensional (3D) methods makes such differentiation much easier and more precise. The determination of noncalcified and hypoechoic portions of the plaques carries an independent risk factor for stroke. 2D along with 3D ultrasound can determine the intima media thickness (IMT) aiding in the detection of preclinical atherosclerotic disease, and subsequent assessment of risk stratification based on the grade of atheroma [3] (Fig. 6.6 atheroma).

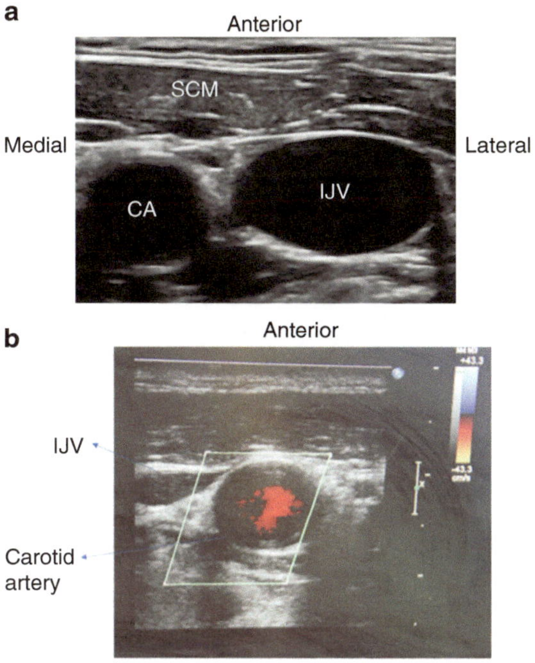

Fig. 6.3 (**a**) US image of carotid artery in short axis. (**b**) Color doppler of carotid artery with compression on IJV

6.2.3 Duplex Ultrasound of Carotid Artery

In addition to the morphological assessment of carotid arteries, US permits measurement of flow based on the reflection of ultrasound waves by utilizing both pulse Doppler US and color flow

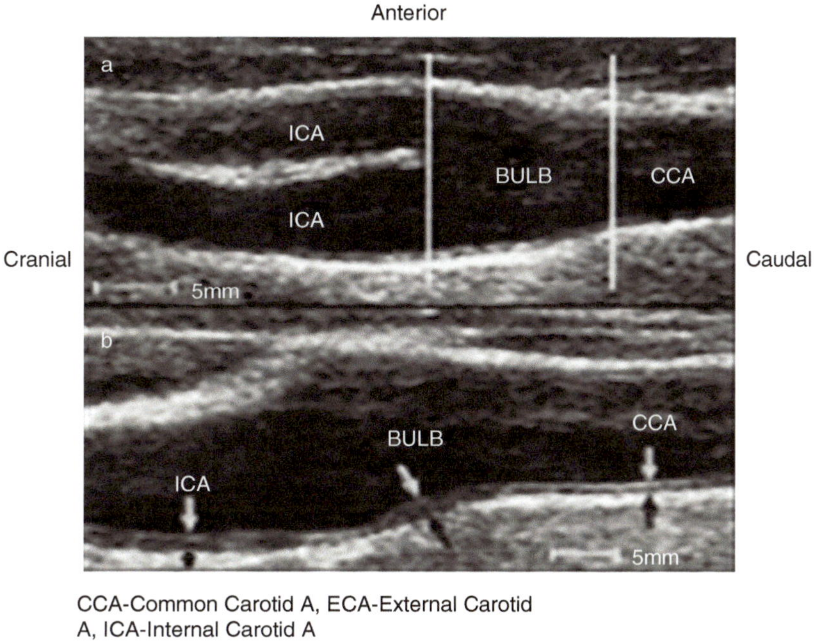

Fig. 6.4 US image of carotid artery in long axis showing bifurcation

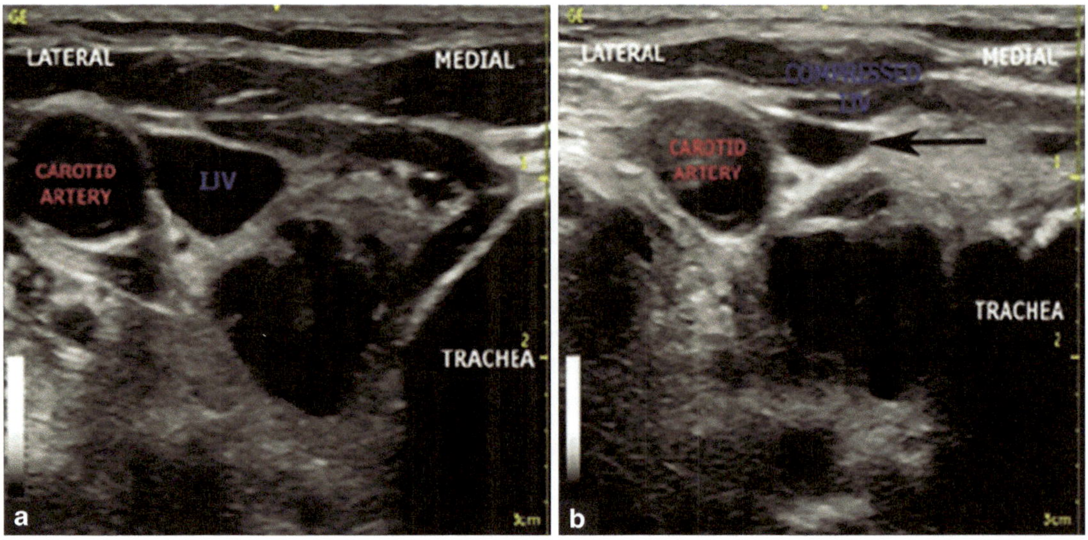

Fig. 6.5 Variants in the course of carotid artery and internal jugular vein

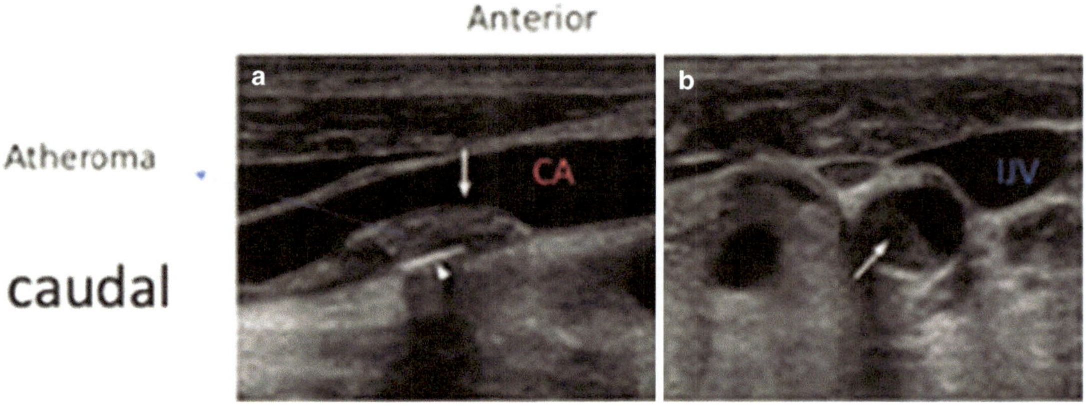

Fig. 6.6 US image of carotid artery in short and long axis with atheromatous plaque

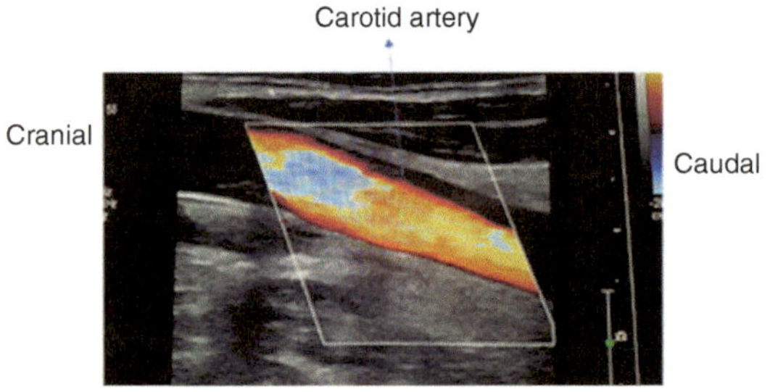

Fig. 6.7 Color doppler of carotid artery in the longitudinal plane

Doppler US. Visualization of color-coded flow provides information about the direction of blood flow (Fig. 6.7). The measurement of velocity superimposed on 2D images can be done with color Doppler US to determine grading of stenotic lesions (Fig. 6.8a, b spectral Doppler). In general, by using color flow Doppler, high-grade stenotic lesions are more easily detected compared with pulse wave Doppler although the latter allows direct estimation of flow velocity. Although the peak systolic velocity (PSV) is commonly used to quantify stenosis, end-diastolic velocity (EDV), carotid index, and spectral waveform analysis are also used for the assessment of stenosis [4]. There are a number of pitfalls when using velocity-based estimation of CA stenosis such as elevated velocities when there is contralateral carotid artery occlusion and

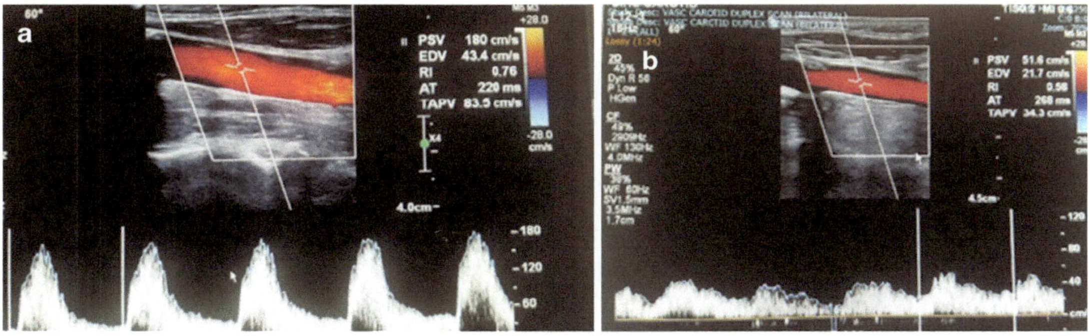

Fig. 6.8 (**a**) Spectral doppler of carotid artery (normal) in the longitudinal plane. (**b**) Spectral doppler of carotid artery with low systolic and diastolic velocity

higher velocities in females. Moreover, DUS is restricted to the cervical portion of the ICA with the option of obtaining added information from transcranial Doppler studies recommended in certain challenging situations. Factors such as severe tortuosity of an artery, high carotid bifurcation, obesity, or extensive calcification of the vasculature might reduce the accuracy of estimation [5]. In spite of these limitations, Duplex ultrasound has many advantages of safety, affordability, and the ability to directly visualize morphology and measure flow compared to other imaging modalities. It is also relatively inexpensive, readily performed at the bedside with no radiation or need for contrast.

6.3 Internal Jugular Vein

6.3.1 Anatomy of Internal Jugular Vein

The internal jugular vein (IJV) is a paired venous structure that receives blood from the brain, face, and neck, and drains it to the right atrium. The internal jugular vein is the continuation of the sigmoid sinus. It arises in the posterior cranial fossa and exits the cranium through the jugular foramen. In the upper part of the neck just underneath the base of the skull, it drains the branches of the facial, retromandibular, and lingual veins. The course of the internal jugular vein is directed caudally in the carotid sheath. It is accompanied by the common carotid artery anteromedially and the vagus nerve posteriorly (Fig. 6.9). It generally lies just lateral and anterior to the internal and common carotid arteries; in rare situation it lies entirely medial to the carotid artery. The IJV combines with the subclavian vein to form the brachiocephalic or innominate vein at the junction of the neck and thorax. The left internal jugular vein is slightly smaller than the right internal jugular vein. Both veins contain valves located a few centimeters before the vessels drain into the subclavian vein. Due to a relatively straighter course, right IJV is preferred over left IJV for central venous cannulation. Familiarity with surface anatomy of IJV is essential for both diagnostic assessment of various disorders and for cannulation.

6.3.2 Ultrasound Assessment of IJV

Both 2D and color Doppler ultrasound are commonly utilized to evaluate the morphology of IJV and its course (Fig. 6.10). Compression US is routinely used to differentiate arterial system from venous structures, especially in significant venous pulsation from adjacent arteries as well as from high central venous pressure (Fig. 6.11). US of IJV helps to identify variants in anatomical course, presence of valves in unusual location, thrombosis, chronic venous insufficiency, and even complete absence of IJV on one or both sides (Video 6.1) (Fig. 6.12). The role of US on IJV has been expanded to measure the changes in the IJV cross-sectional area CSA during the cardiac cycle simi-

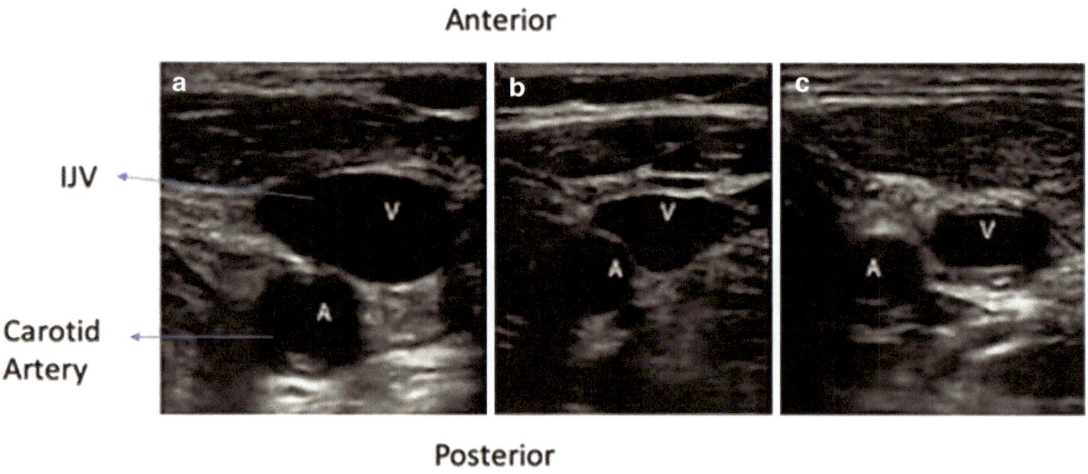

Fig. 6.9 Relationship between IJV and carotid artery. (**a**) IJV anterior to CA, (**b**) IJV anterolateral to CA and (**c**) IJV lateral to CA

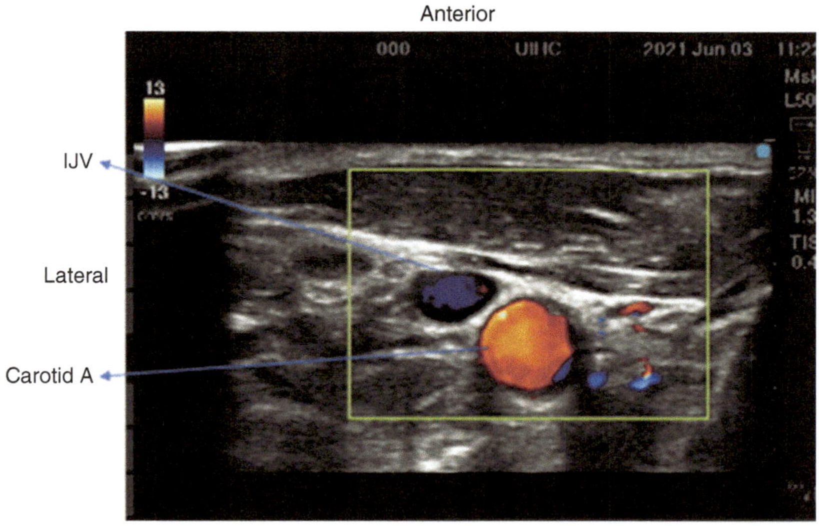

Fig. 6.10 Color flow doppler of IJV

lar to caval index in inferior vena cava, and can estimate the jugular venous pulse and right atrial pressure [6]. Despite potential inaccuracies, the DS observation of the IJV pulsatility remains an acceptable method of central venous pressure monitoring in various clinical settings [7]. It also helps to predict fluid responsiveness in mechanically ventilated patients after cardiac surgeries similar to IVC variability [8]. In addition to regular assessment of IJV for cannulation and fluid status, Spectral DS analysis of the IJVs is an emerging new concept in examining their physiological hemodynamic ranges. Many studies have shown abnormal extracranial venous flow in a variety of central nervous system disorders, such as multiple sclerosis, migraine, Parkinson's disorders, Meniere syndrome, and obstructive sleep apnea [9–12]. An accurate and reproducible DS venous blood flow volume (BFV) method is essential to diagnose those conditions.

6.3.2.1 Anatomy of Subclavian Vessels

The subclavian vein is the continuation of the axillary vein as it courses beneath the clavicle. At the lateral border of the first rib, it travels superiorly then under the clavicle travels medially until

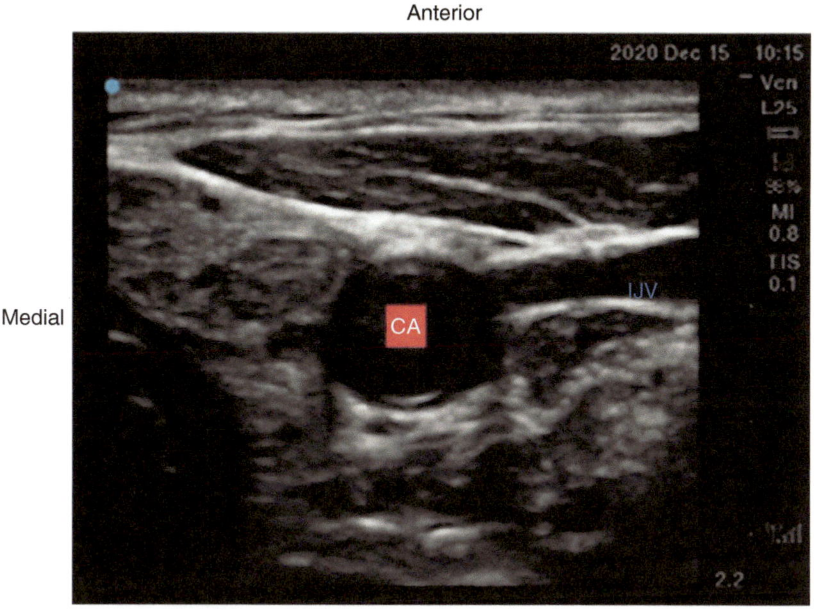

Fig. 6.11 Compression USG of IJV

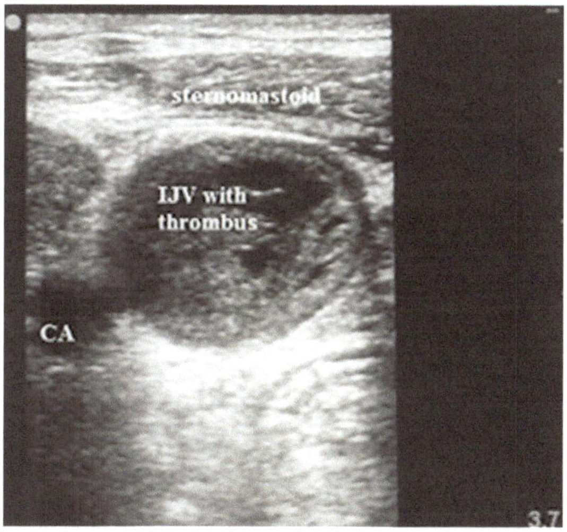

Fig. 6.12 Thrombosis of IJV

it joins the internal jugular vein to form an innominate vein. The subclavian artery runs posterior and superior to the subclavian vein. The brachial plexus courses superiorly and deep to the medial portion of the subclavian artery. On the left side, the thoracic duct lies close to the subclavian vessels. Most importantly, the lung and pleural cavity lie inferior and deeper to the subclavian vein and are particularly vulnerable to accidental puncture more often on the left chest where the apex of the lung can extend just above the first rib. Familiarity with anatomical variants of subclavian vessels are essential prior to any interventional procedures or cannulation of both vein and artery.

6.3.2.2 Ultrasound Assessment of Subclavian Vessels

Similar to IJV, 2D and color Doppler US are utilized to assess the morphology, patency, anatomical variants, and certain pathological conditions such as aneurysm, stenosis, or thrombosis of the vessels (Video 6.2) (Fig. 6.13). Compared to US-guided cannulation of IJV there is limited data on the utilization of US for SV cannulation. Meta-analysis of over 2000 patients from nine studies showed that the use of US resulted in a reduced rate of accidental arterial puncture (0.8% vs 5.9%); and hematoma formation (1.2% vs 6.6%). However, there was no statistically significant difference between the use of US and the conventional landmark technique in the total complication rate, the overall success rate, the number of attempts until success, the time to successful cannulation, and the success rate with the first attempt [13, 14]. Currently, there is no strong evidence of using the US for SV cannulation from different societies.

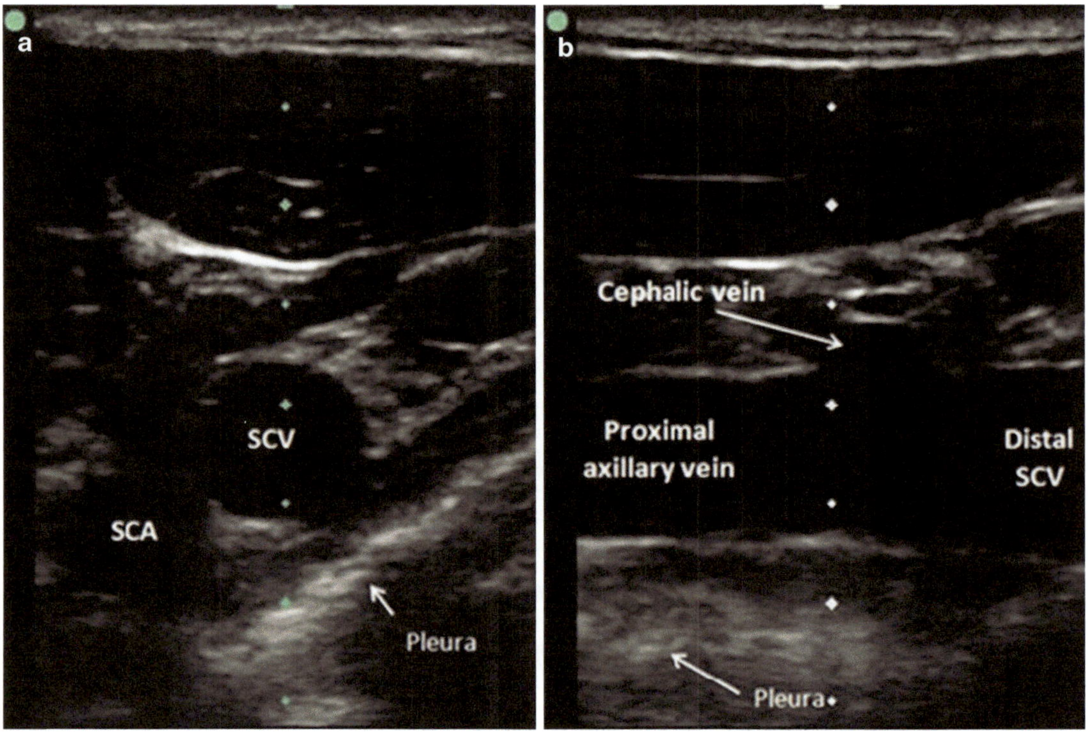

Fig. 6.13 US image of subclavian vessels (infraclavicular approach—short axis and long axis)

6.4 Anatomy of Inferior Vena Cava

The inferior vena cava is formed by the confluence of the two common iliac veins at the L5 vertebral level. The IVC has a retroperitoneal course within the abdominal cavity. It runs along the right side of the vertebral column with the aorta lying laterally on the left. Various other veins drain into the IVC along its course before it passes through the diaphragm at the caval hiatus at the T8 level. Hepatic veins are the last tributaries of IVC before it enters into the thoracic cavity and drains into the right atrium at the inferior cavo-atrial junction.

6.4.1 Ultrasound Assessment of IVC

Ultrasound evaluation of the IVC provides a rapid, noninvasive assessment of a patient's hemodynamic status at the bedside. Structurally, the IVC is a thin-walled, highly compliant vessel and its capacity to distend is not unlimited and is restricted by connective tissue in its walls and surrounding structures. Its size and dynamics vary with respiration and changes in intravascular volume. The size of the IVC and its respiratory variability has been shown to correlate with right atrial pressure (RAP) and intravascular volume. (Table 6.1) These observations are valuable in estimating RAP, detecting changes in intravascular volume, and monitoring a patient's response to volume resuscitation [15]. The development of negative intrathoracic pressure during inspiration increases the venous blood return from the extrathoracic veins into the right heart. This leads to an increase in the blood flow through the IVC and a subsequent decrease in its blood volume, resulting in a reduction in intraluminal pressure. These

Table 6.1 Correlation between size of IVC and estimated central venous pressure (CVP)

Maximum diameter of IVC(cm)	CI (%)	CVP (mmHg)
<1.5	100	0–5
1–5–2.5	>50	6–10
1.5–2.5	<50	11–15
>2.5	<50	16–20
>2.5	0	>20

changes decrease the diameter of the IVC during inspiration relative to expiration. These observations are reversed with positive pressure ventilation in which IVC diameter increases during inspiration. In extremely hypovolemic status, IVC nearly collapses completely with inspiration during spontaneous breathing. Generally, respiratory phasic changes are easily appreciable in relatively hypovolemic status compared to high intravascular volume status.

Traditionally, central venous pressure (CVP) and volume status in the acute care setting have been measured by placing a central line. Central lines are invasive, time-consuming to insert, and may cause significant complications. US of IVC is a relatively inexpensive bedside tool. Clinicians can perform serial IVC measurements on a critically ill patient to guide their decision in providing more intravenous fluids or to administer more aggressive medication therapy [16].

6.4.2 Assessment of IVC with Ultrasound

Various acoustic windows to visualize the IVC and it depends on the clinician's ability to acquire those views. Most commonly subcostal-subxiphoid site is used to view the IVC, especially from intra-hepatic part to IVC—right atrial junction. This view is the part of point-of-care cardiac ultrasound (POCUS) described in detail in trans thoracic echocardiography chapter. Other views to visualize IVC are from transabdominal short axis and right lateral transabdominal coronal long axis commonly referred to as "rescue view." Short-axis view was obtained by placing US in the mid-epigastric region with the orientation marker towards the patient's right. By gently fanning the probe up and down, one can visualize IVC and the aorta anterior to the central shadowing from the vertebral body (Fig. 6.14a, b). By

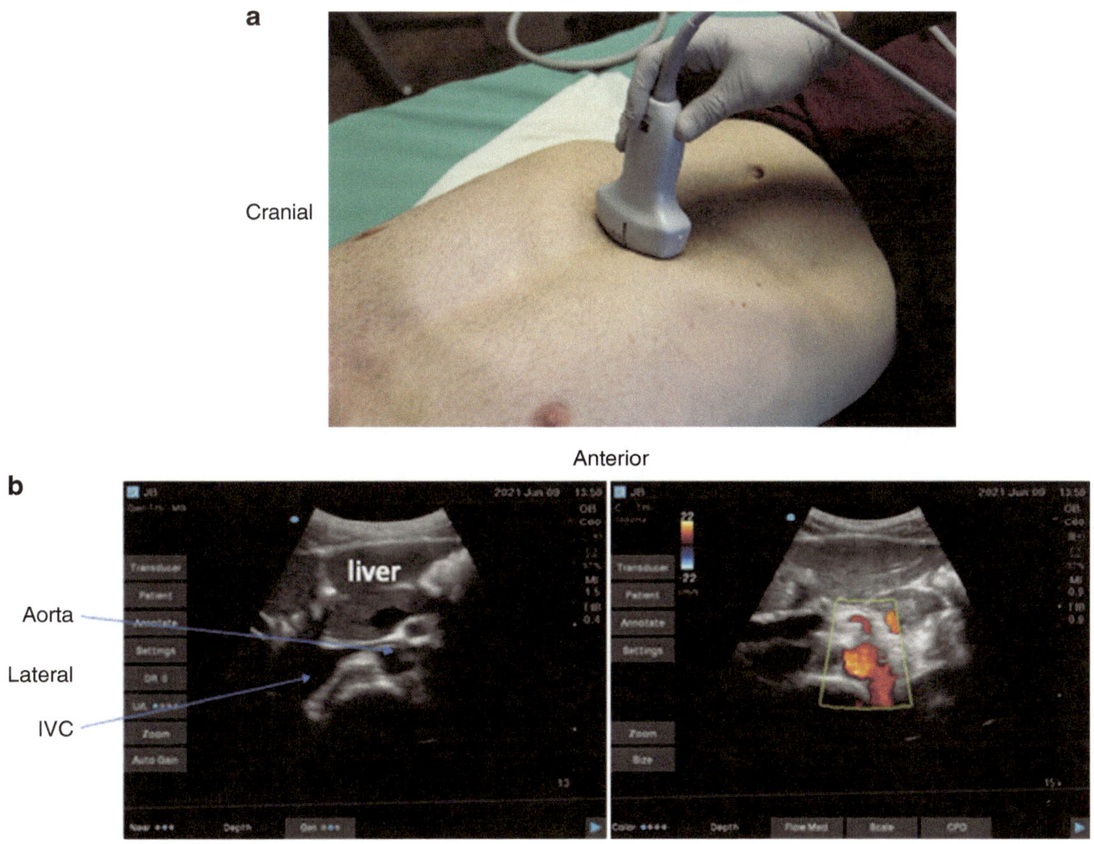

Fig. 6.14 (**a**) Trans abdominal SAX approach for IVC (probe position pointer towards right). (**b**) Trans abdominal SAX approach for IVC

fanning further cranially towards the chest, hepatic veins joining the IVC come into view. Longitudinal view of IVC is typically obtained from subcostal view however in certain clinical situations due to surgical dressings, distended abdomen, etc., longitudinal view of the IVC is acquired through the right lateral transabdominal coronal approach, also known as the "rescue view." The probe is placed in the right anterior to midaxillary line similar to the placement for evaluating pleural effusion with the orientation marker towards cranially (Video 6.3). By scanning more anteriorly, the IVC can be visualized running adjacent to the liver and crossing the diaphragm and joining the right atrium (Fig. 6.15a, b). Aorta is often seen parallel to it and it is essential to differentiate between these two structures by using color flow or spectral Doppler. Pulsatility is not a great way to differentiate between IVC and aorta because IVC frequently demonstrates transmitted pulsations. Moreover, in moderate to severe tricuspid regurgitation, IVC can be very pulsatile mimicking the aorta. Irrespective of the approach, a phased-array (frequency of 2.0–4.0 MHz) or curvilinear probe (frequency of 3.5–5.0 MHz) should be used to visualize IVC. These relatively low-frequency probes provide better penetration and visualization of deep structures. Literature favors B-mode, subxiphoid Lax view as the most reliable means of IVC acquisition. IVC measurement is less reliable in M-mode when compared to B-mode. This discrepancy is augmented when calculating IVC collapsibility index to determine fluid responsiveness [17, 18].

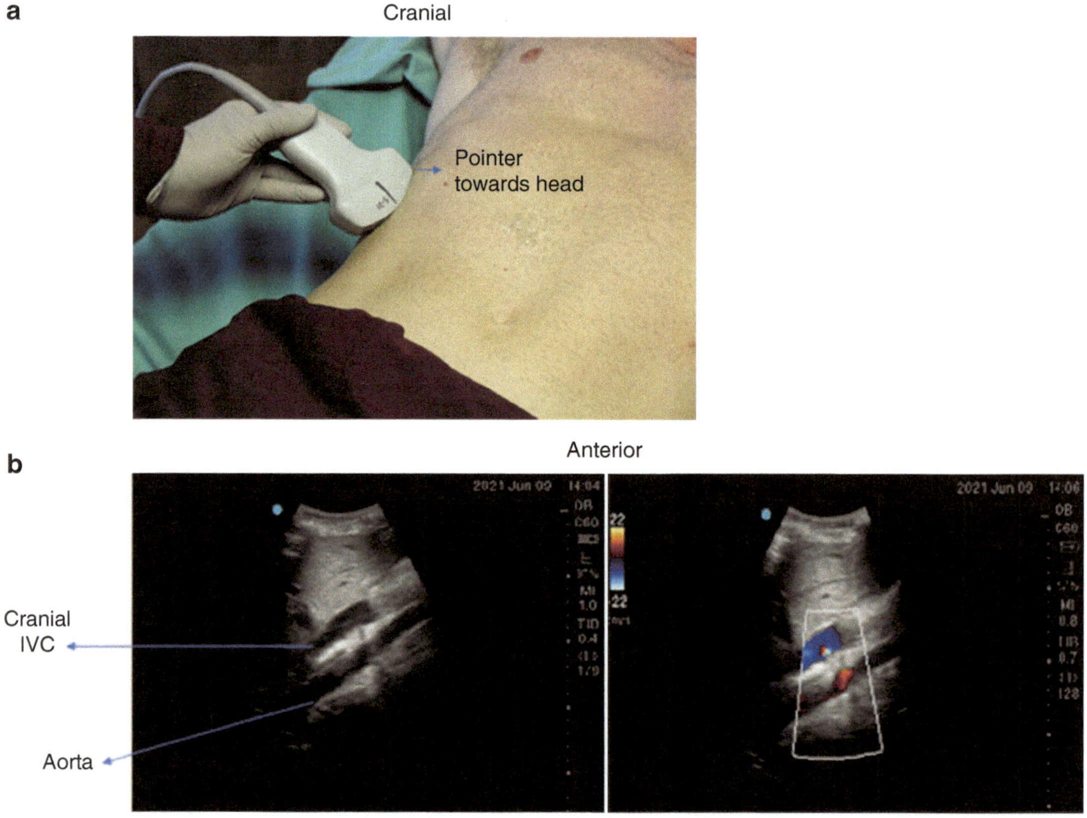

Fig. 6.15 (**a**) Right lateral trans-abdominal coronal approach (rescue view) probe position pointer towards head. (**b**) Right lateral trans-abdominal coronal approach (rescue view) with color flow doppler

6.4.3 Clinical Applications and Limitations of IVC as a Tool for Predicting Fluid Responsiveness

An IVC collapsibility index (IVCCI), which correlates with RAP and CVP, can be calculated with the following formula: (IVCmax − IVCmin)/IVCmax. It is the common measurements use to estimate CVP as well as predict fluid responsiveness in a critically ill patient. Systemic review from 21 studies including over 1400 patients showed a medium to strong correlation between IVC diameter and IVCCI and estimated CVP in spontaneously breathing patients however weak correlation in mechanically ventilated patients, especially with PEEP [19]. Another meta-analysis for caval index with 20 studies showed a wide range of heterogeneity with sensitivity and specificity of 0.71 (95% CI: 0.62–0.80) and 0.75 (95% CI: 0.64–0.85), respectively. Inconsistency results are not in favor of reliable methods in predicting fluid responsiveness [20]. From a single center study in mechanically ventilated patients, Yao et al. proposed IVC ADI (area distensibility index) calculated as: (maximum IVC area − minimum IVC area)/minimum IVC area × 100% and IVC DR(diameter ratio) calculated as: long axis IVC parameter/short axis IVC parameter have more value than IVC diameter distensibility index for predicting fluid responsiveness in mechanically ventilated patients [21]. In spite of various available tools in IVC, one should evaluate ten common pathophysiologic conditions (Table 6.2) that influence measurements [22].

Table 6.2 Factors influencing fluid responsiveness indices

Pathophysiological factor affecting fluid responsiveness	Cause for inaccuracy
Mechanical ventilation with high PEEP and/or low tidal volumes	Larger IVC size due to systemic venous congestion and low respiratory variations
Assisted ventilation modalities, noninvasive ventilation, CPAP	Spontaneous breathing makes IVC variation unpredictable
Spontaneous breathing with varying respiratory pattern	Deep inspiratory effort, producing markedly negative intrathoracic pressures that induce collapsibility even in the absence of FR. On the other hand shallow breathing creates minimal intrathoracic pressure changes, may induce absence of collapsibility even in presence of FR
Acute exacerbation of COPD or asthma	Lung hyperinflation and auto PEEP decrease venous return falsely induces distension of IVC
RV dysfunction	RV dilatation and systemic venous congestion causing large IVC may be associated with FR
Moderate to severe tricuspid regurgitation	Chronic enlargement of IVC and reduced collapsibility may erroneously rule out FR
Cardiac tamponade	Hindrance of venous return influences FR prediction
Increased intra-abdominal pressure	IVC collapses or IVC gets distended depending on the types and mode of ventilation
Local factors	Mass, thrombosis, IVC filters or ECMO cannula might influence size and collapsibility
Anatomical factors	Significant displacement of IVC might cause an error in diameter as well as other indices

6.5 Abdominal Aorta

6.5.1 Anatomy of Abdominal Aorta

The abdominal aorta (AA) is a continuation of the thoracic aorta beginning at the level of the T12 vertebrae. It is approximately 13 cm long and bifurcates into the left and right common iliac arteries at the level of the L4 vertebra. There are many branches that arise from AA (Fig. 6.16) and for US assessment knowing the origin and course of celiac, superior mesenteric, renal, and inferior mesenteric arteries is essential. Celiac artery arises at the level of T12 and supplies the liver, stomach, abdominal esophagus, spleen, the superior duodenum, and the superior pancreas. Superior mesenteric artery arises at T1 just below the celiac artery and supplies the distal duodenum, jejuno-ileum, ascending colon, and part of the transverse colon. Renal arteries are the paired visceral arteries that arise laterally at the level between L1 and L2 and supply the kidneys. Inferior mesenteric artery arises at the level of L3 and supply the large intestine from the splenic flexure to the upper part of the rectum.

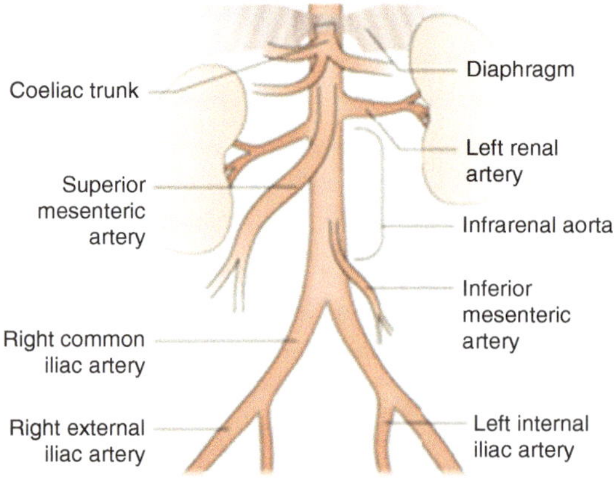

Fig. 6.16 Course and branches of abdominal aorta

6.5.2 Ultrasound Assessment of Abdominal Aorta

Ultrasonography of the AA is primarily performed to detect or exclude an abdominal aortic aneurysm (AAA). By periodic screening, the occurrence of aneurysm rupture can generally be reduced in otherwise symptom-free patients. In addition, US of AA is helpful to detect other aortic diseases/disorders such as stenosis, embolism caused by thrombosis in peripheral occlusion, dissection, and aortitis [23]. Compared with gold standard CT measurement errors and measured value discrepancies occur due to failure to use standardized measurement methods. Multiple sources of error are due to differences in choosing between outer-to-outer (OTO) or inner-to-inner (ITI) diameter, systole or diastole, axial or orthogonal measurement plane [24]. ECG gated measurements are generally advisable to minimize errors.

6.5.3 Ultrasound Technique of Abdominal Aorta

2D ultrasound is generally used to assess the patency and course of AA. Color flow Doppler is required in certain technically challenged

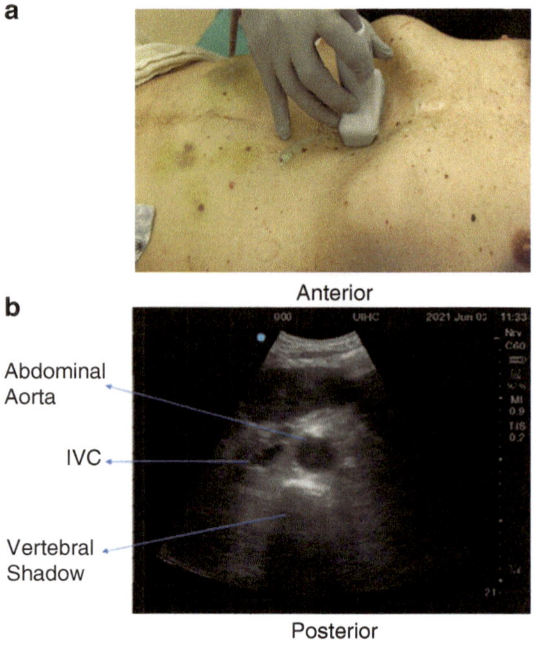

Fig. 6.17 (**a**) US probe position at the sub xiphoid region. (**b**) US at the sub xiphoid region showing abdominal aorta and IVC

patients to differentiate from adjacent great vessels such as IVC. Low frequency (2–5 MHz) with higher penetration is preferred over high-frequency probes. Place the US transducer in the subxiphoid region, apply gentle pressure and adjust the depth to visualize the blood vessels and vertebra. Displacing intra-abdominal air is essential to improve the image quality. Both IVC and aorta are viewed in short axis in front of the vertebra (Video 6.4) (Fig. 6.17a, b). By moving the transducer gradually along the AA towards caudally major branches such as celiac trunk, superior mesenteric, renal arteries, and inferior mesenteric will be visualized (Fig. 6.18). Appropriate angle of incidence is essential to accurately measure the size of AA [25]. Being a relatively less expensive bedside tool, assessing AA with ultrasound is the quickest way prior to extensive evaluation with other imaging modalities such as CT or 3D print.

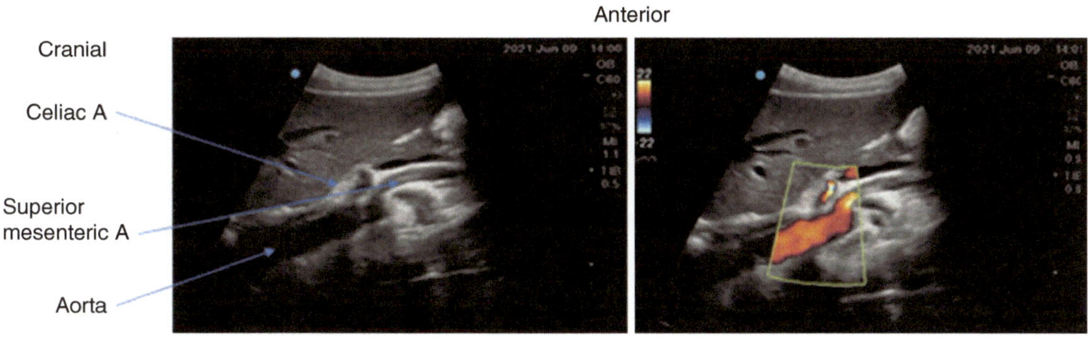

Fig. 6.18 US abdominal aorta shows origin of celiac trunk and superior mesenteric artery with color flow doppler

6.6 Role of Ultrasound in the Deep Vein Thrombosis (DVT)

6.6.1 Anatomy of Upper Limb Veins

The upper extremity venous system comprises superficial and deep veins based on their relations to the deep fascia. The major superficial veins of the upper limb are the cephalic and basilic veins. They are located within the subcutaneous tissue of the upper limb. The basilic vein originates from the dorsal venous network of the hand and ascends to the medial aspect of the upper limb. At the border of the teres major, the vein moves deep into the arm. Here, it combines with the brachial veins from the deep venous system to form the axillary vein. The cephalic vein also arises from the dorsal venous network of the hand. It ascends the anterolateral aspect of the upper limb, passing anteriorly at the elbow. At the shoulder, the cephalic vein travels between the deltoid and pectoralis major muscles and enters the axilla region via the clavipectoral triangle. Within the axilla, the cephalic vein empties into the axillary vein (Fig. 6.19).

6.6.2 Ultrasound Assessment of Upper Limb Veins for DVT

US of upper limb can be performed from proximal to distal or from distal to proximal primarily to assess the patency, anatomical variants, and certain pathological conditions including thrombosis (Fig. 6.20). 2D and color Doppler US are used for the assessment although spectral Doppler might be needed in certain challenging conditions to differentiate between veins and arteries. It is advisable to do a complete evaluation of veins on both arms. In addition to the assessment of IJ and subclavian veins as described in the previous section, the patient's arm should be partially abducted to assess the axillary vein. Axillary vein is generally visualized from infraclavicular portion to axilla, where confluence of cephalic vein into the axillary vein can be observed (Fig. 6.13). On further moving the probe distally on the medial aspect basilic vein along with brachial veins adjacent to brachial artery can be viewed. Compression ultrasonography is recommended to differentiate blood vessels as often noticed vessels are close to each other in this specific part of the arm (Fig. 6.21). On the lateral aspect of the arm, cephalic vein which is generally superficial compared to basilic vein can be visualized. Assessment of veins at the cubital fossa is essential as often noticed thrombophlebitis in this area due to prior cannulation. By moving the probe caudally from the cubital fossa, ulnar and radial veins can be viewed. High-frequency probes are used for UL assessment although low frequency might require in certain obese patients with excess fat tissue in the arm and forearm.

Color Doppler sonography is a rapid, accurate, and noninvasive technique in the evaluation of venous disease in the upper extremity and is

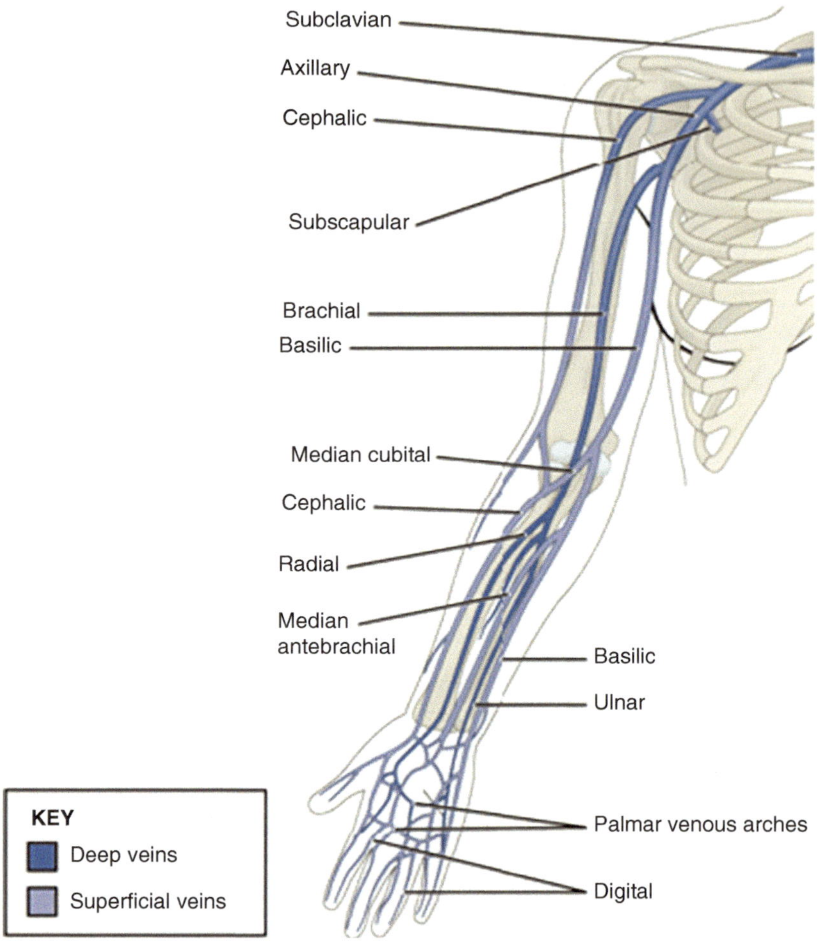

Fig. 6.19 Upper limb venous system

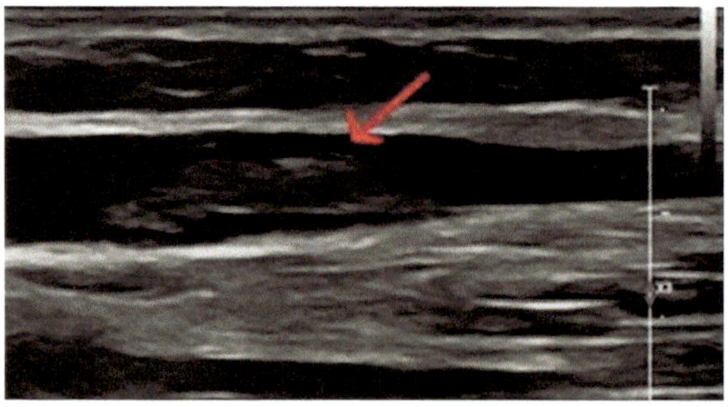

Fig. 6.20 Basilic vein thrombosis

the modality of choice in screening for UEDVT [26]. However, contrast venography, CT, or MRI may be necessary in select cases in which sonographic findings are nondiagnostic or equivocal or when clinical suspicion for UEDVT remains high despite normal Doppler findings.

6.6.3 Anatomy of Lower Limb Vessels

Lower extremity venous system comprises deep veins and superficial veins. The deep veins are located beneath the muscular fascia and drain the surrounding muscles, whereas the superficial veins are above the deep fascia and drain the cutaneous tissues. Both deep and superficial veins have one-way valves inside the vessels that contribute to unidirectional flow from distal to proximal portion of the vein. In order from the groin to the calf, deep veins consist of the common femoral vein (CFV), the deep femoral vein, the femoral vein (FV), the popliteal vein (PV), and three tributaries of the PV (the anterior tibial vein, posterior tibial vein, and peroneal vein)

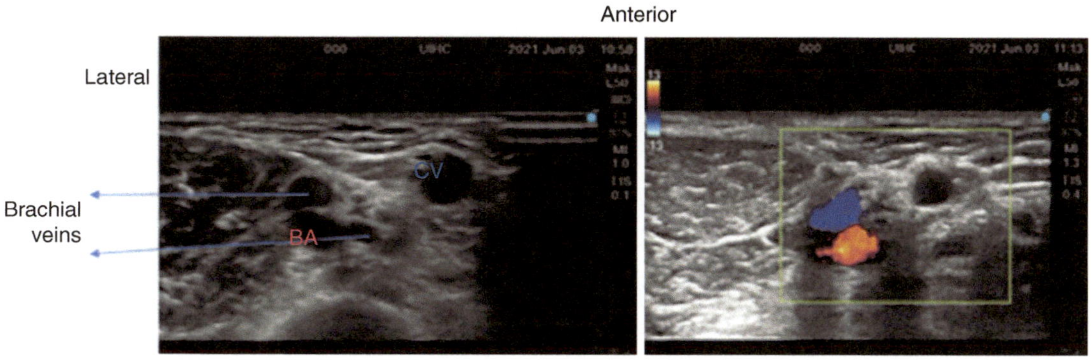

Fig. 6.21 US at the mid arm medial aspect showing brachial vessels and basilic vein. *BA* brachial artery, *CV* Cephalic vein

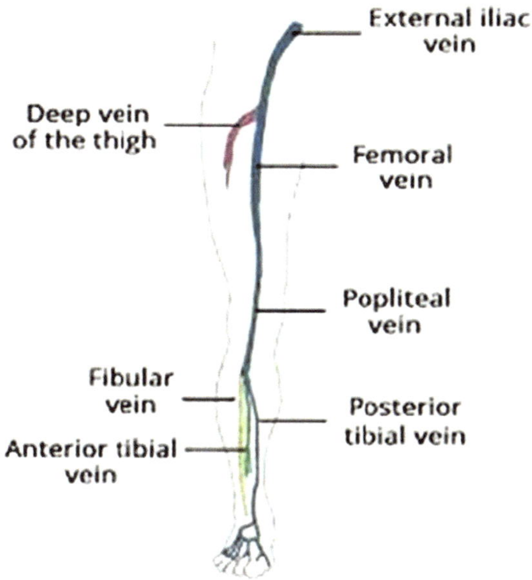

Fig. 6.22 Venous system of lower limb

(Fig. 6.22). These deep veins are generally accompanied by an artery, and the veins are generally larger in diameter than the accompanying artery. The FV was previously named as the superficial femoral vein. However, the term "superficial" has been removed to avoid confusion as the vein is actually a part of a deep venous system. There are numerous anatomical variants in the superficial venous system. Unlike deep veins, superficial veins do not have an accompanying artery. The principal vein of the superficial veins is the great saphenous vein (GSV) that is the longest vein in the human body and joins the CFV at the saphenofemoral junction. Venous duplication of the lower extremities is a common anatomical variant. The prevalence of venous duplication varies depending on the location of the veins. The most common vessels are the FV and the PV, and a retrospective study on the use of ultrasonography for the detection of deep venous thrombosis (DVT) shows a 10.1% prevalence of duplication within the femoral-popliteal venous system [27].

Femoral artery (FA) is the continuation of the external iliac artery, terminal branch of abdominal aorta. The external iliac artery becomes the femoral artery when it crosses the inguinal ligament which is an important anatomical structure to determine cannulation or interventional site for femoral artery (Fig. 6.23). Profunda femoris artery (PFA) is the first branch that arises from FA and there are variants in the origin of PFA. Clinicians should differentiate between PFA from FA before placing catheters.

6.6.4 Ultrasound Evaluation of Femoral Vessels

The ultrasonographic assessment should be performed with the patient in a supine position. The head elevated up to 30 degrees with reverse trendelenburg position is preferable because it can pool the blood in the veins of the lower extremities and help the visualization. External rotation of the examining leg with slight knee flexion is

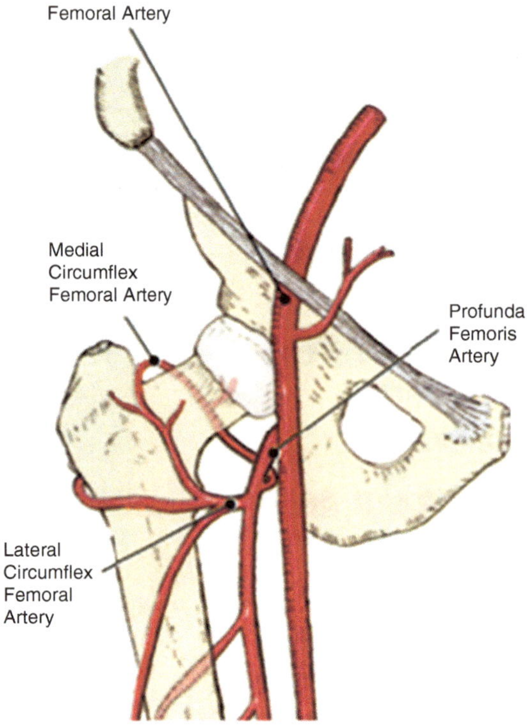

Fig. 6.23 Course of Femoral artery

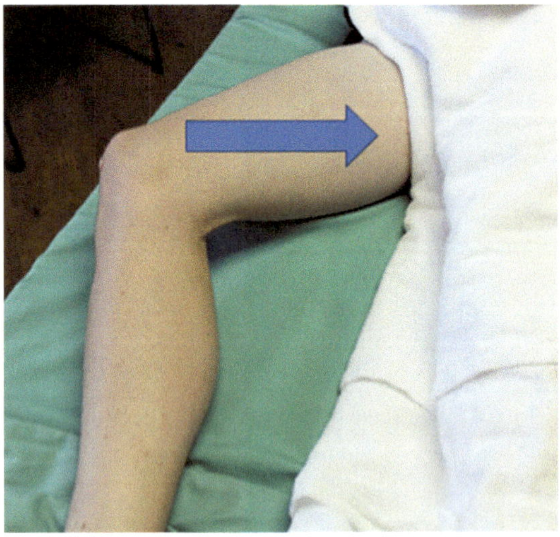

Fig. 6.24 External rotation of the examining leg with slight knee flexion

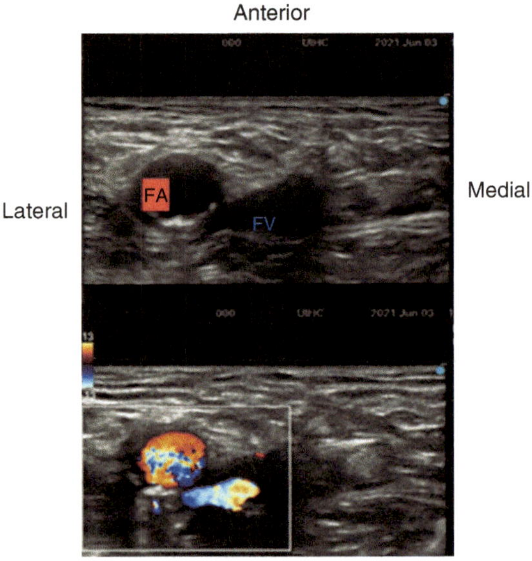

Fig. 6.25 US of femoral vessels with color doppler at the inguinal crease

recommended as it could further enlarge the veins and decrease the depth of the target structures [28]. This position also allows the smooth transition when a sonographer moves the probe from the thigh to the popliteal fossa without repositioning the patient (Fig. 6.24). A linear ultrasound probe with a high-resolution 5–12 MHz is usually chosen to assess the vessels of the lower extremities; however, a lower frequency curved probe may be needed in an obese patient to ensure adequate penetration (Video 6.5).

The CFV is the most proximal vein and to be scanned in the beginning during the sonographic assessment of the lower extremities. By placing the probe along the inguinal ligament between the anterior superior iliac spine and the pubic symphysis, the transverse view of the CFV is obtained. The CFV is medial to the common femoral artery and is usually larger in size (Fig. 6.25). For CVC placement in the FV, the use of US compared with the landmark technique increased the overall success rate (US-89.0% vs landmark 78.9%); and the success rate with the first attempt (85.0% vs 48.7%). Similar to subclavian cannulation there is no strong evidence of routine use of US for FV cannulation; however, authors suggested to utilize US for certain challenging population such as morbid obesity with deeper structures. From the inguinal crease by rotating the probe 90 degrees, the longitudinal view of CFV is visualized. While keeping the CFV centered on the transverse view's image, the probe is moved distally 1–2 cm to reach the saphenofemoral junction where the GSV joins the CFV (Fig. 6.26). By further moving the probe 1–2 cm distally, then the bifurcation of the CFV into the deep femoral vein and FV is observed (Fig. 6.27). The deep femoral vein dives deeper into the thigh after the bifurcation, whereas the FV travels along with the femoral artery through the adductor canal in the distal thigh and emerges as the PV at the popliteal fossa. By placing the probe along the posterior crease of the knee, the transverse view of the PV is visualized. In this view, the PV is posterior to the accompanying artery (the PV is closer to the skin, and the accompanying artery is located deep in the vein) (Fig. 6.28). By further moving the probe distally to the level of the calf, the trifurcation is observed where the PV gives rise to three tributaries (Fig. 6.29).

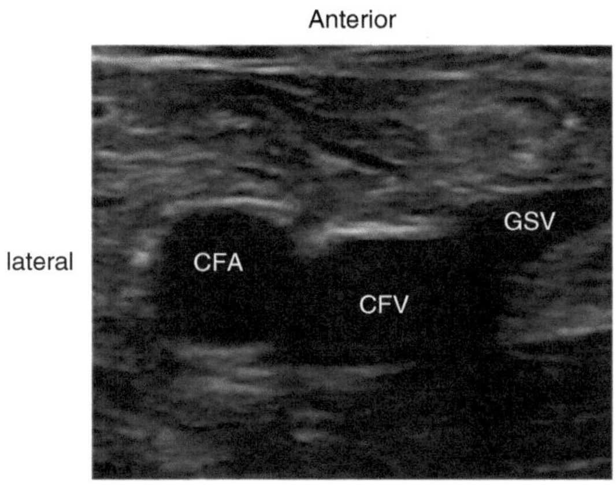

Fig. 6.26 Common femoral vein at the saphenofemoral vein junction

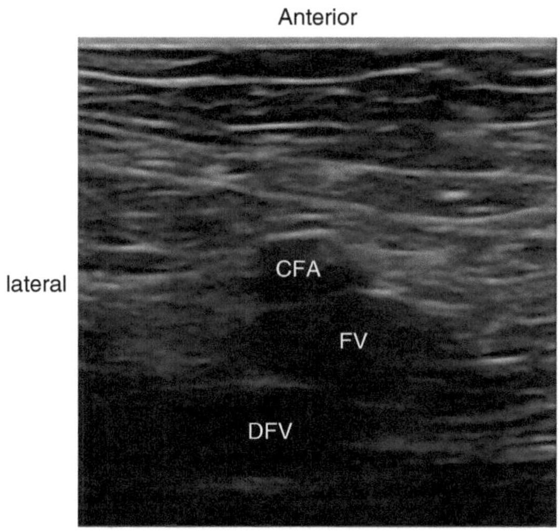

Fig. 6.27 US of common femoral vein (CFV) at its bifurcation into deep femoral vein (DFV) and femoral vein (FV)

6.6.5 Role of Ultrasound in the Evaluation for Deep Vein Thrombosis

Deep vein thrombosis is generally diagnosed by symptoms of swelling and pain of the affected leg

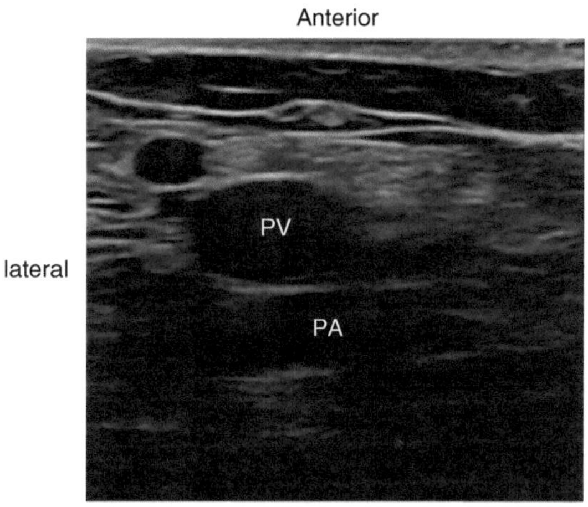

Fig. 6.28 US of the popliteal vein in transverse view. *PA* popliteal artery, *PV* popliteal vein

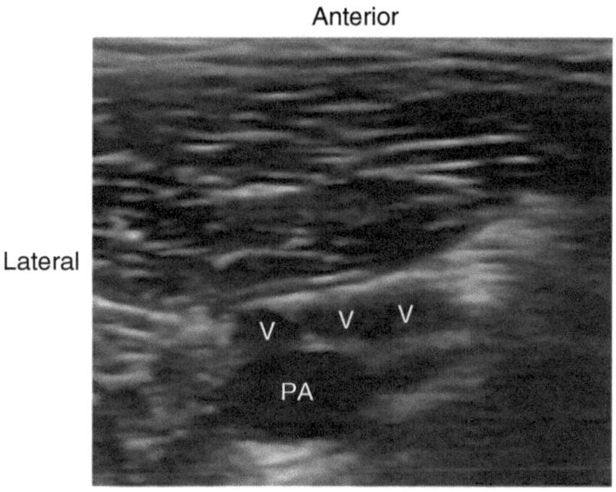

Fig. 6.29 US of poplital vein inthe proximal part of the calf

and tenderness by physical examination. However, individuals with DVT can also be asymptomatic. Nevertheless, unrecognized DVT could cause a life-threatening condition, such as pulmonary embolism; therefore, early detection and treatment are of utmost importance. Ultrasonography is the most appropriate initial diagnostic tool for detecting DVT. Although it requires knowledge of the vascular anatomy and experience with scanning technique, ultrasonography has numerous advantages compared with the other imaging modalities, such as contrast venography, CT, and MRI. These advantages include portability, low cost, noninvasiveness, and avoidance of radiation or nephrotoxic contrast exposure. When DVT is suspected at the lower extremities, the deep venous system should be scanned routinely from the level just above the inguinal ligament to at least the level of the popliteal fossa. There has been a controversy on the role of the routine evaluation of the three tributaries of the PV at the level of the calf because isolated thrombus in the tributaries often spontaneously resolves, and the risk of the antithrombotic therapy may exceed the risk of pulmonary embolism [29]. In addition, evaluating the calf veins increases the complexity and time required to perform ultrasonography. Of note, although the GSV is not a deep vein, investigating thrombus in the proximal GSV adjacent to the saphenofemoral junction is necessary because of the high risk of thrombus dislodgement into the deep venous system and may warrant anticoagulation therapy [30].

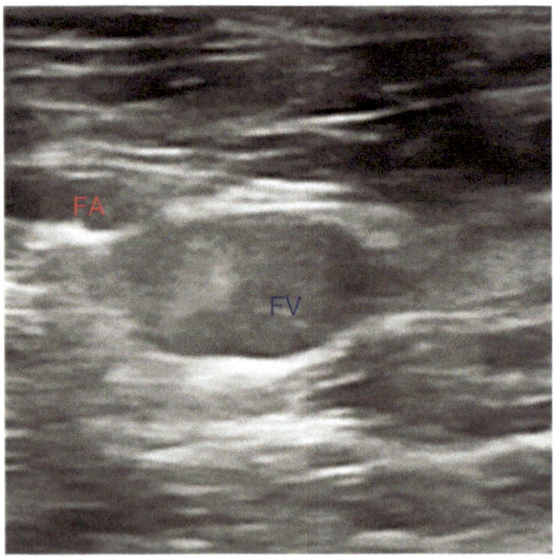

Fig. 6.30 Direct visualization of the DVT hyperechoic material is seen in the common femoral vein

During an ultrasonographic examination, direct visualization of thrombus is a promising way to detect DVT. It can be clearly observed when the thrombus is echogenic (Fig. 6.30). However, the presence of a thrombus is often ambiguous under direct visualization. For example, anechoic or hypoechoic thrombus may not be apparent. In contrast, slowly flowing blood or blood stasis inside a vein mimics the image of a thrombus. Therefore, direct visualization is not sufficient enough to detect or rule out DVT. Applying color flow Doppler ultrasonography aids to identify thrombus as color flow inside the vein is reduced or lost when the vein is partially or completely occluded with thrombus (Fig. 6.31). Furthermore, the compressibility of

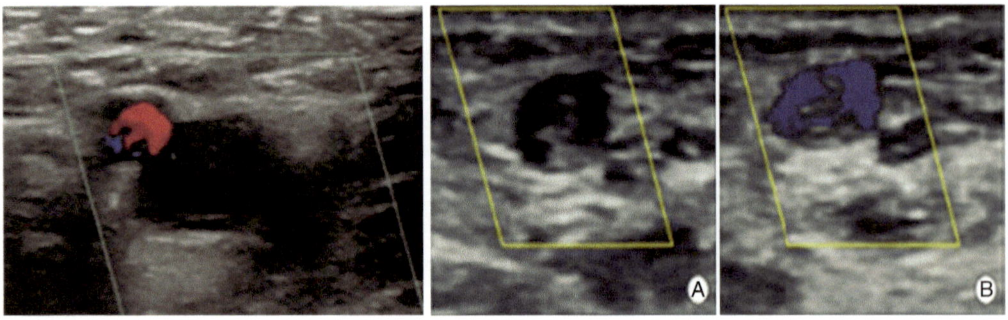

Fig. 6.31 Complete and partial occlusion of femoral vein due to thrombosis

the venous segment should be routinely tested on the target vein as it provides high sensitivity and specificity to diagnose DVT. Inability to compress a vein while applying pressure by the probe is the hallmark finding of thrombus in the venous segment (Fig. 6.32). On the other hand, the complete collapse of a vein rules out thrombus in that region (Fig. 6.33). This compression technique provides only regional information; thus, it may need to apply every 2–3 cm on a targeted vein. Lastly, the patency of a vein can be examined by squeezing the distal part of the vein, often by performing calf compression. Augmented flow during the maneuver is observed by color and pulse Doppler ultrasonography in the normal vein. On the contrary, venous occlusion is likely if there is no increase in the venous flow. Of note, venous compression must be carefully performed as there is a potential risk of dislodging thrombus and causing a catastrophic complication.

6.6.6 Ultrasound Evaluation of Chronic Venous Insufficiency

Clinical symptoms of venous insufficiency are similar to those of DVT. The symptoms include leg pain, swelling, and skin manifestations such as discoloration, induration, and ulceration.

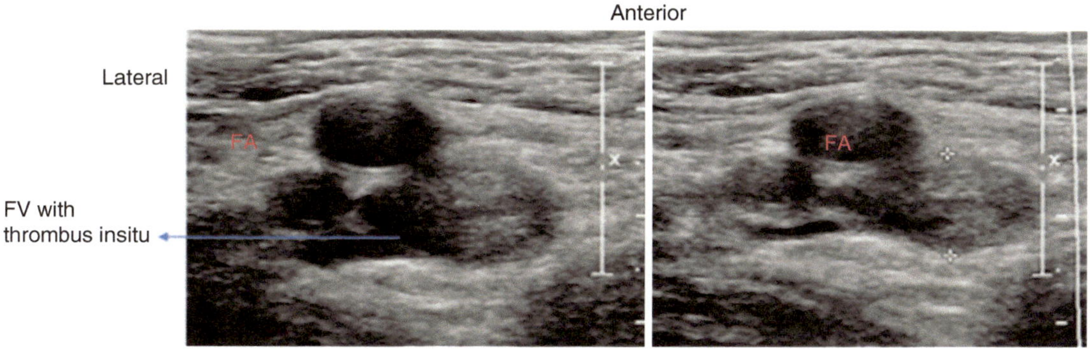

Fig. 6.32 DVT in the common femoral vein noncompressible thrombosed vein in short axis

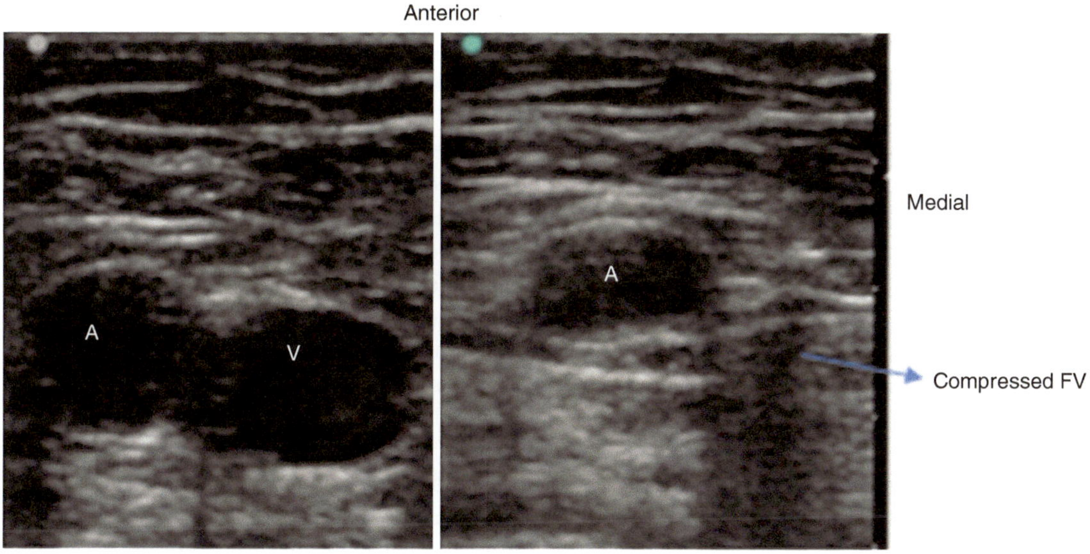

Fig. 6.33 US compression test to exclude deep vein thrombus (DVT)

Although the immediate concern is ruling out acute DVT and its potentially life-threatening condition, venous insufficiency should not be overlooked, especially in patients with persistent or recurrent symptoms. Normally, venous blood flow from a superficial venous system of the lower extremities is directed towards the deep venous system and ultimately moves to the IVC. Reversal of the venous blood flow is prevented by numerous valves in the veins and muscle contraction of the leg. However, when venous valves become incompetent, venous blood flow can be reversed. Venous blood pooling and venous dilation caused by the flow reversal will further accelerate valve failure at the distal portion of the leg. The disease process can be triggered and worsened by existing venous obstruction caused by DVT or congestive heart failure. Unlike a deep venous system, a superficial venous system is not surrounded by muscles; thus, superficial veins are more vulnerable to elevated venous pressure.

Ultrasonographic assessment of venous insufficiency is preferably performed with the patient in the standing position because it induces hemodynamics where venous reflux is significant (Fig. 6.34). Detecting flow reversal with color and pulse Doppler ultrasonography is the most useful method for localizing valvular incompetence and evaluating the severity of the disease (Fig. 6.35). When the venous valve is incompetent, prolonged flow reversal is observed during elevated intra-abdominal pressure by the Valsalva maneuver. This is a reliable technique for the proximal veins; however, venous insufficiency at the distal legs cannot be detected by this method when the valve is competent at the proximal veins. Thus, venous flow augmentation by squeezing the leg is applied when evaluating the venous reflux at the distal legs. Additionally, venous dilation and valvular structure assessed by ultrasonography aid the diagnosis.

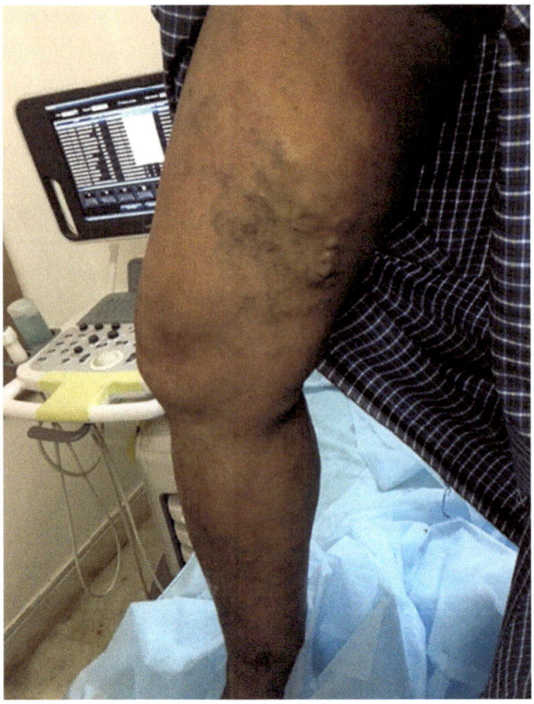

Fig. 6.34 US evaluation of chronic venous insufficiency in standing position

6.6.7 Pitfalls and Artifacts of Using Ultrasound for DVT

Despite the high diagnostic accuracy of ultrasonography, there are a few pitfalls and limitations that one should always keep in mind to avoid misdiagnosis when evaluating patients with suspected DVT. A false-negative result may delay or deprive the patient of appropriate anticoagulation therapy and increase the risk of serious complications such as pulmonary embolism, whereas a false-positive result may put the patient at unnecessary risk of anticoagulation therapy. Firstly, gain and the other imaging parameters must be properly adjusted prior to the examination because improper settings lead to a false interpretation. For example, improperly high gain produces artifactual echo images that can be mistaken for thrombus. Color artifacts generated by improperly high color scales also lead to a false interpretation as it can obscure the image of thrombus. Although testing the venous compressibility is a useful diagnostic method, inadequate venous compression can lead to a false-positive result for DVT. Pressure must be firmly applied to the targeted venous segment until the adjacent artery is slightly compressed. Anatomical variants can also lead to misdiagnosis. Venous duplication is one of the commonest

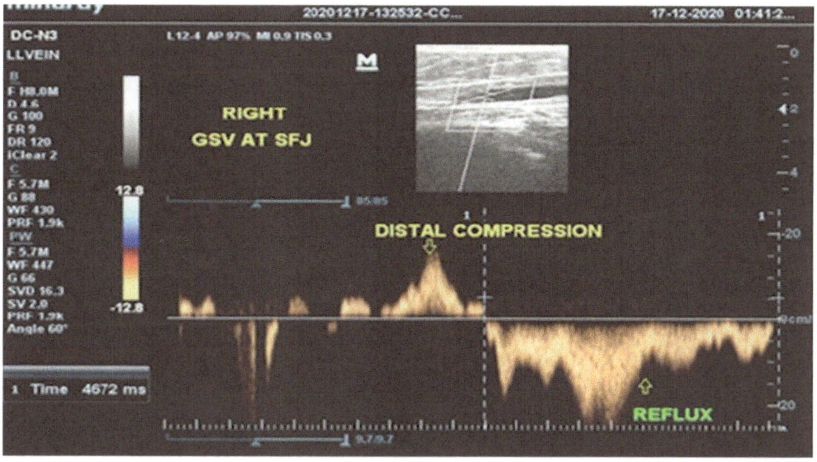

Fig. 6.35 Reflux of blood flow with distal compression in venous insufficiency

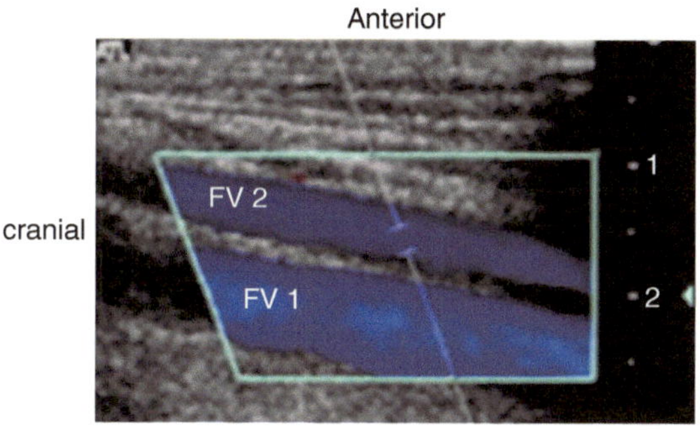

Fig. 6.36 Duplicated femoral vein—Color Doppler ultrasonography in longitudinal view

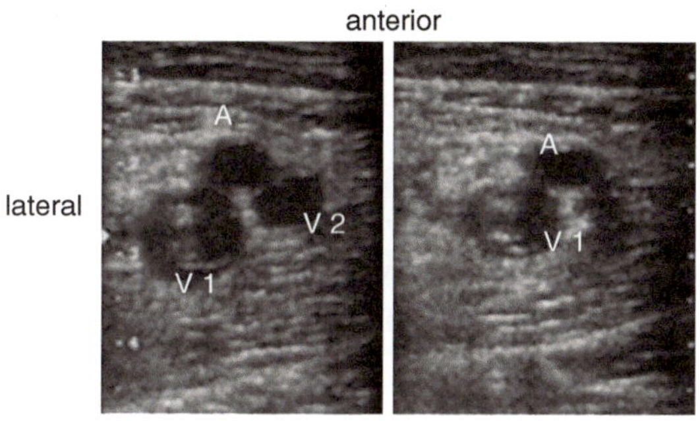

Fig. 6.37 DVT in the duplicated femoral vein noncompressible thrombosed vein (V1) in transverse view

causes of a false-negative result for DVT diagnosis as an occluded duplicated vein can be overlooked (Figs. 6.36 and 6.37) [31]. The femoral-popliteal venous system is a common site of venous duplication, and it should be suspected when a vein is smaller than normal or when the location is unusual. Experience and careful attention to the anatomical variant could prevent the false-negative result. One should be aware that various other abnormalities at the lower extremities can be easily mistaken for DVT because clinical symptoms are similar and many of the images resemble noncompressible vessels. These abnormalities include Baker's cyst (a fluid-filled cyst behind the knee), pseudoaneurysms, hematomas, cellulitis, muscle tears, soft tissue tumors, enlarged lymph nodes, chronic venous insufficiency, and superficial thrombophlebitis. Thrombus in a superficial vein can also be mistaken as DVT, especially in a patient with excess weight or enlarged superficial veins. One of the key things that differentiate DVT from the other abnormalities is identifying the adjacent artery as deep veins are almost always accompanied by an artery. In addition, unlike many other abnormal tissues, veins are often circular in the transverse view and tubular in the longitudinal view. Lastly, the differentiation between acute and chronic DVT by ultrasonography can be challenging, although the differentiation is clinically relevant as the treatment of the two conditions often differs. As thrombus ages, it tends to be more echogenic; however, the age of thrombus cannot be precisely determined by the echogenicity alone as significant variation is observed. Therefore, attention needs to be paid to some other observations that may help in the differentiation. For

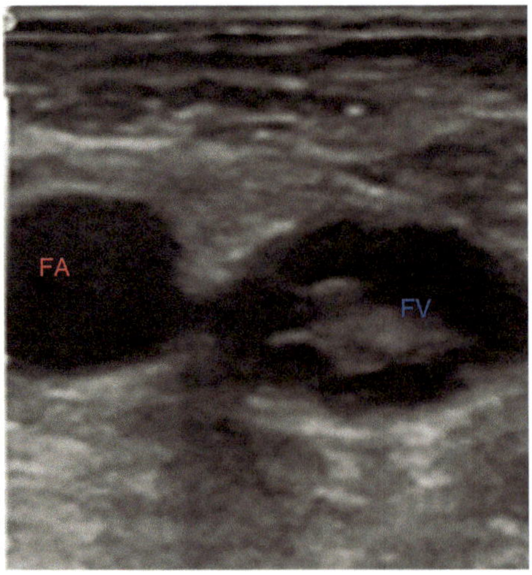

Fig. 6.38 A free-floating thrombus in the common femoral vein in transverse view

example, the size of the affected vein is useful information as acute DVT often dilates the vein, whereas chronic DVT usually diminishes the venous size. Development of the collateral vessels is also an important finding as it is suggestive of chronic DVT. Additionally, a free-floating thrombus (Fig. 6.38) often suggests an acute etiology, and this poses a high risk of pulmonary embolism.

6.6.8 Limitations of Ultrasound for the Diagnosis of DVT

Some of the limitations of ultrasonography for DVT diagnosis are its dependency on the sonographer's skill and its limited visualization of the pelvic veins and calf veins (the tributaries of the PV). The image acquisition is technically more challenging in a patient with excess weight or marked soft tissue edema. A more penetrating, lower frequency probe (less than 5 MHz) may be necessary for some obese patients to visualize the veins in the deep region of the leg, although it reduces the image quality. Another limitation is that ultrasonography is not always feasible to evaluate the entire course of the targeted vein when a patient has an open wound or external orthopedic hardware in the area where the probe needs to be applied on. Further evaluation with alternative imaging modalities such as CT venography and MR venography is necessary when the acquisition of ultrasonographic images is technically challenging or when ultrasonographic results are nondiagnostic or equivocal. However, these alternative modalities are expensive and associated with complications of radiation and contrast exposure.

6.7 Outcome Studies Related to DVT Assessment with Ultrasonography

Over the past decades, many articles were published establishing ultrasonography as the modality of choice for the DVT diagnosis when investigating the patient upon initial presentation. The sensitivity and specificity of ultrasonography for symptomatic DVT are high, reaching 90–99% in many studies [32]. However, one should be aware of the unreliability when evaluating DVT in the pelvic veins and the calf veins because, as described earlier, these veins are less well visualized on ultrasonography. There has been a controversy on performing a limited ultrasonographic examination. Examples of a limited examination include 2-point ultrasonography where compression examination is only applied on the CFV and the PV (Fig. 6.39). A large prospective study shows that 2-point ultrasonography plus D-dimer is equivalent to a

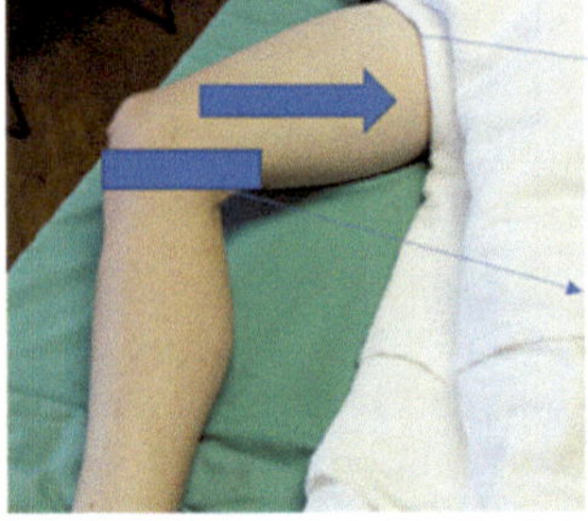

Fig. 6.39 Two point ultrasonography compression examination is applied on the common femoral vein and the popliteal vein

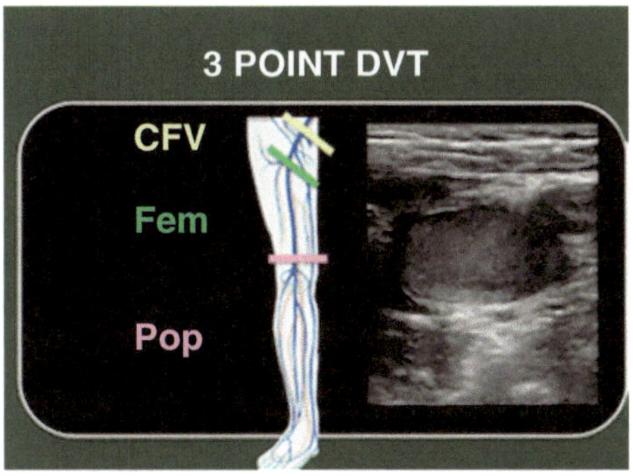

Fig. 6.40 US of deep veins- three point scan

whole-leg/complete ultrasonography for diagnosing suspected symptomatic DVT [33]. Several studies favor the use of 3-point limited ultrasonographic examination by adding the FV to the 2-point limited examination (Fig. 6.40), which may increase the sensitivity for DVT diagnosis [34, 35]. The advantage of limited ultrasonographic examination is a significant reduction of the time required for the examination. In addition, it requires less technical expertise and can be easily performed at the bedside by front-line healthcare professionals with minimum training. On the other hand, whole-leg/complete ultrasonography requires more technical expertise as well as time to perform and is often conducted by an experienced sonographer (often by a vascular technologist) and interpreted by a radiologist. It involves scanning the entire lower extremities, including the calf veins with color Doppler, pulse wave Doppler, and compression examination at every 2 cm interval. Although it is ideal, the complete examination may not be readily performed within a clinically acceptable time frame in many institutions, and it could result in suboptimal patient outcomes as a prompt DVT diagnosis at the bedside may decrease morbidity and mortality. An understanding of lower extremity venous anatomy and its common variations is essential for the performance of duplex ultrasound, interpretation of the images, decision for surgery, and, ultimately, the execution of radiofrequency ablation. In recent years, the nomenclature of the lower extremity venous system has been modified to eliminate confusion.

Questions

1. The most commonly utilized duplex ultrasound feature in the diagnosis of carotid artery stenosis is
   A. End diastolic velocity
   B. Carotid index
   C. Peak systolic velocity
   D. Continuous wave Doppler
2. The role of ultrasound in the assessment of internal jugular vein includes all except
   A. Assessing patency of IJV
   B. To determine its relationship with carotid artery
   C. To identify vagus nerve
   D. To estimate central venous pressure based on change in the cross-sectional area
3. The following is true based on the ultrasound image

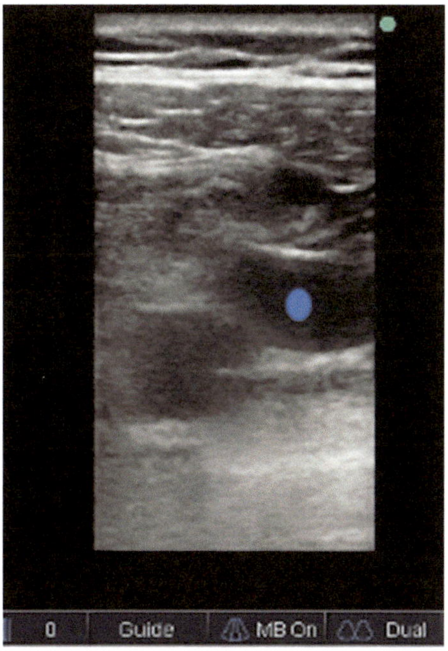

   A. It denotes ultrasound assessment of right IJV and carotid artery
   B. The highlighted structure represents left common carotid artery
   C. The highlighted structure represents right subclavian vein
   D. It denotes supraclavicular approach of subclavian vessels

4. The probe position indicates following assessment and view

Cranial

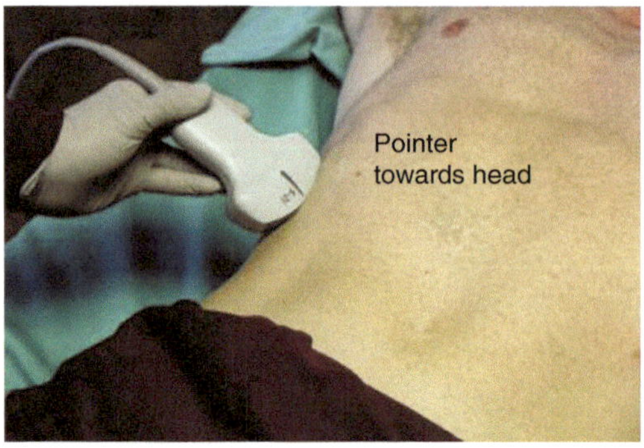

   A. Abdominal aorta in short axis
   B. IVC in short axis
   C. Superior mesenteric artery in long axis
   D. IVC in long axis as rescue view
5. All are true in the utilization of IVC as tool to predict fluid responsiveness except
   A. Strong correlation between IVC diameter and collapsibility index in spontaneously breathing patients
   B. RV dysfunction influences the diameter of IVC by causing large IVC
   C. Significant displacement of IVC due to various abdominal factors will cause an error in the diameter of IVC
   D. Caval index shows consistent results from multiple studies
6. The following branches of aorta are visualized relatively easy with ultrasonography except
   A. Superior mesenteric artery
   B. Gastric artery
   C. Celiac artery
   D. Inferior mesenteric artery
7. The following is true in relation to the given ultrasound image

Anterior

Lateral

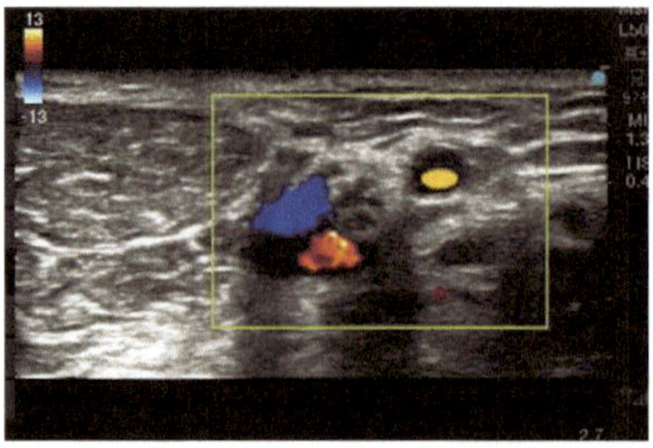

   A. It denotes ultrasound assessment of upper limb veins at the mid-forearm level
   B. Highlighted structure in the yellow indicates brachial vein
   C. Highlighted structure in the yellow indicates cephalic vein
   D. Highlighted structure in the yellow indicates basilic vein
8. With inspiration in spontaneously breathing, which of the following is true?
   A. Abdominal pressure decreases and intrathoracic pressure increases
   B. Abdominal pressure increases and intrathoracic pressure decreases
   C. Abdominal pressure increases and intrathoracic pressure increases
   D. Abdominal pressure decreases and intrathoracic pressure decreases
9. Which of the following would not increase doppler velocities within a vessel?
   A. Enlarged segment of the vessel at the level of the carotid bulb
   B. Narrowing of a normal stented internal carotid artery
   C. Intraluminal 50–69% diameter stenosis within the internal carotid artery
   D. Intraluminal 70–99% diameter stenosis within the internal carotid artery
10. The ultrasound image represents following view

Anterior

Lateral

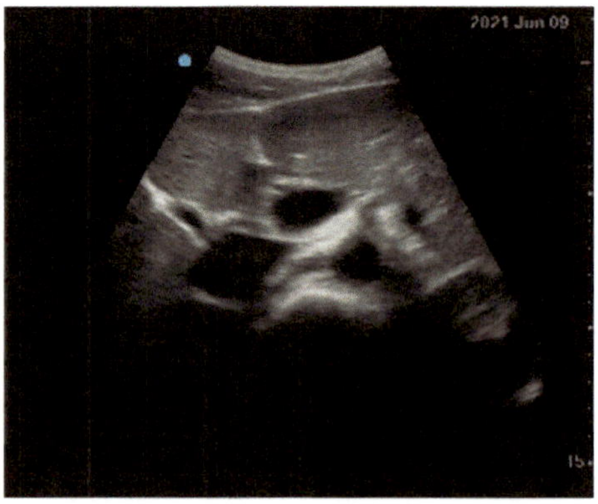

   A. Subxiphoid view for IVC assessment
   B. Transabdominal longitudinal view for IVC
   C. Transabdominal short-axis view of IVC and aorta
   D. Transabdominal longitudinal view of hepatic vein

11. The deep venous system of the lower extremity consists of the following veins except
    A. Common femoral vein
    B. Great saphenous vein
    C. Deep femoral vein
    D. Femoral vein
    E. Popliteal vein
12. The following veins are generally accompanied by an artery except
    A. Common femoral vein
    B. Great saphenous vein
    C. Deep femoral vein
    D. Femoral vein
    E. Popliteal vein
13. When evaluating the deep veins of the lower extremity, the better image quality of ultrasonography can be achieved by
    A. The head elevated at 30 degrees in a reverse Trendelenburg position
    B. External rotation of the examining leg with slight knee flexion
    C. A linear ultrasound probe with a high-resolution 5–12 MHz
    D. All of the above
14. The ultrasonographic findings of thrombus in the venous segment include
    A. Inability to compress the vein while applying pressure by the probe
    B. Complete collapse of the vein while applying pressure by the probe
    C. Augmented venous flow by squeezing the distal part of the vein
    D. None of the above
    E. All of the above
15. All of the following statements are true expect
    A. Clinical symptoms of venous insufficiency are similar to those of DVT
    B. Venous insufficiency can be triggered and worsened by existing venous obstruction caused by DVT or congestive heart failure
    C. Venous blood flow from a superficial venous system is normally directed towards the deep venous system
    D. The deep veins are more vulnerable to the elevated venous pressure compared with the superficial veins
16. All the following potentially leads to false-positive or false-negative results for DVT except
    A. Improperly high gain setting
    B. Color artifact generated by improper high color scale
    C. Inadequate venous compression while testing the venous compressibility
    D. None of the above
    E. All of the above
17. Clinical symptoms and/or ultrasonographic images of DVT can be similar to those of
    A. Baker's cyst
    B. Cellulitis
    C. Enlarged lymph node
    D. Superficial thrombophlebitis
    E. All of the above
18. All of the following statements are true except
    A. Most of the deep veins are accompanied by an artery
    B. The age of thrombus can be easily determined by the echogenicity alone
    C. A free-floating thrombus poses a high risk of pulmonary embolism
    D. Acute DVT often dilates the affected vein
    E. Chronic DVT usually diminishes the venous size
19. The limitations of ultrasonography for DVT diagnosis include
    A. Dependency on the sonographies' skill
    B. Limited visualization of the pelvic veins and calf veins
    C. Technical difficulties in a patient with excess weight or marked soft tissue edema
    D. None of the above
    E. All of the above
20. Compared with whole-leg/complete ultrasonography, a limited ultrasonographic examination requires
    A. More time
    B. More technical expertise
    C. Scanning the popliteal vein and its tributaries
    D. None of the above
    E. All of the above

References

1. Choi IS. Functional vascular anatomy of the head and neck. Interv Neuroradiol. 2003;9(Suppl 2):29–30.
2. Devadas D, Pillay M, Sukumaran TT. A cadaveric study on variations in branching pattern of external carotid artery. Anat Cell Biol. 2018;51(4):225–31.
3. Johri AM, Nambi V, Naqvi TZ, Feinstein SB, Kim ESH, Park MM, et al. Recommendations for the Assessment of Carotid Arterial Plaque by Ultrasound for the Characterization of Atherosclerosis and Evaluation of Cardiovascular Risk: From the American Society of Echocardiography. J Am Soc Echocardiogr. 2020;33(8):917–33.
4. Lee W. General principles of carotid Doppler ultrasonography. Ultrasonography. 2014;33(1):11–7.
5. Jahromi AS, Cinà CS, Liu Y, Clase CM. Sensitivity and specificity of color duplex ultrasound measurement in the estimation of internal carotid artery stenosis: a systematic review and meta-analysis. J Vasc Surg. 2005;41(6):962–72.
6. Sisini F, Toro E, Gambaccini M, Zamboni P. The oscillating component of the internal jugular vein flow: the overlooked element of cerebral circulation. Behav Neurol. 2015;2015:170756.
7. Constant J. Using internal jugular pulsations as a manometer for right atrial pressure measurements. Cardiology. 2000;93(1–2):26–30.
8. Ma GG, Hao GW, Yang XM, Zhu DM, Liu L, Liu H, Tu GW, Luo Z. Internal jugular vein variability predicts fluid responsiveness in cardiac surgical patients with mechanical ventilation. Ann Intensive Care. 2018;8(1):6.
9. Chung CP, Chao AC, Hsu HY, Lin SJ, Hu HH. Decreased jugular venous distensibility in migraine. Ultrasound Med Biol. 2010;36(1):11–6.
10. Chi HY, Lin CS, Hsu MH, Chan PC, Hu HH. Chronic influences of obstructive sleep apnea on cerebral venous flow. J Ultrasound Med. 2015;34(11):2043–8.
11. Liu M, Xu H, Wang Y, Zhong Y, Xia S, Utriainen D, Wang T, Haacke EM. Patterns of chronic venous insufficiency in the dural sinuses and extracranial draining veins and their relationship with white matter hyperintensities for patients with Parkinson's disease. J Vasc Surg. 2015;61(6):1511–20.
12. Zivadinov R, Ramanathan M, Dolic K, Marr K, Karmon Y, Siddiqui AH, Benedict RH, Weinstock-Guttman B. Chronic cerebrospinal venous insufficiency in multiple sclerosis: diagnostic, pathogenetic, clinical and treatment perspectives. Expert Rev Neurother. 2011;11(9):1277–94.
13. Brass P, Hellmich M, Kolodziej L, Schick G, Smith AF. Ultrasound guidance versus anatomical landmarks for subclavian or femoral vein catheterization. Cochrane Database Syst Rev. 2015;1:Cd011447.
14. Lalu MM, Fayad A, Ahmed O, Bryson GL, Fergusson DA, Barron CC, Sullivan P, Thompson C. Ultrasound-guided subclavian vein catheterization: a systematic review and meta-analysis. Crit Care Med. 2015;43:1498–507.
15. Moreno FL, Hagan AD, Holmen JR, et al. Evaluation of size and dynamics of the inferior vena cava as an index of right-sided cardiac function. Am J Cardiol. 1984;53(4):579–85.
16. Feissel M, Michard F, Faller JP, et al. The respiratory variation in inferior vena cava diameter as a guide to fluid therapy. Intensive Care Med. 2004;30(9):1834–7.
17. Finnerty NM, Panchal AR, Boulger C, et al. Inferior vena cava measurement with ultrasound: what is the best view and best mode? West J Emerg Med. 2017;18(3):496–501.
18. Lang RM, Badano LP, Mor-Avi V, Afilalo J, Armstrong A, Ernande L, Flachskampf FA, Foster E, Goldstein SA, Kuznetsova T, Lancellotti P, Muraru D, Picard MH, Rietzschel ER, Rudski L, Spencer KT, Tsang W, Voigt JU. Recommendations for cardiac chamber quantification by echocardiography in adults: an update from the American Society of Echocardiography and the European Association of Cardiovascular Imaging. J Am Soc Echocardiogr. 2015;28(1):1–39.
19. Ciozda W, Kedan I, Kehl DW, Zimmer R, Khandwalla R, Kimchi A. The efficacy of sonographic measurement of inferior vena cava diameter as an estimate of central venous pressure. Cardiovasc Ultrasound. 2016;14(1):33.
20. Orso D, Paoli I, Piani T, Cilenti FL, Cristiani L, Guglielmo N. Accuracy of ultrasonographic measurements of inferior vena cava to determine fluid responsiveness: a systematic review and meta-analysis. J Intensive Care Med. 2020;35(4):354–63.
21. Yao B, Liu J-y, Sun Y-b, Zhao Y-x, Li L. The value of the inferior vena cava area distensibility index and its diameter ratio for predicting fluid responsiveness in mechanically ventilated patients. Shock. 2019;52:37–42.
22. Via G, Tavazzi G, Ten Price S. situations where inferior vena cava ultrasound may fail to accurately predict fluid responsiveness: a physiologically based point of view. Intensive Care Med. 2016;42:1164–7.
23. Schäberle W. Ultrasonography in vascular diagnosis. 2nd ed. Heidelberg: Springer; 2011. p. 18, 400–403, 441
24. Chiu KW, Ling L, Tripathi V, Ahmed M, Shrivastava V. Ultrasound measurement for abdominal aortic aneurysm screening: a direct comparison of the three leading methods. Eur J Vasc Endovasc Surg. 2014;47(4):367–73.
25. Schäberle W, Leyerer L, Schierling W, Pfister K. Ultrasound diagnostics of the abdominal aorta: English version. Gefasschirurgie. 2015;20(Suppl 1):22–7.
26. Joffe HV, Goldhaber SZ. Upper-extremity deep vein thrombosis. Circulation. 2002;106:1874–80.
27. Simpson WL, Krakowsi DM. Prevalence of lower extremity venous duplication. Indian J Radiol Imaging. 2010;20(3):230–4.

28. Read H, Holdgate A, Watkins S. Simple external rotation of the leg increases the size and accessibility of the femoral vein. Emerg Med Australas. 2012;24(4):408–13.
29. Robert-Ebadi H, Righini M. Should we diagnose and treat distal deep vein thrombosis? Hematology Am Soc Hematol Educ Program. 2017;2017(1):231–6.
30. Scott G, Mahdi AJ, Alikhan R. Superficial vein thrombosis: a current approach to management. Br J Haematol. 2015;168(5):639–45.
31. Screaton NJ, Gillard JH, Berman LH, Kemp PM. Duplicated superficial femoral veins: a source of error in the sonographic investigation of deep vein thrombosis. Radiology. 1998;206(2):397–401.
32. Bhatt M, Braun C, Patel P, Patel P, Begum H, Wiercioch W, et al. Diagnosis of deep vein thrombosis of the lower extremity: a systematic review and meta-analysis of test accuracy. Blood Adv. 2020;4(7):1250–64.
33. Bernardi E, Camporese G, Buller HR, Siragusa S, Imberti D, Berchio A, et al. Serial 2-point ultrasonography plus D-dimer vs whole-leg color-coded Doppler ultrasonography for diagnosing suspected symptomatic deep vein thrombosis: a randomized controlled trial. JAMA. 2008;300(14):1653–9.
34. Zuker-Herman R, Ayalon Dangur I, Berant R, Sitt EC, Baskin L, Shaya Y, et al. Comparison between two-point and three-point compression ultrasound for the diagnosis of deep vein thrombosis. J Thromb Thrombolysis. 2018;45(1):99–105.
35. Pedraza Garcia J, Valle Alonso J, Ceballos Garcia P, Rico Rodriguez F, Aguayo Lopez MA, Munoz-Villanueva MDC. Comparison of the accuracy of emergency department-performed point-of-care-ultrasound (POCUS) in the diagnosis of lower-extremity deep vein thrombosis. J Emerg Med. 2018;54(5):656–64.

Focused Assessment with Sonography in Trauma (FAST) Exam

7

Vishakha Prasad Erasu and Priyadarshini Marathe

7.1 Definition

The Focused Assessment with Sonography in Trauma (FAST) exam is a point of care Ultrasound exam to assess the presence of pathological fluid within the intraperitoneal, intrathoracic, and pericardial spaces in patients presenting with blunt or penetrating trauma to the torso region.

7.2 Introduction/Background

7.2.1 History of the FAST Exam

The term FAST representing "focused assessment by sonographic examination of the trauma patient" was first used towards the end of the twentieth century to describe the use of ultrasound in abdominal trauma. In 1996 Rozycki described the FAST exam consisting of three views of the abdomen to rule out bleeding in abdominal trauma [1]. The widely used "focused assessment with sonography in trauma" or FAST scan as it has come to be known today was developed based on this and has four views of the torso. Studies that looked at the impact of focused ultrasound in trauma patients showed a decrease in the delay times from admission to operating theatre [2, 3] and a benefit in performing the FAST exam in hypotensive patients with blunt truncal trauma [4]. The newer protocol of e-FAST exam or Extended Focused Assessment with Sonography in Trauma was proposed by Kirkpatrick et al. in a paper in the Journal of Trauma in 2004 [5]. The extended FAST exam includes two additional views of the anterior most areas of the chest to look for the presence of a pneumothorax. As it gained popularity, the FAST exam has been compared to the diagnostic peritoneal lavage (DPL) and the CT scan performed on the trauma patient (Table 7.1) [6, 7]. The FAST exam has been recommended in the assessment of trauma patients as part of the Advanced Trauma Life Support (ATLS) training since 1997 [8]. It has become part of the management of trauma patients in most trauma centers in many parts of the world.

7.2.2 Anatomy and Physiology of Fluid Collection in Body Cavities

In the trauma patient with internal bleeding, blood (as does fluid) tends to collect in the dependent regions based on the position of the patient

V. P. Erasu (✉)
Oxford University Hospitals NHS Foundation Trust, Oxford, UK

Emergency Medicine Research in Oxford, Oxford, UK
e-mail: Vishakha.Prasad@ouh.nhs.uk

P. Marathe
Oxford University Hospitals NHS Foundation Trust, Oxford, UK
https://www.linkedin.com/in/dr-priyadarshini-marathe-56519677/

A. Chakraborty, B. Ashokka (eds.), *A Practical Guide to Point of Care Ultrasound (POCUS)*,
https://doi.org/10.1007/978-981-16-7687-1_7

Table 7.1 Comparison of DPL vs. FAST exam vs. CT scan. This table compares the salient features of the FAST exam, DPL, and CT scan in the trauma patient

Feature	DPL	FAST exam	CT scan
Bedside test	Yes	Yes	No
Needs transport	No	No	Yes
Ease of performing test in an unstable patient	Can be done	Can be done	Not without risk of transfer and time
Performed simultaneously with clinical assessment	Yes	Yes	No
Invasive procedure	Yes	No	No
Radiation exposure	No	No	Yes
Ease of a repeat test	Cumbersome	Easily done	Increases radiation risk
Operator dependent	Yes	Yes	No
Affected by previous surgery	Yes (if altered anatomy like adhesions, etc.)	Yes (if altered anatomy)	No
Time to perform test	Time to instill lavage fluid and aspirate—Average of 10–15 min	Few minutes	10–15 min excluding transfer times
Cost of test	Low	Low	Higher

and the site of bleeding. As these patients are usually positioned supine, the dependent regions become the hepatorenal recess, splenorenal recess, and pelvis within the peritoneal cavity. In the pleural cavity, the fluid settles posteriorly and inferiorly within each pleural space. If the patient assumes a sitting posture, free fluid would collect in the pelvis as this would become the most dependent area of the peritoneal cavity. The FAST exam takes advantage of this phenomenon to rapidly detect fluid (i.e., blood, urine, or faecal matter) in these dependent spaces by only focusing on these regions. The FAST exam can detect a minimum of 200–250 mls of fluid in the peritoneal cavity.

The hepatorenal recess is the potential space in the right upper quadrant of the peritoneal cavity. It lies between the liver and the right kidney and in physiological conditions appears as a hyperechoic line on ultrasound where the fascial layers adjoin each other. The splenorenal recess is the potential space in the left upper quadrant of the peritoneal cavity and lies between the spleen and the left kidney. In physiological situations when there is no fluid or blood in this space, it appears as a hyperechoic line on ultrasound representing the adjoining fascia of the spleen and left kidney. The anatomy of the pelvis varies in male and female patient. In the female patient, the bladder lies anterior to the uterus, with the rectum lying most posteriorly. The vescicovaginal or Douglas pouch is the dependent region formed between the fascia overlying the bladder and uterus. In the male patient, the rectovescical pouch is the space between the bladder and rectum. The vescicovaginal and rectovescical pouches, form the most dependent pockets for fluid collection in the female and male pelvis, respectively.

The site of injury and hence the location of the bleeding point influences the collection of blood in the dependent regions of the peritoneal cavity. Injury in the right upper quadrant will cause blood to collect in Morrison's pouch and then flow into the subdiaphragmatic and pelvic spaces. The left upper quadrant differs from the right upper quadrant as blood tends to collect in the subdiaphragmatic space more often than in the splenorenal space. Injury to the pelvic region will cause blood to collect in the pelvis but large pelvic bleeds can cause blood to flow into the Morrison's pouch as well.

In the pleural cavity, fluid or blood in the supine patient tends to collect in the dependent regions. In each hemithorax fluid will collect in the posterior and inferior parts with the lung floating in the free fluid. Air does the opposite by rising to occupy the nondependent regions and will collect above the respective lung. In the upright patient, this will be the upper part of the hemithorax while in the supine patient this will correspond to the anterior most part of the hemithorax.

The pericardial space lies within the two layers of the pericardium, creating a potential space for fluid to collect around the heart. This potential space has a much smaller capacity than the pleural and peritoneal cavities and fluid here tends to surround the heart forming a thin film and then expanding as more fluid collects.

7.2.3 Diagnostic Peritoneal Lavage

Diagnostic Peritoneal Lavage (DPL) in trauma patients was first described by Root in 1965 [9] but over the years has been replaced by the FAST exam and CT scan. This procedure consists of an initial diagnostic tap which consists of aspirating for fluid from the abdominal cavity to confirm the presence of blood. The lavage can be performed as the second step and is very sensitive in detecting blood in the peritoneal cavity. The diagnostic peritoneal lavage test is considered positive when blood is aspirated from the peritoneal cavity on direct tap or lavage. Detailed explanation of DPL is out of scope of this chapter.

7.2.4 CT Scan in the Trauma Patient

The diagnostic imaging of choice in the trauma patient depends on the findings of the ATLS primary survey in addition to the mechanism of injury and patient characteristics. When assessing the patient with blunt or penetrating trauma to the torso region, a CT scan is the imaging of choice which may be done as part of a pan scan (consisting of CT scans of the head, cervical spine, and torso) or regional scan of the chest, abdomen, and pelvis independently [10, 11].

7.3 Focused Question in FAST Exam

The objective of the FAST exam is to answer the question—"is there fluid?" within the pericardial, pleural, and peritoneal spaces by obtaining the right upper quadrant, left upper quadrant, pelvic and subcostal views using a low-frequency probe.

FAST scan pearls
1. ONE Question—Is there free fluid?
2. TWO Possible answers—Yes or no (if unclear view then cannot determine)
3. THREE Body cavities—Pericardium, peritoneum and pleural
4. FOUR Views—RUQ, LUQ, pelvic, and subcostal
5. FIVE MHz or less- frequency of probe

7.4 Indications of FAST Exam

The indications for the FAST exam in the trauma patient are:

- Blunt or penetrating trauma to the chest.
- Blunt or penetrating trauma to the abdomen/pelvis.
- Any unexplained shock—to look for a possible cause.

The FAST exam can be used outside the context of trauma and in unstable patients without a clear history of trauma to assess for the presence of fluid in the body cavities. In this case, the scan is called a FAFF (focussed assessment for free fluid) scan.

7.5 Contraindications

A FAST exam should never delay or hinder the resuscitation of the trauma patient. This is the only situation-based contraindication for a FAST exam and there are no other absolute contraindications to performing a FAST exam.

7.6 Preparation

The FAST exam is performed as an adjunct of the primary survey in trauma patients. The general recommendation is to position the ultrasound machine to the right side of the patient if the operator is right-handed and to the left side if the operator is left-handed. This allows the dominant hand to be used for scanning and the nondominant hand to manage the controls on the machine. It is recommended to use necessary personal protective equipment and probe or device covers for infection control as per local policy. Ideally, sterile gel sachets should be used for each scan to reduce the risk of contamination.

7.7 Position of Patient

The trauma patient is usually positioned supine and this position facilitates the accumulation of fluid in the potential body spaces as discussed above. Occasionally, if the injury permits, the trauma patient may be in the sitting position, and in such instances, fluid will gravitate to the dependent portions of the body cavities, i.e., the lower parts of the pleural cavities or the pelvis. If the patient is sitting up then in a patient with a pneumothorax air will collect superiorly and underlie the upper anterior ribs, in contrast to the lower anterior chest when the patient is examined in the supine position. This should be considered while performing an e-FAST (Extended FAST) exam.

7.8 Probe and Machine Preset

A low-frequency probe of 2–5 Hz is preferred for the FAST exam to visualize structures in depth. If a wider footprint is preferred the curvilinear probe is used whereas the phased array probe can be used to enhance visualization between the ribs given its narrower footprint.

Newer Ultrasound machines have the option to select a preset for the probe. The Abdominal Exam or FAST Exam preset is the recommended choice with the marker on the screen placed on the left. If the marker is placed unconventionally on the right, the images received will be reversed to those shown in this chapter.

7.9 Scanning Technique

The order of scanning to obtain the four views of the FAST exam (Fig. 7.1) is determined by the region injured and on the clinical suspicion of finding blood. For example, in case of a penetrating injury to the left torso, the FAST exam can begin with the pericardial view followed by the splenorenal recess and then the other abdominal views. Similarly, in a patient with an injury to the pelvic region, the FAST exam can begin with the pelvic views. When the site of injury is unclear it is reasonable to begin by scanning the hepatorenal recess moving on to the splenorenal recess, followed by the pelvic and cardiac views. Irrespective of the order of scanning the operator must ensure that all areas have been assessed to complete the FAST exam.

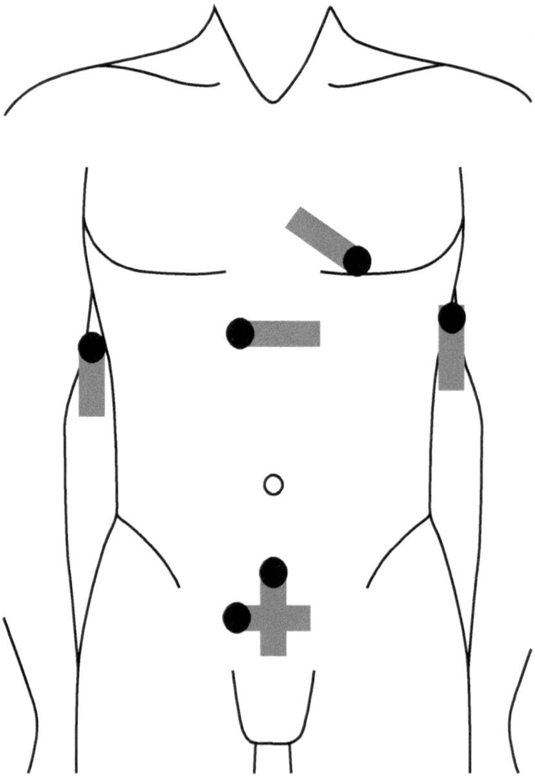

Fig. 7.1 Standard FAST views—Probe positions

7.10 Views

7.10.1 Right Upper Quadrant View

The probe is placed between the anterior and midaxillary lines in the 10th–11th intercostal space, orienting the marker or probe indicator towards the patient's head (Fig. 7.2). The probe is aimed towards the patient's vertebral column starting with a depth selection of more than 20 cm, and then adjusting to get the optimum image. Identifying the liver with its hepatic sinusoids is the first step before proceeding to identify other structures. Then sliding the probe up and down a rib space or more, while fanning the probe, continue to look for an anechoic stripe of fluid in the hemithorax above the diaphragm (suggestive of hemothorax) or in the peritoneal cavity below the diaphragm (suggestive of hemoperitoneum). The structures that are visualized craniocaudally in this view are:

Lung
Diaphragm
Liver (including tip of liver)
Morison's pouch
Right kidney (both upper and lower poles)
Right psoas major muscle

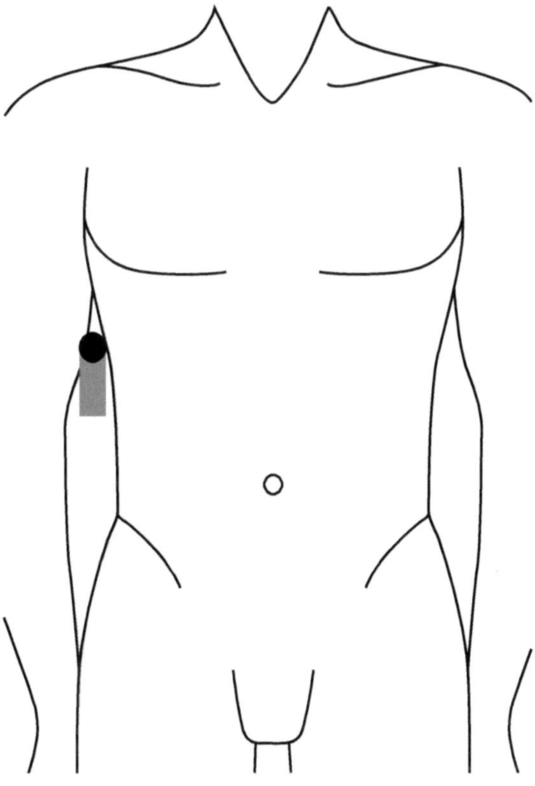

Fig. 7.2 The probe placement for the right upper quadrant view

Characteristic features of this view (Fig. 7.3):

- The lung contains air which is a poor conductor of sound while the liver provides a good sonographic window. The diaphragm acts as a specular reflector at this tissue-air interface and hence a normal lung appears as a mirror image of the liver.
- If there is fluid in the pleural cavity this appears as an anechoic black area (Fig. 7.4). Fluid is a good conductor of sound and the thoracic vertebral bodies that are not normally visible above the diaphragm due to air in the lungs can now be visualized. This is known as the thoracic spine sign or spine sign.
- When a significant amount of fluid collects in the pleural cavity, the lung becomes atelectatic and collapses. This collapsed lung dances with respiration in the anechoic fluid, giving the appearance of a whale tail or a jellyfish sign.
- The diaphragm appears as a curved bright white line due to specular reflection.
- The liver is identified by its homogenous appearance and sinusoids. It is a good conductor of sound providing an acoustic window for visualizing the other structures in the region.
- Morison's pouch or hepatorenal recess is normally collapsed and appears as a hyperechoic white line between the liver and right kidney. When fluid collects in this recess, it appears as a black anechoic stripe between the liver and the right kidney.
- The right kidney is identified by its characteristic shape and the presence of an outer cortex and inner medulla.
- It is important to fan the probe and slide up and down the ribs to visualize the liver and kidney in entirety. The tip of the liver and both poles of the kidney should be looked for and it should be documented if unable to obtain a clear view of these structures.

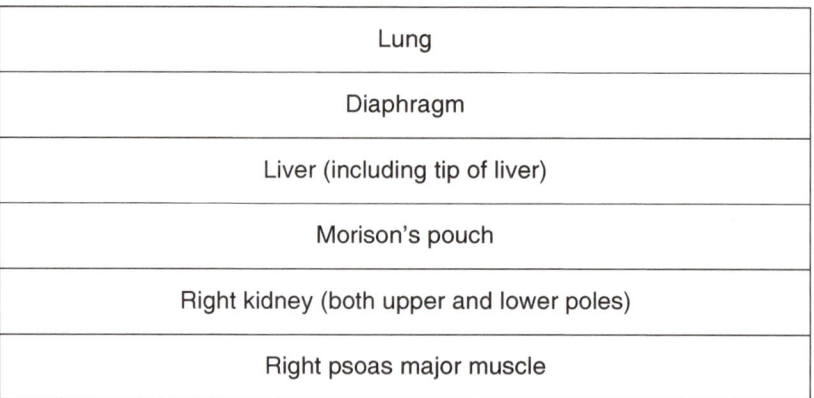

Lung
Diaphragm
Liver (including tip of liver)
Morison's pouch
Right kidney (both upper and lower poles)
Right psoas major muscle

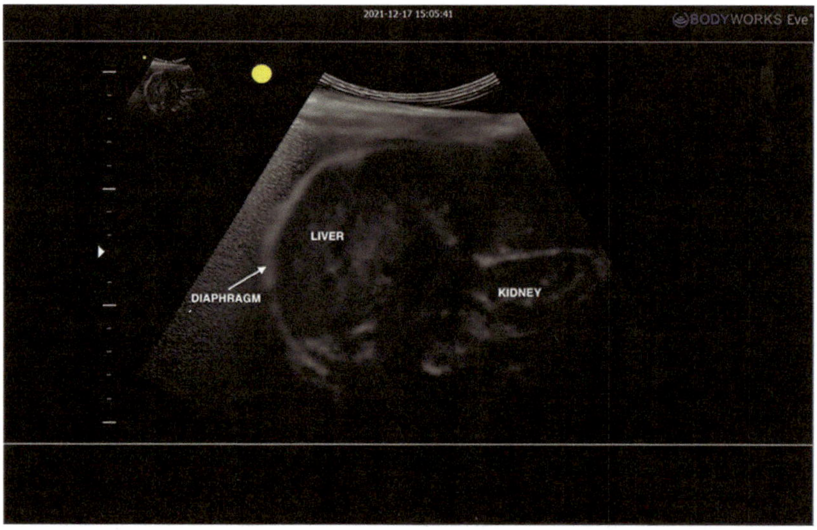

Fig. 7.3 The right upper quadrant view showing a section of the liver and the right kidney. There is no pathological fluid seen in this image

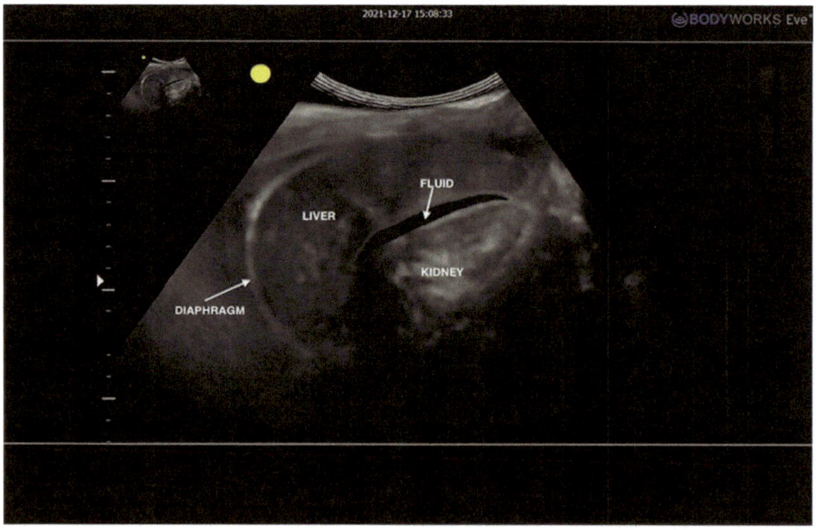

Fig. 7.4 Shows free fluid in the space between the liver and right kidney as a black anechoic stripe

- The psoas muscle is located posterior to the kidney and fluid can collect anterior to it in some instances.
- The patient can be requested to take a deep breath, which helps move the above structures caudally for better visualization. During deep inspiration the side of the chest opens up, placing the ribs in a more horizontal position and increasing the space between the ribs thus improving the image by reducing rib shadows. The patient can be asked to move their arm out of the way by placing their hand near their head which again makes the ribs more horizontal while opening up the space between the ribs.
- Rib shadows can cause hindrance in visualizing structures, leaving the operator with an unclear picture. In such instances, it helps to remember the anatomy of the rib cage and rotate the Ultrasound probe to position it parallel to and in between the ribs. Posteriorly the ribs leave the transverse processes and travel downwards and laterally and, in the front, they travel upwards and medially to join the sternum.

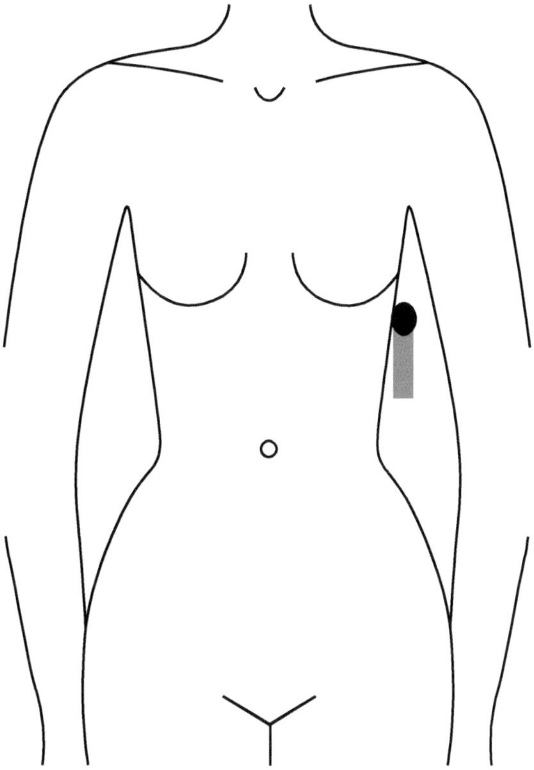

Fig. 7.5 The probe placement for the left upper quadrant view

7.10.2 Left Upper Quadrant View

The probe is placed in the 7–9th intercostal space in the posterior axillary line with the operator's hand almost resting on the surface that the patient is lying on (Fig. 7.5). The probe marker is towards the patient's head and the probe tilted to look slightly anteriorly towards the vertebral column with a depth selection of more than 20 cm, adjusting later to get the optimum image. The spleen has a similar echotexture to the liver but is located more posteriorly, hidden under the ribs. The structures visualized in this view are:

Lung
Diaphragm
Spleen
Splenorenal recess
Left kidney (both upper and lower poles)
Left psoas major muscle

Characteristic features of this view (Fig. 7.6):

- The lung is difficult to visualize in this view. It may be seen as a curtain that comes across the screen as the patient breathes.
- The diaphragm is visualized as a hyperechoic semilunar structure and the space between the diaphragm and spleen is a common site for blood to collect in case of splenic lacerations (Fig. 7.7).
- The splenorenal recess and left kidney should be visualized in entirety, fanning the probe to look for fluid. Fluid will appear as an anechoic black stripe between the spleen and the left kidney.
- The psoas muscle is located posterior to the kidney and fluid can collect anterior to it in some instances.
- Rib shadows can cause hindrance in visualizing structures and the tips given above (right upper quadrant view) can be used to mitigate these.

Lung
Diaphragm
Spleen
Splenorenal recess
Left Kidney (both upper and lower poles)
Left psoas major muscle

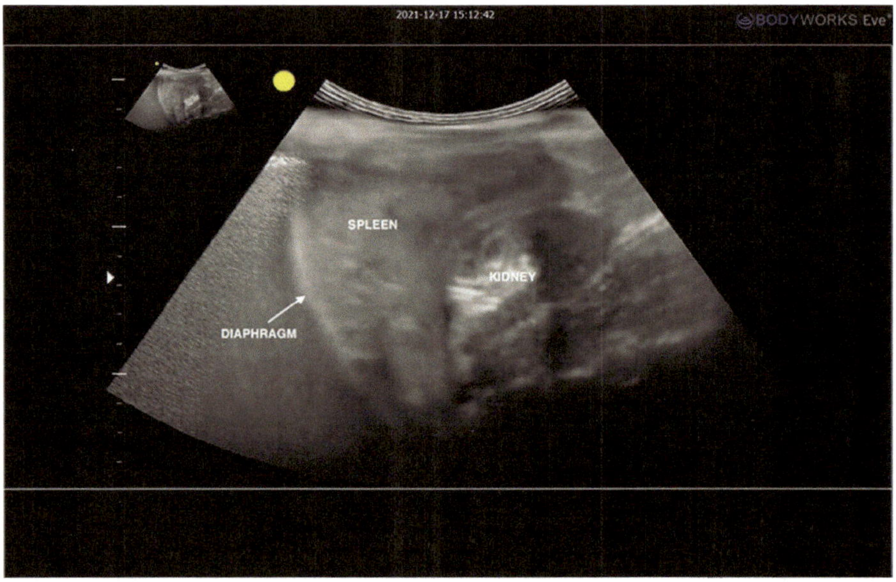

Fig. 7.6 The left upper quadrant view showing the diaphragm, a section of the spleen, and the left kidney. There is no pathological fluid seen in this image

7.10.3 Pelvic Cavity: Sagittal and Transverse Views

The pelvic cavity is assessed in both transverse and longitudinal sections. Begin with the probe in the suprapubic region with the probe marker to the right of the patient. Slide the probe caudally to almost touch the pubic symphysis and then angle the probe away from the patient's feet, to look into the pelvic cavity with a depth selection of 15 cm. Fan the probe, cranio-caudally to look for fluid that appears as an anechoic black line behind the bladder or behind the uterus in a female patient. Rotate the probe 90° clockwise so that the probe marker is now pointing towards the patient's head, maintaining the tilt to look into the pelvic cavity (Fig. 7.8). Now fan or slide the probe from side to side to look for fluid in the pelvis. The structures visualized in this view are:

Female patient:
Urinary bladder
Vesicouterine pouch/pouch of Douglas
Uterus
Rectouterine space
Rectum

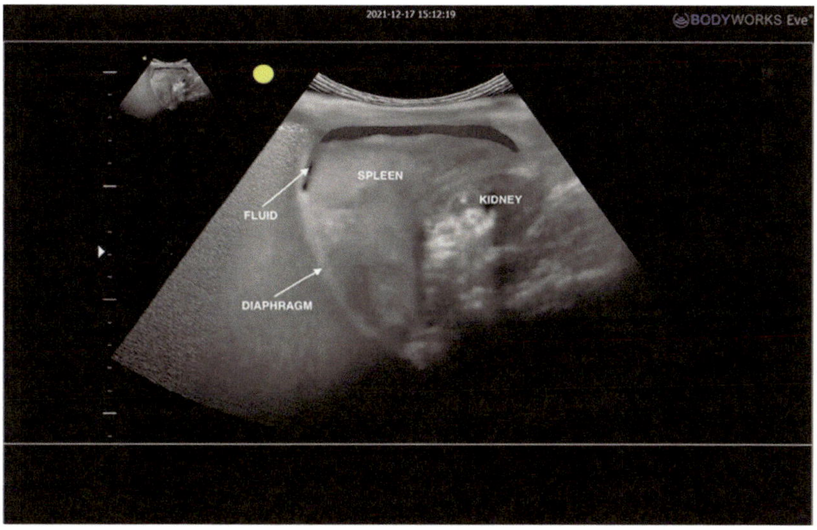

Fig. 7.7 Shows free fluid as a black anechoic stripe between the diaphragm and spleen in the left upper quadrant view

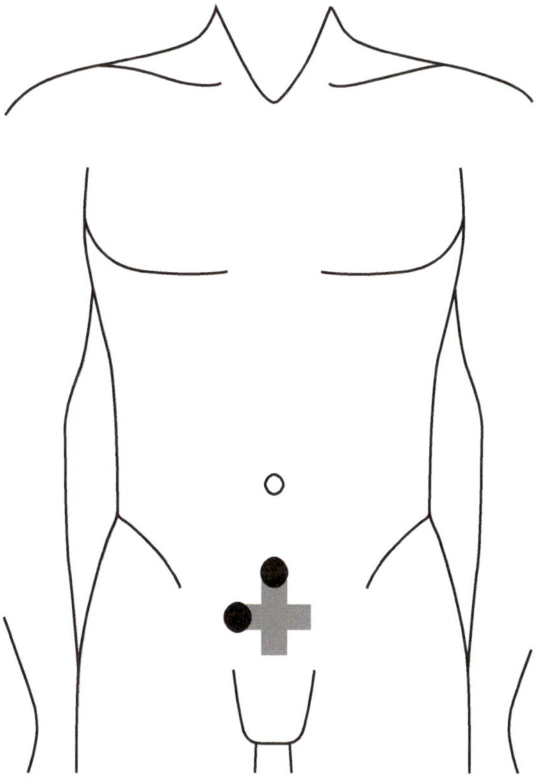

Fig. 7.8 The probe placement for the 2 pelvic views

Male patient:
Urinary bladder
Rectovesical space
Rectum

Characteristic features of this view (Figs. 7.9 and 7.10):

- When empty, the urinary bladder lies collapsed within the pelvis and when full, it can rise all the way up to the umbilicus. The urinary bladder is better visualized when containing urine and provides an acoustic window to assess the space behind the bladder where fluid can potentially collect.
- If the bladder is full, then an enhancement of the structures posterior to the bladder may cause them to appear hyperechoic. The TGC (time-gain-compensation) can be adjusted to get around this artifact.
- The vesicouterine and rectouterine spaces in the female patient and the rectovesical space in the male patient are normally collapsed. When fluid collects in them, they appear as anechoic black areas on ultrasound (Figs. 7.11 and 7.12).
- Small pockets of fluid may be easily missed; hence, it is important to fan the probe to look for fluid in all areas of the pelvis.
- Physiological fluid in the pelvis of the young female patient is common and can mimic a positive FAST scan in trauma. Clinical presentation, patient's hemodynamic status and surgical opinion along with further imaging with CT should be considered to confirm the cause of the fluid on a case-to-case basis.

Female patient:
Urinary bladder
Vesicouterine pouch / pouch of Douglas
Uterus
Rectouterine space
Rectum
Male patient:
Urinary bladder
Rectovesical space
Rectum

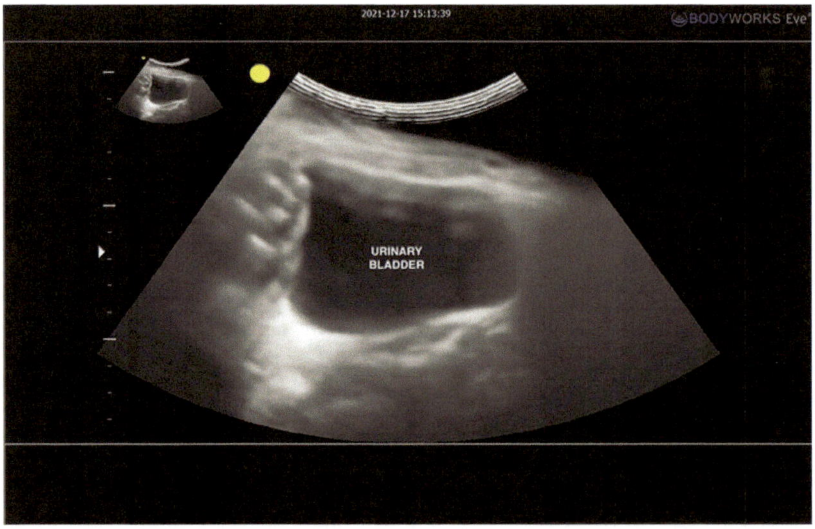

Fig. 7.9 The transverse view of the pelvis showing a well-filled urinary bladder. There is no pathological fluid in this image

- Occasionally, fluid in the rectum may be mistaken as fluid in the pelvis. In such cases, tilting the patient while maintaining necessary spinal precautions, to see if the fluid remains in the same place or moves into the paracolic gutters helps to differentiate between the two.

7.10.4 Pericardium

The subcostal view is usually used to access the heart, but if a clear view is not obtained due to abdominal viscera obstructing the view, the parasternal long-axis view can be used instead. The subcostal view can be accessed using the curvi-

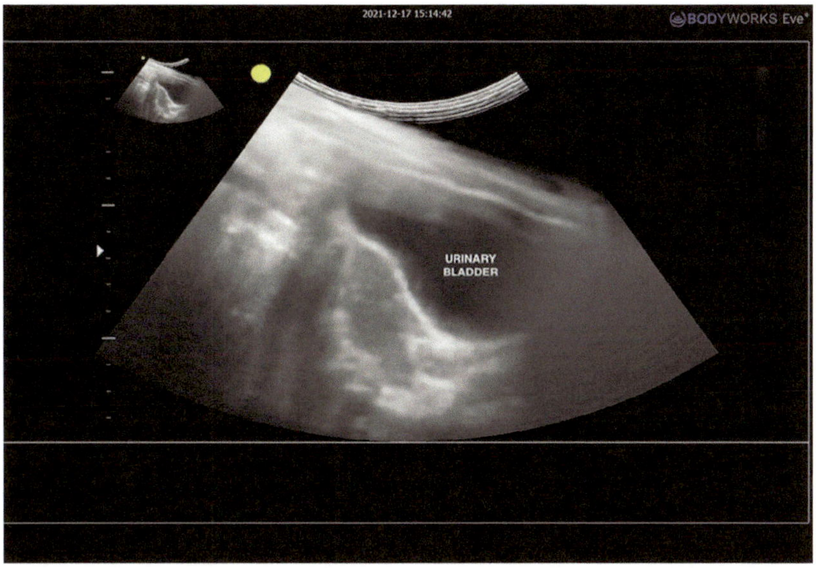

Fig. 7.10 The sagittal view of the pelvis showing a well-filled urinary bladder. There is no pathological fluid in this image

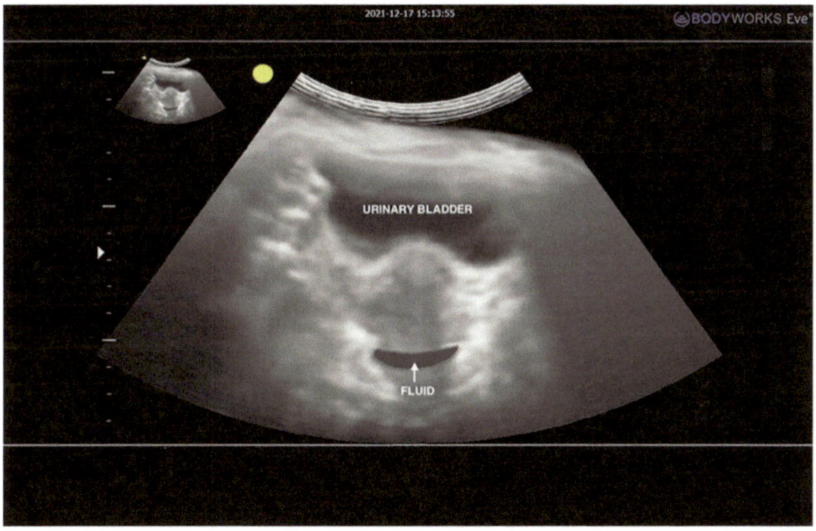

Fig. 7.11 Shows free fluid in the pelvis in transverse view

linear probe or the phased array probe. The marker on the screen for the phased array probe is conventionally placed to the right of the screen in the cardiac preset. If the probe marker is to the right of the patient in cardiac preset, the structures on the patient's right will appear on the left of the screen and vice versa. The probe marker may be placed to the left of the patient if the operator would like to obtain images with the right side of the patient corresponding to the right side of the screen while using the phased array probe in cardiac preset. This should be kept in mind when using this probe as the images will be mirrored accordingly. Alternatively, newer machines will have an abdominal preset option with the cardiac probe which can be selected for the subcostal views of the FAST exam.

Before placing the probe on the patient, the depth should be increased to 20 cm as the structures to be visualized are situated at a considerable distance from the probe. Place the probe in the epigastrium of the patient and slide up to almost touch the xiphisternum. Now tilt the probe to aim the probe towards the patient's left shoulder, attempt-

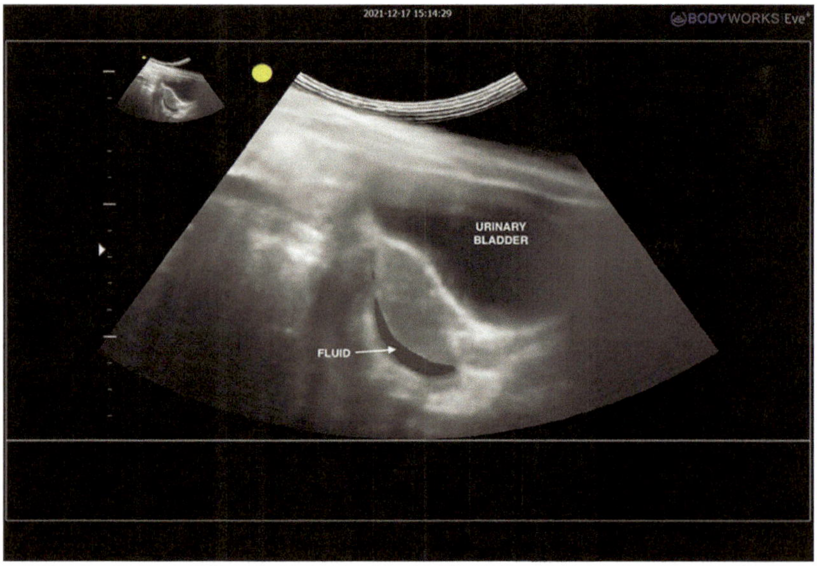

Fig. 7.12 Shows free fluid in the pelvis in sagittal view

ing to look just beneath the ribs to locate the heart through the acoustic window of the liver. If this view is unclear then proceed to attempt the parasternal long-axis view. This view is obtained by placing the probe on the left sternal border in the third or fourth intercostal space with the probe marker towards the right shoulder. Alternatively, the probe marker can be towards the left hip to obtain images with the patient's right corresponding to the right side of the screen (Fig. 7.13). Structures visualized in this view:

Subcostal view:
Liver
Heart
Parasternal long-axis view:
Heart
Descending aorta

Characteristic features of the subcostal view (Fig 7.14):

- The liver provides an acoustic window for visualizing the heart in the subcostal view and is the structure seen closest to the probe. The closest chamber to the liver is the right ventricle. and all four chambers of the heart can be visualized in this view.
- Pericardial fluid (Fig. 7.15) in small amounts tends to collect posteriorly and as the quantity increases it surrounds the heart and is detected anteriorly. Therefore, it is important to look for any anechoic shadow behind the heart to avoid missing a small pericardial collection. This is done by fanning through the heart in an anteroposterior direction.

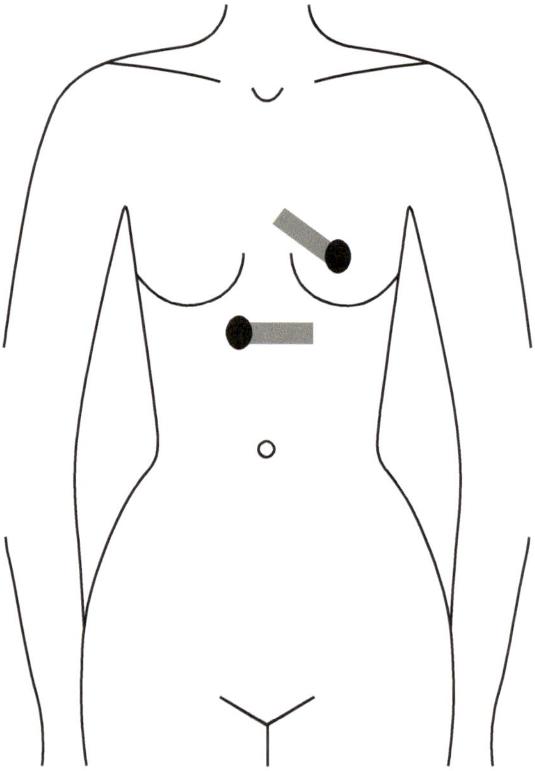

Fig. 7.13 The probe placement for the subcostal and parasternal views

Subcostal view:
Liver
Heart
Parasternal long axis view:
Heart
Descending aorta

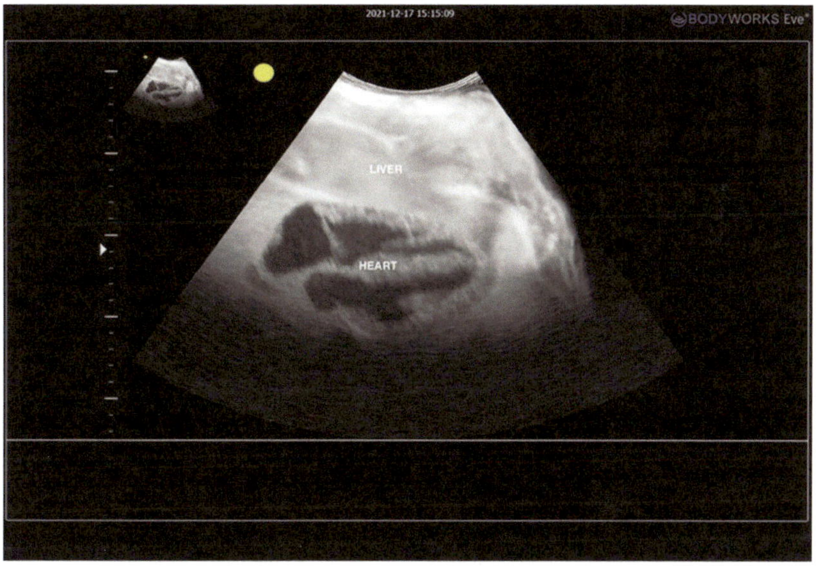

Fig. 7.14 The subcostal view showing the liver (structure closer to the probe) and the heart

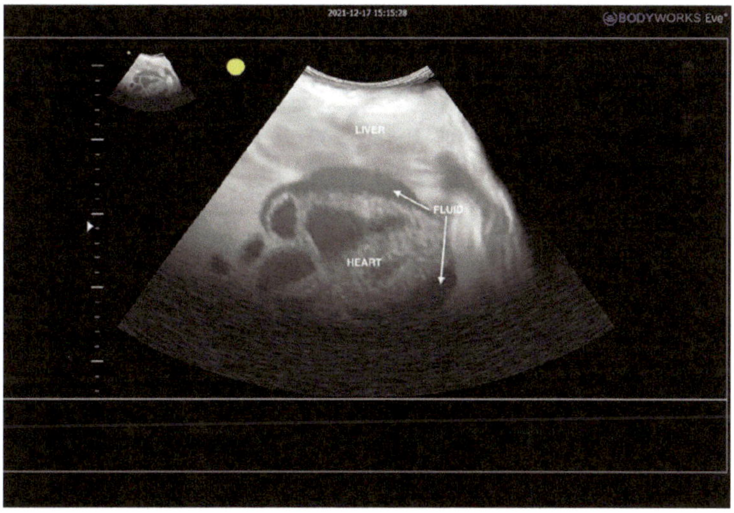

Fig. 7.15 Free fluid is seen in the pericardial cavity on subcostal view

- While attempting to look for the heart beneath the ribs the probe is placed tangentially on the skin. Care must be exercised to keep the probe in contact with the patient's skin at all times to avoid compromising on the image quality. A generous amount of ultrasound gel will help maintain good probe-to-skin contact.
- Occasionally the subcostal view may not provide a clear image due to a barrel chest or abdominal viscera obstructing or a tender abdomen. In such instances, the parasternal long-axis view (Fig. 7.16) can be obtained and the depth setting should be decreased to 10–15 cm before proceeding with this view.
- In the parasternal long-axis view the descending aorta is posterior to the heart. This is used as a landmark to differentiate whether the anechoic black shadow seen posterior to the heart is a pericardial or pleural collection. A pericardial collection (Fig. 7.17) will be situated anterior to the aorta whereas pleural fluid is located posterior to the descending aorta. If any fluid is detected in the subcostal view it is recommended to confirm it on a parasternal long-axis view because the subcostal view may mistake pleural fluid for pericardial fluid.
- Other views that can be used to supplement imaging of the heart for fluid in the pericardial

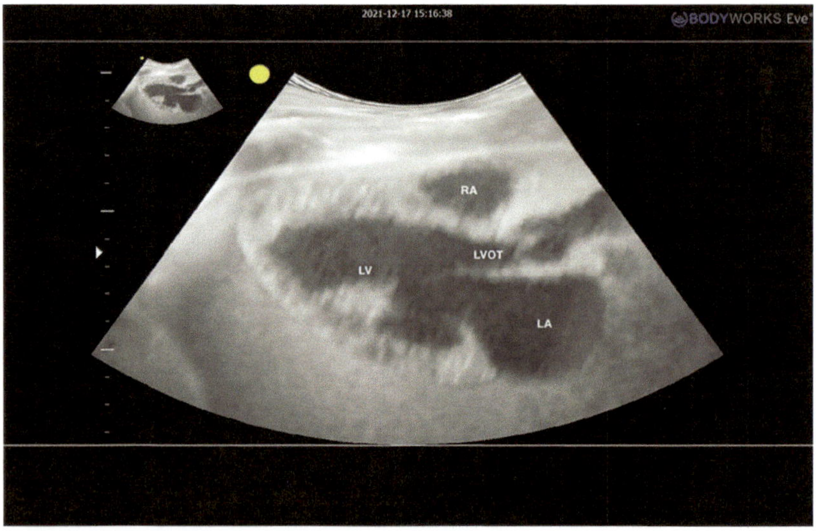

Fig. 7.16 The parasternal long-axis (PLAX) view showing the heart

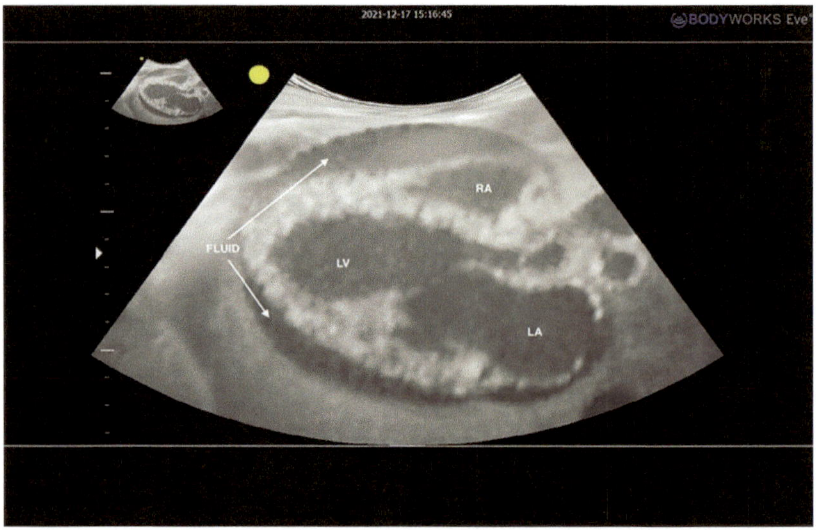

Fig. 7.17 Free fluid is seen around the heart both anteriorly and posteriorly in the parasternal long-axis view

cavity are the parasternal short-axis view and the apical four-chamber view (please refer to chapter on ECHO for this).

- When performing a FAST scan, the operator must be aware of the features of cardiac tamponade to differentiate it from a pericardial effusion sans tamponade. Identification of the features of cardiac tamponade in the hemodynamically unstable trauma patient necessitates immediate emergency management. The features on ultrasound that indicate cardiac tamponade are pericardial effusion plus:
- Right ventricular (RV) collapse in diastole.
- Right atrial (RA) collapse in systole.
- Plethoric IVC with minimal respiratory variation.

The collapse of the RA/RV due to cardiac tamponade appears as a wavy seesaw on ultrasound and it has been referred to as the "little man jumping on the trampoline" sign.

7.11 Extended FAST or e-FAST Scan

The extended FAST exam was first proposed in 2004 and included bilateral chest ultrasound exams to detect the presence of a pneumothorax in addition to the four views of the FAST exam. Ideally, the high-frequency linear probe is used for assessing the chest for features of a pneumothorax as the pleura is a superficial structure. If this probe is not available the scan can be performed with the low-frequency probes. In the supine trauma, patient air collects in the anterior-most part of the thorax, whereas in an upright trauma patient the air will collect in the apical regions of the thorax. The anterior-most rib space is different for each patient and is usually between the fourth to sixth intercostal spaces. The operator may face difficulty in obtaining a good view if the patient's breast tissue interferes with the imaging.

The exam is performed by placing the probe in the second intercostal space in the mid-clavicular line in a linear fashion with the probe marker pointing towards the patient's head. The structures towards the head end of the patient will appear on the left side of the screen. Once a certain rib space is examined in both 2D mode and M-mode, the probe is moved caudally to cover most of the rib spaces, repeating the assessment for features of a pneumothorax bilaterally. The structures visualized in this view are:

Skin
Subcutaneous tissues
Adjoining ribs with intercostal muscles
Parietal pleura and lung sliding
Superficial lung parenchyma

Characteristic features of this view:

- The focus of the image obtained is the bright pleural line in the middle of the screen with the two adjoining ribs and their shadows on either side.
- Lung sliding is the gliding of the parietal pleura on the visceral pleura during breathing and is appreciated as "ants marching" on the white pleural line. This movement has to be appreciated in real time and is absent when there is air between the two pleural surfaces as in a pneumothorax.
- Occasionally a lung point is appreciated at the junction of the pneumothorax and normal lung where lung sliding abruptly ends. The normal lung parenchyma may show a few B lines or comet tails which may also end abruptly at the lung point.
- The M-mode is then used to complement the findings of the 2D mode. The line of the M-mode is placed over the pleural line and the obtained image is analyzed. If the upper half of the image shows horizontal lines with a grainy bottom half, the appearance is called a sandy beach sign and indicates a normal lung. If the entire image shows lines throughout, without the sandy granular appearance, it is known as the barcode or stratosphere sign and is characteristic of a pneumothorax.
- It is important to look in multiple intercostal spaces for a pneumothorax.
- The presence of subcutaneous emphysema hinders the use of ultrasound to assess for a

pneumothorax (air is a poor conductor of sound) and in such instances other imaging modalities should be used.
(Also see chapter on lung for more information)

7.12 Limitations of FAST Scan

1. Amount of fluid—There has to be a significant amount of fluid in the potential spaces for detection via ultrasound. This amount is estimated at 200–250 mL in the peritoneal cavity. In the pericardial space, effusions as small as 50 mL can cause pericardial tamponade [12].
2. Rule-in (vs.) Rule-out—The FAST exam should always be used as a Rule-in test and should not be used to rule out pathology. A patient who has a negative FAST scan can still have an injury [13] but has not yet collected enough blood in the peritoneal cavity for it to be detected on ultrasound.
3. Retroperitoneal fluid—A FAST scan cannot detect fluid in the retroperitoneal space and this should always be considered as an area of potential bleed in the unstable trauma patient.
4. Subcutaneous emphysema—Air is a poor conductor of sound hence the presence of subcutaneous emphysema will hinder visualization of any underlying pathology.
5. Operator dependent—The speed and accuracy of the FAST exam is dependent on the training and experience of the operator.
6. Equipment—In many areas of the world, an ultrasound machine is not available for the management of the trauma patient leaving a void in the service that can be delivered in such cases.
7. Training—As with the availability of equipment the access to training may limit the use of the FAST scan in some parts of the world. The availability of virtual learning platforms can help overcome this problem.

7.13 FAST Scan Flowchart (Fig. 7.18)

7.14 Reporting a FAST Scan

The FAST exam is always reported for the particular time at which it was performed and can change as the clinical status of the patient progresses. Therefore, FAST exam reports should mention the time at which the exam was performed. Images of the FAST exam should be saved on the device and serve as a baseline scan for clinical correlation at a later time.

A report on a FAST exam should indicate whether all views were clearly visualized and whether any fluid was present in any of those views. If certain regions of a view were not clearly visualized this must be commented on. A FAST report should also recommend the next clinical management, e.g., no further imaging, repeat FAST scan in certain time, proceed to CT or urgent management in theatre. Below is a sample template for the FAST exam used at the Oxford University Hospitals, UK.

POCUS FAST

(Focused Assessment by Sonography in Trauma)

OPERATOR		SUPERVISOR		OBSERVER	
DATE:		TIME:		LOCATION:	

Before scan:

What is the indication for this scan?	
Patient consent obtained?	
Procedure explained?	

FAST scan location	Comment on clarity of views obtained Please use C=clear P=Partial N=not seen	Free fluid seen? Please say YES or NO	Any other comments?
RIGHT UPPER QUADRANT VIEWS			
Right Hemithorax			
Right side of diaphragm			
Liver			
Morrisons space			
Tip of the liver			
Upper pole of right kidney			
Lower pole of right kidney			
Right psoas muscle			
LEFT UPPER QUADRANT VIEWS			
Left Hemithorax			
Left side of the diaphragm			
Spleen			
Splenorenal space			
Upper pole of left kidney			
Lower pole of left kidney			
Left psoas muscle			
PELVIC VIEWS			
Transverse			
Longitudinal			
PERICARDIAL VIEWS			
View used?			

Any other scans done? Extended – FAST? e.g. Lungs, MSK, eye etc – please write your findings below.

After scan:

Images saved?	
Patient informed of scan findings?	
POCUS machine cleaned and plugged in safely at designated area?	

Summary of FAST scan	
Clinical decision taken post scan?	

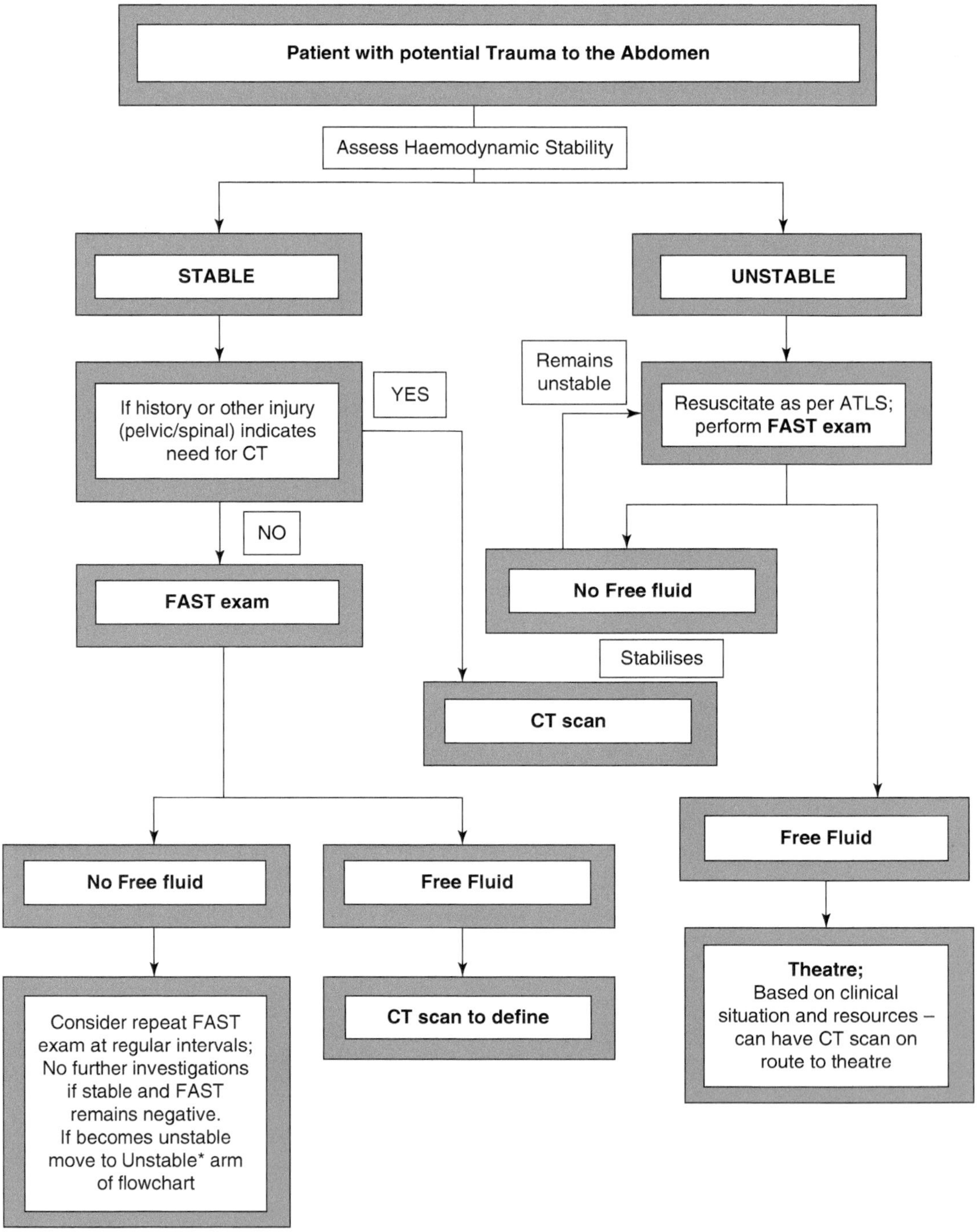

Fig. 7.18 This flowchart shows possible clinical pathways for the trauma patient with an abdominal injury based on the patient's hemodynamic stability and FAST exam results

7.15 FAST Scan vs. US Abdomen

A FAST exam is clearly different from an ultrasound abdomen exam with regards to the purpose and procedure of the scan. A FAST exam is performed in trauma and focuses on the question of whether there is fluid in the peritoneal cavity (along with pleural and pericardial spaces). It does not comment on any of the internal organs while an ultrasound abdomen assesses all abdominal structures looking for pathology that can explain the presenting symptoms. A FAST scan is easier to learn and recommended as part of training for emergency physicians, critical care physicians, and prehospital medical personnel.

7.16 Caution

Do NOT delay resuscitation to perform a FAST exam.
Always report the FAST scan for a particular time in the patient's journey.
Always use the FAST exam as a rule-in test and not to rule out pathology.
Do NOT clear a region as negative for fluid unless all areas are clearly visualized.

7.17 Summary

The FAST exam is a useful tool in unstable trauma patient and should be used as part of the primary survey when available. A clear understanding of the physiology of pathological fluid collection within potential body spaces and the effect of gravity on the location of this fluid is necessary before attempting the FAST scan. The FAST exam is performed with a low-frequency probe and attempts to answer the question of whether there is any fluid within the three body spaces. These are the peritoneal, pleural, and pericardial spaces and are examined in four views, namely the right upper quadrant, left upper quadrant, pelvic, and cardiac. It is absolutely vital to visualize the four views clearly before reporting a negative scan. A useful advantage of the FAST scan is that it can be performed simultaneously during the clinical examination as a bedside test and can be repeated as needed. A FAST scan should never delay or interrupt resuscitation measures.

Self-Assessment Questions: Chose the Single Best Answer

1. The FAST scan includes all of the following views EXCEPT:
   A. Right upper quadrant
   B. Left upper quadrant
   C. Pelvic
   D. Longitudinal view of the aorta
2. You are going to begin your FAST scan with the abdominal exam. The probe that can be used for this exam is:
   A. The curvilinear probe with abdominal/FAST preset
   B. The cardiac probe with abdominal preset
   C. Both of the above
   D. Only the linear probe
3. You are going to perform the extended FAST scan. Which probe is best suited for visualizing the pleura and why?
   A. Linear probe because of its high frequency
   B. Linear probe because of its low frequency
   C. Phased array probe because of its low frequency
   D. None of the above
4. The Morison's pouch is the most dependent area in the abdomen of the supine patient. This lies between the:
   A. Spleen and left kidney
   B. Liver and right kidney
   C. Urinary bladder and rectum
   D. Urinary bladder and uterus
5. All of the following are expected to be visualized on the left upper quadrant view EXCEPT:
   A. Heart
   B. Diaphragm
   C. Spleen
   D. Left kidney

6. The FAST exam on a hemodynamically unstable young gentleman involved in a significant motor vehicle collision is positive. What would be the next step in the management of this patient (ATLS management ongoing)
   A. DPL to check if the fluid in the abdomen is blood
   B. Observe and repeat FAST scan when patient becomes stable
   C. CT scan if stabilizes by resuscitation, else emergency exploratory laparotomy in theatre
   D. Repeat FAST scan every 5 min till the patient is stable
7. The FAST exam on a hemodynamically stable young lady who fell down a flight of stairs after a few drinks is negative. She is tender in the abdomen and confused. What would be the most appropriate next step in the management of this patient?
   A. Repeat a FAST scan if clinical picture changes
   B. Pan CT to exclude injuries from head to pelvis
   C. Discharge home to sober up
   D. Get a radiologist to perform a bedside abdominal ultrasound
8. The following non-trauma patients benefit from having a FAST/FAFF scan:
   A. Suspected ruptured ectopic pregnancy
   B. Medical patient with unexplained hypotension
   C. Both
   D. None
9. The following are normal findings while performing an extended FAST scan EXCEPT:
   A. A-lines
   B. Occasional B-lines
   C. Lung Sliding
   D. Lung point
10. The full bladder can enhance structures situated posterior to it and make them appear hyperechoic. The adjustment that can help to make the image better is:
    A. Increase depth
    B. Time-gain-compensation
    C. Increase gain
    D. All of the above
11. Physiological fluid is commonly found in the following space in the FAST scan:
    A. Hepatorenal recess
    B. Splenorenal recess
    C. Pelvis of the female patient
    D. Pleural spaces
12. The next step when unable to obtain a subcostal view of the pericardium is to:
    A. Press harder while pointing to the right shoulder
    B. Obtain the parasternal long-axis view
    C. Proceed with other views of the FAST scan
    D. Perform a transthoracic echocardiography
13. The direction of the probe when obtaining the subcostal view is pointing towards the:
    A. Left shoulder
    B. Right shoulder
    C. Suprasternal notch
    D. Umbilicus
14. The depth setting for obtaining the subcostal view is:
    A. 2 cm
    B. 5 cm
    C. 10 cm
    D. 20 cm
15. While performing the extended FAST exam, the sign that signifies the presence of a pneumothorax in the M-mode is called:
    A. Seashore/Sandy beach sign
    B. Barcode/Stratosphere sign
    C. Trampoline sign
    D. Fishtail sign
16. The FAST exam should be performed:
    A. To look for pathological fluid in the unstable trauma patient
    B. To rule out any abdominal pathology in the trauma patient
    C. In every trauma patient irrespective of hemodynamic status and injury
    D. By the senior-most clinician available
17. Signs of Cardiac Tamponade are:
    A. Large pericardial effusion
    B. Right ventricular (RV) collapse in diastole
    C. Right atrial (RA) collapse in systole
    D. All of the above

18. The presence of fluid in the thorax, e.g., Hemothorax on a FAST scan is seen as:
    A. Anechoic shadow above the diaphragm
    B. Vertebral bodies become visible above the diaphragm (Spine sign)
    C. Collapsed lung dances in the fluid (Whale tail or Jellyfish sign)
    D. All of the above
19. A posterior pericardial effusion in the PLAX view is located:
    A. Anterior to the descending aorta
    B. Posterior to the descending aorta
    C. Anterior to the IVC
    D. Posterior to the IVC
20. Your colleague performed a FAST scan in a stable trauma patient that was negative, after which the patient went on to have a CT scan that showed small lacerations of the right kidney and right lobe of the liver with minimal intra-abdominal fluid. Your colleague feels upset that they recorded a negative FAST exam. What advice will you give your colleague?
    A. Advise them that they need more practice in FAST scans as their FAST report was incorrect
    B. Advise them that the FAST exam has low sensitivity in detecting small amounts of fluid and the fluid may have started collecting after the FAST was done, so the FAST they did was valid for that time
    C. Advise them to get a second opinion on the CT report as it cannot be correct
    D. Advise them to arrange for an exploratory laparotomy

References

1. Rozycki GS, Ochsner MG, Schmidt JA, Frankel HL, Davis TP, Wang D, et al. A prospective study of surgeon-performed ultrasound as the primary adjuvant modality for injured patient assessment. J Trauma. 1995;39(3):492–8; discussion 8–500
2. Rozycki GS, Feliciano DV, Schmidt JA, Cushman JG, Sisley AC, Ingram W, et al. The role of surgeon-performed ultrasound in patients with possible cardiac wounds. Ann Surg. 1996;223(6):737–44; discussion 44–6
3. Melniker LA, Leibner E, McKenney MG, Lopez P, Briggs WM, Mancuso CA. Randomized controlled clinical trial of point-of-care, limited ultrasonography for trauma in the emergency department: the first sonography outcomes assessment program trial. Ann Emerg Med. 2006;48(3):227–35.
4. Rozycki GS, Ballard RB, Feliciano DV, Schmidt JA, Pennington SD. Surgeon-performed ultrasound for the assessment of truncal injuries: lessons learned from 1540 patients. Ann Surg. 1998;228(4):557–67.
5. Kirkpatrick AW, Sirois M, Laupland KB, Liu D, Rowan K, Ball CG, et al. Hand-held thoracic sonography for detecting post-traumatic pneumothoraces: the extended focused assessment with sonography for trauma (EFAST). J Trauma. 2004;57(2):288–95.
6. Quinn AC, Sinert R. What is the utility of the focused assessment with sonography in trauma (FAST) exam in penetrating torso trauma? Injury. 2011;42(5):482–7.
7. Griffin XL, Pullinger R. Are diagnostic peritoneal lavage or focused abdominal sonography for trauma safe screening investigations for hemodynamically stable patients after blunt abdominal trauma? A review of the literature. J Trauma. 2007;62(3):779–84.
8. ATLS. Advanced Trauma Life Support. Advanced Trauma Life Support® Student Course Manual. 10 ed: Library of Congress Control Number: 2017907997; 2018.
9. Root HD, Hauser CW, McKinley CR, Lafave JW, Mendiola RP Jr. Diagnostic peritoneal lavage. Surgery. 1965;57:633–7.
10. Gupta M, Schriger DL, Hiatt JR, Cryer HG, Tillou A, Hoffman JR, et al. Selective use of computed tomography compared with routine whole body imaging in patients with blunt trauma. Ann Emerg Med. 2011;58(5):407–16.e15.
11. Salim A, Sangthong B, Martin M, Brown C, Plurad D, Demetriades D. Whole body imaging in blunt multisystem trauma patients without obvious signs of injury: results of a prospective study. Arch Surg. 2006;141(5):468–75.
12. Goodman A, Perera P, Mailhot T, Mandavia D. The role of bedside ultrasound in the diagnosis of pericardial effusion and cardiac tamponade. J Emerg Trauma Shock. 2012;5(1):72–5.
13. Nishijima DK, Simel DL, Wisner DH, Holmes JF. Does this adult patient have a blunt intra-abdominal injury? JAMA. 2012;307(14):1517–27.

8 Miscellaneous POCUS: Gastric Ultrasound, Urinary Bladder Ultrasound, Ocular Ultrasound, Obstetric POCUS

Chetan Mehra and Amit Dikshit

8.1 Introduction

The presence of the ultrasound machine in the operation theater has led to chance usage of the modality and incidental development of the fields such as gastric, urinary bladder, and ophthalmic ultrasound, which is probably performed only by the anesthesiologists. These techniques have unique indications and they provide valuable clinical insight at the *point of care* in a timely manner.

In this chapter, we will discuss gastric ultrasound, ultrasonic assessment of the urinary bladder, ocular ultrasound, and point-of-care ultrasound of the gravid uterus. For the benefit of the readers, there is a Video 8.1 linked with this chapter that will guide the readers through the new and interesting modalities of miscellaneous POCUS.

Supplementary Information The online version contains supplementary material available at [https://doi.org/10.1007/978-981-16-7687-1_8].

C. Mehra (✉)
Department of Anaesthesiology, Critical Care and Pain, Indraprastha Apollo Hospital, New Delhi, India

A. Dikshit
Ruby Hall Clinic and Hospital, Pune, India

8.2 Gastric Ultrasound

8.2.1 Introduction

- Preoperative fasting guidelines help limit the aspiration risk in patients undergoing elective surgical procedures. However, fasting intervals are not applicable or reliable in urgent or emergency surgeries or for patients with delayed gastric emptying [1].
- Gastric ultrasound is a point-of-care tool for the assessment of antral gastric volume, which is an indirect correlate for risk of aspiration of gastric contents. It can help to determine the nature and volume of gastric contents (empty, clear fluid, thick fluid/solid) [2].

8.2.2 Indications [3]

Potential advantage of gastric ultrasound can be seen in the following patient population:

- Suspected delay in gastric emptying:
  - Pregnancy.
- Suspected gastro-paresis.
  - Diabetes Mellitus.
  - Chronic hepatic/renal dysfunction.
  - Neuromuscular disorders.
- Lack of adherence to fasting instructions:
  - Emergency/urgent procedure.

A. Chakraborty, B. Ashokka (eds.), *A Practical Guide to Point of Care Ultrasound (POCUS)*,
https://doi.org/10.1007/978-981-16-7687-1_8

- Unreliable fasting history, because of.
    - Language barrier.
    - Altered sensorium.
    - Cognitive dysfunction.

8.2.3 Limitations

Gastric ultrasound findings may be inaccurate in subjects with abnormal underlying gastric anatomy (e.g., previous gastric resection or bypass, gastric band in situ, previous fundoplication, large hiatus hernia) [4].

8.2.4 Scanning Technique

- Patient position:
    - Start scanning with the patient in supine position, followed by examination with patient in right lateral decubitus position. Final assessment of gastric antral volume/contents should be based on examination in both positions [2].
- Transducer selection:
    - Curved array/low-frequency (2–5 MHz).
    - Select abdominal settings for scan.
- Probe position:
    - Start scanning epigastrium in mid-sagittal plane, just caudal to xiphisternum.
- Sweep the transducer both ways, from left to right subcostal margins (Fig. 8.1).
- Identification of relevant structures is based on characteristic ultrasound images as discussed ahead (Fig. 8.2).

8.2.5 Applied Anatomy

8.2.5.1 Gastric Antrum

- Gastric antrum, as a part of stomach, is easily amenable to sonographic examination. It accurately reflects the content of the entire stomach.
- It appears as a hollow viscus with a prominent multilayered wall.
- Antrum is sandwiched between liver (anteriorly) and pancreas (posteriorly).
- Landmarks for identification of gastric antrum are [1] left lobe of liver, [2] Pancreas, [3] Aorta, [4] Inferior vena cava, and [5] Superior mesenteric artery and vein.
- It is usually located superficially at a depth of 3–4 cm.

8.2.5.2 Gastric Wall

- It appears as a characteristic five-layered wall and sets the organ apart from other hollow viscus.

8.2.6 Ultrasound Image Correlation (Table 8.1)

Ultrasound appearance of antrum can be graded based on antral shape, antral wall appearance, and antral content, as follows [2]:

8.2.6.1 Empty Stomach

- Antrum has no appreciable content in both supine and RLD position (Grade 0 antrum).
- Bull's eye or Target Pattern: It appears flat and collapsed or with a round-to-ovoid shape.

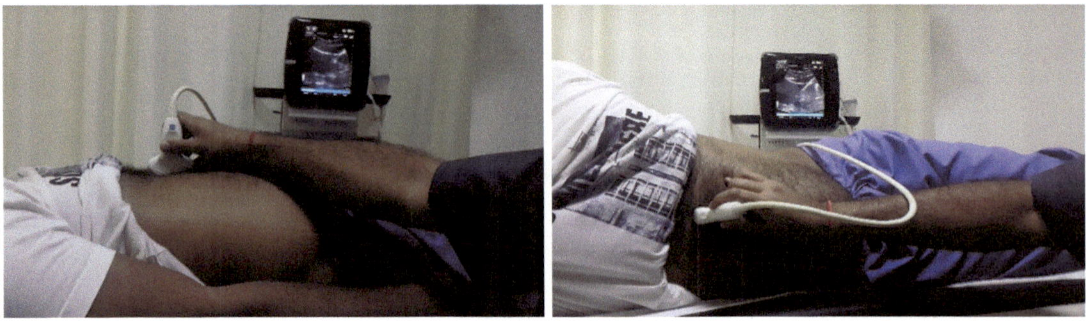

Fig. 8.1 Probe placement in supine and right lateral decubitus position

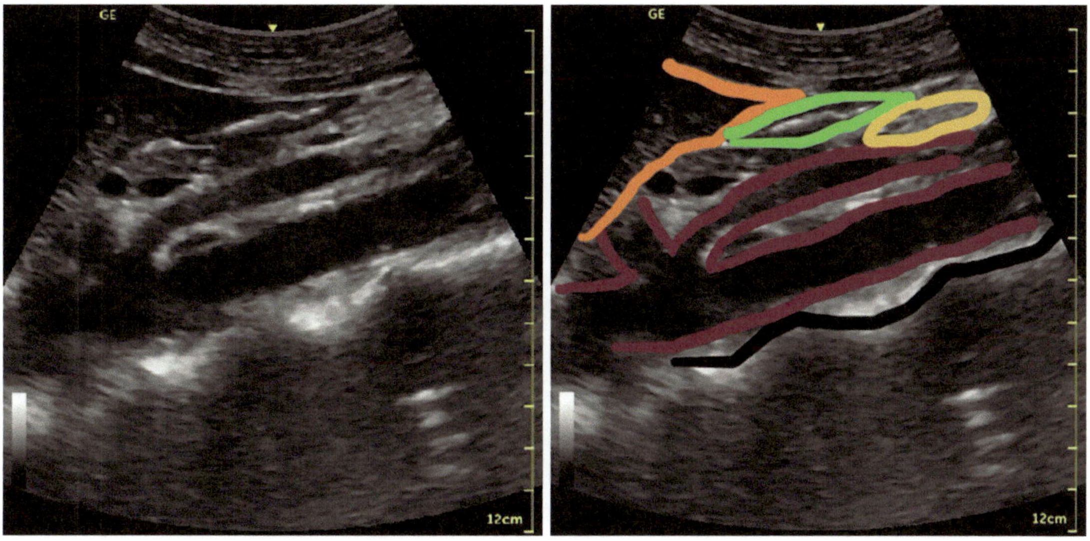

Fig. 8.2 Gastric Antrum ultrasound image with schematic representation of anatomic structures *(Black—vertebral column, dark red—aorta with celiac and superior mesenteric branches, orange—liver, yellow—pancreatic body, green—flat empty antrum). *left side of image is cranial and right side of image is caudal end*

Table 8.1 Appearance of Antrum and antral wall with contents

Grade	Antral shape	Antral wall	Content
Empty	Flat and collapsed or round (Bull's eye)	Thick with prominent muscularis propriae	None (grade 0) OR small amount of hypoechoic content (grade 1)
Solid	Round/distended	Thin	Heterogenous, particulate, mixed with air
Clear fluid	Round/distended	Thin	Hypoechoic
Milk/ suspensions	Round/distended	Thin	Hyperechoic

8.2.6.2 Solid Early Stage

- Antrum appears distended with thin walls.
- The content is of high or mixed echogenicity.
- Specific pattern: "Frosted-glass" pattern (usually shortly after a solid meal). It is due to a mix of air and solid along the anterior wall, blurring the posterior wall and deeper structures (Fig. 8.3).

8.2.6.3 Solid Late Stage

- Heterogeneous, particulate content (usually after 1–2 h following a solid meal).
- Homogeneous hyperechoic content: characteristic of dairy products or particulate fluids.

8.2.6.4 Clear Fluid

- Antrum appears round and distended with thin walls.
- The content appears anechoic or hypoechoic.
- The size of antrum is proportional to gastric volume.
- Antrum will appear larger in RLD position compared to supine position (Fig. 8.4).

8.2.6.5 Fluid with Air Bubbles

- Starry night pattern (multiple air bubbles on a hypoechoic background) usually seen shortly after ingestion of clear fluids or effervescent drinks.

8.2.7 Gastric Volume Assessment (Clear Fluids)

- Volume assessment can differentiate a low (normal) quantity of baseline gastric secretions from a higher (non-fasting) volume.
- Cross-sectional area of the antrum (CSA) has a linear correlation with the gastric volume (Figs. 8.3 and 8.4: marked by yellow dotted lines).

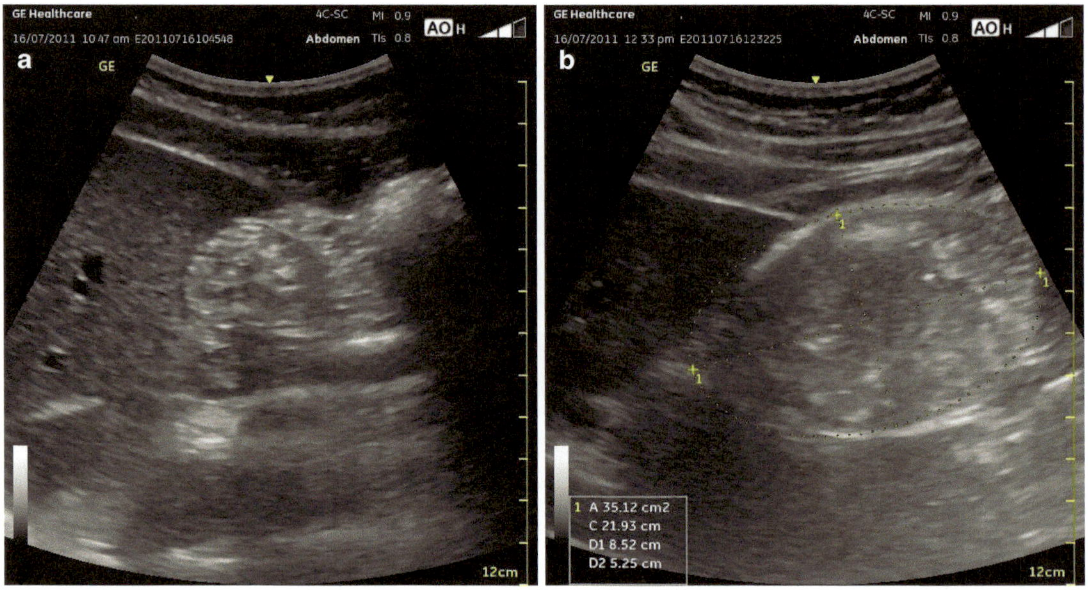

Fig. 8.3 Gastric antrum image acquired 150 min after meal. (**a**) Supine and (**b**) Right lateral decubitus position

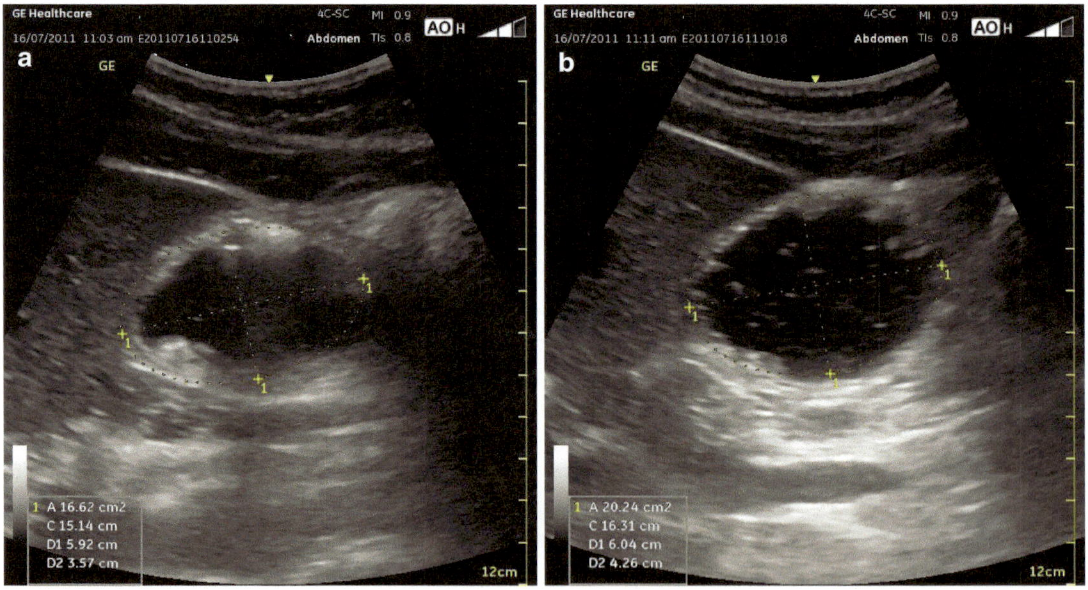

Fig. 8.4 Gastric antrum image acquired 15 min after drinking clear water. Image (**a**) Patient in supine position; Image (**b**) Patient in right lateral decubitus position; Image (**c**) Image acquired 2 h after water intake *(Measurements: A—area, C—circumference, D1 and D2—diameters in two perpendicular planes)*

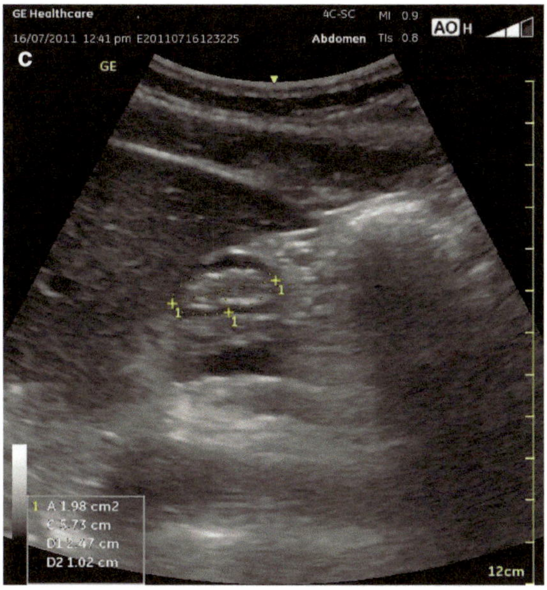

Fig. 8.4 (continued)

Table 8.2 Antral grading system (Grades 0–2)

Grade	Antral presentation	Volume implications	Aspiration risk
0	Empty in both supine and RLD position	Minimal	Low risk
1	Empty in supine, clear fluid visible in RLD position	≤1.5 ml/kg, compatible with baseline gastric secretions	Low risk
2	Clear fluid visible in both positions	>1.5 ml/kg, likely in excess of baseline gastric secretions	High risk

- Measurement of CSA: [4]
  - Identify antrum at the level of aorta in RLD position.
  - Obtain a still image of antrum at rest (between peristaltic contractions).
  - Use the free-tracing tool of ultrasound machine to measure the CSA including the full thickness of gastric wall (serosa to serosa).
  - Volume (ml) = 27.0 + 14.6 × CSA (RLD position) – 1.28 × age

8.2.7.1 Antral Grading System (Grades 0–2) [5] (Table 8.2)

8.2.8 Qualitative Versus Quantitative Assessment

- Qualitative assessment determines the appearance of the antrum, wall and its contents.
- Quantitative assessment determines aspiration risk derived from calculated gastric volume using a mathematical model.

Clinical data suggest that a volume of up to 1.5 mL/kg (100 mL for the average adult) is normal in fasted patients [1].

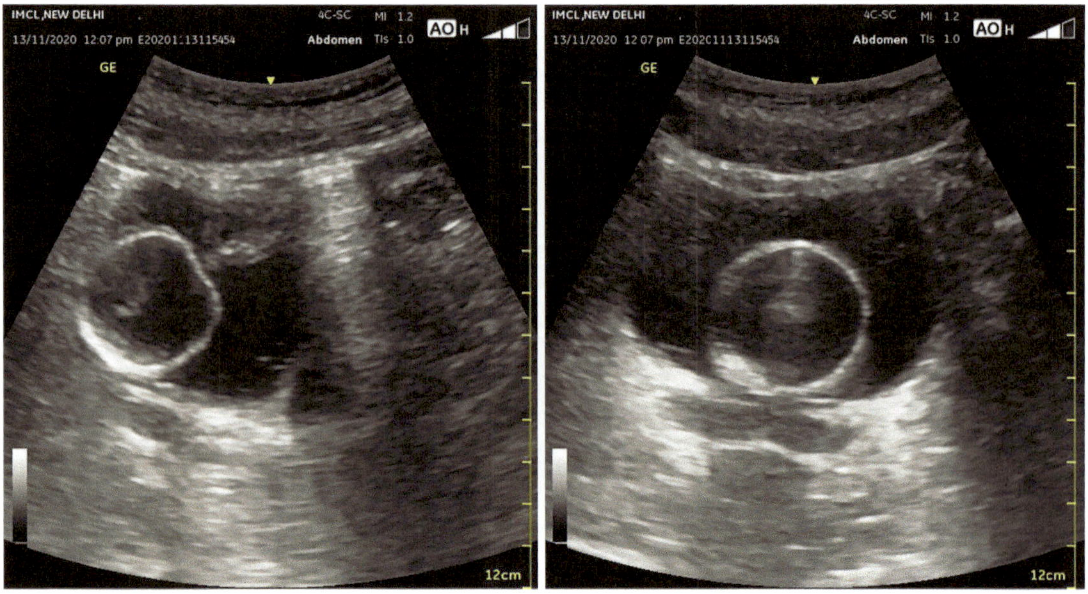

Fig. 8.5 Urinary bladder with foley's catheter in situ (Longitudinal and transverse probe orientation) left image depicts longitudinall scan and right image depicts transverse scan

8.3 Point-of-Care Ultrasound Examination of Urinary Bladder

8.3.1 Introduction

Ultrasound examination of the urinary bladder is an easy, quick, and accurate way to directly visualize and assess the bladder at the bedside.

8.3.2 Indications

1. Assess bladder volume (pre and post-void residual) [6, 7].
2. Confirmation of proper urinary foley catheter placement/troubleshooting malfunctioning foley catheter (Fig. 8.5) [8].
3. Assess bladder pathologies such as bladder stones, ureteral jets (Fig. 8.6), and bladder masses and other causes of hematuria.
4. It is helpful for quick assessment in patients with concern for postrenal acute kidney injury, dilated collecting system, and patients with frequent urinary tract infections.

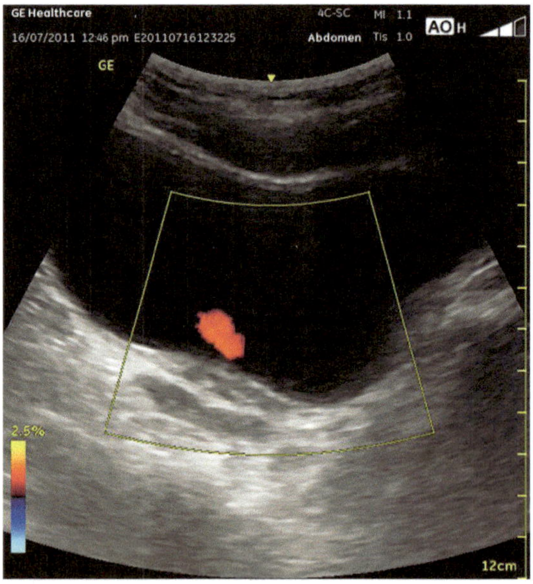

Fig. 8.6 Bladder Ultrasound showing Ureteric jet

8.3.3 Following Topics Will Be Covered in this Description

Use Point-of-Care Bladder ultrasound to:

1. Perform Bladder Ultrasound in a Step-by-Step Fashion.
2. Measure Bladder Volume.
3. Recognize Common Bladder Ultrasound Pathology.

8.3.4 Patient Position

Patient placed in supine position with suprapubic area exposed. Knees can be flexed to soften the anterior abdominal wall.

8.3.5 Ultrasound Probe Selection

Curvilinear Ultrasound Probe with abdominal or renal preset: With its wider footprint, it allows full visualization of the bladder.

8.3.6 Technique [7]

1. Longitudinal view: Place the probe longitudinally in mid-line above the pubic symphysis (Fig. 8.7).
2. The probe marker should point cranially in order to obtain a sagittal view of the bladder.
3. Sweep the probe on either side to examine the lateral borders of the bladder.
4. As the bladder is directly posterior to the pubic symphysis, the ultrasound beam should be directed towards the pelvis, so as to identify the bladder underneath the bone.
5. Transverse view: Rotate the probe 90° to obtain a transverse view and sweep it superior to inferior, so as to image the bladder completely (Fig. 8.7).
6. The shape of the bladder varies depending on anatomical differences and filled-up status of bladder. Its shape can be thought of as spherical, a triangular prism, cylinder (ellipsoid), or cuboid.
7. Surrounding structures including the pubic bone, abdominal cavity, rectum (or bowel gas), uterus (in females), and prostate (in males) are important ultrasound landmarks for the identification and assessment of bladder volume.

8.3.7 Calculation of Bladder Volume

Bladder volume can be estimated using the formula: Height × Width × Length × 0.7

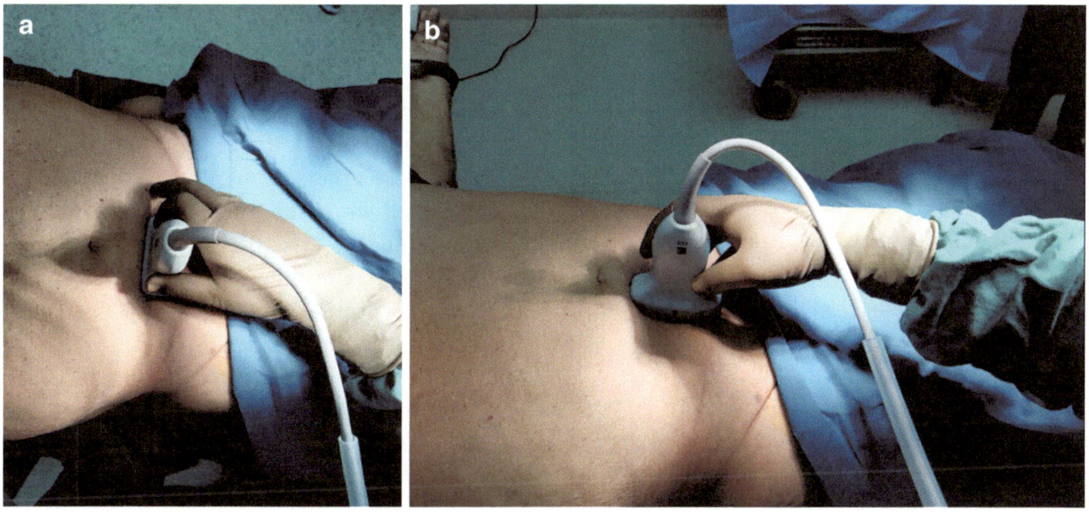

Fig. 8.7 Bladder ultrasound. (**a**) Transverse probe orientation and (**b**) Transverse probe orientation

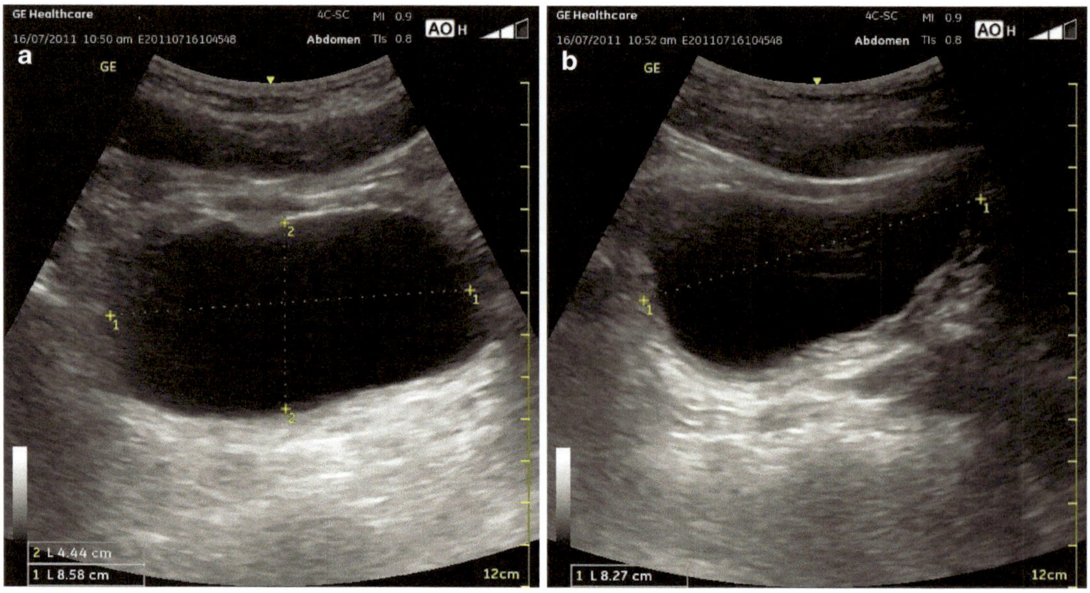

Fig. 8.8 Bladder ultrasound. (**a**) Transverse and (**b**) Longitudinal Views with transverse, longitudinal, and vertical lengths measurements

1. The factor (0.7) in the formula refers to the correction coefficient, that varies with the proposed shape of bladder (unknown–0.72, triangular prism–0.66, ellipsoid–0.81, cuboid–0.89, spherical–0.52).
2. Width and Depth of the bladder are measured in the transverse view (Fig. 8.8).
3. Height (vertical dimension) is measured in the longitudinal view.
4. Both pre- and post-void measurements should be taken to diagnose urinary retention.

   Point-of-care ultrasound can detect foley's catheter, bladder mass, bladder calculus, enlarged prostate, or hematoma.

   Kinking of foley's catheter can cause falsely low urine output which can be easily ruled out using bedside bladder ultrasound.

   Use of color Doppler interrogation at the base of the urinary bladder can show ureteric jets of urine. In the author's opinion, this technique can also be utilized in the differential diagnosis of an oliguric patient.

   This technique is beneficial in the postoperative assessment of renal transplant recipient patients.

8.4 Point-of-Care Ultrasound Examination of Eye

8.4.1 Optic Nerve Sheath Diameter (ONSD)

8.4.1.1 Introduction

1. An elevation of intracranial pressure (ICP) secondary to cerebral edema is a major contributor to morbidity and mortality in trauma, neurosurgical patients, and acute liver failure (ALF) [9].
2. Geriatric surgical populations with multiple comorbidities undergo robotic surgeries with steep Trendelenburg position. Impaired cerebral autoregulation may be compounded by alterations in cerebral homeostasis in this population, due to prolonged duration of surgery in steep head low positioning.
3. ONSD measurement can be a valuable surrogate for invasive monitoring for assessment of ICP in such patients who present with coagulopathy and high ICP [9, 10].
4. Perioperative ICP monitoring may be beneficial for guiding the administration of targeted therapy (i.e., mannitol, hypertonic saline,

hyperventilation, and reverse Trendelenburg positioning) to prevent brain herniation.

5. Ultrasonographic ONSD assessment has proven to be useful for monitoring high ICP in patients with brain injury, idiopathic intracranial hypertension, and spontaneous intracranial hemorrhage [9, 10].

It has proven to be more than 80% sensitive and more than 80% specific in detecting raised ICP by many authors.

Papilledema can be detected as an optic disc bulge into the retina (Fig. 8.11b).

8.4.1.2 Anatomic Correlation

Optic nerve sheath is contiguous with dura mater and its contents are contiguous with the subarachnoid space. Thus, raised ICP leads to an increase in the optic nerve sheath diameter and hence can be used as an indirect correlate for ICP assessment.

It is measured at a point 3.0 mm behind the globe which is believed to be an area of greatest ultrasound contrast. A measurement of up to 5.0 mm is considered a normal ONSD. Elevated ICP should be suspected with an ONSD of more than 5.0 mm.

In patients with suspected raised ICP presenting with symptoms like agitation, sedation, confusion, blurring of vision, conjunctival or periorbital edema, or delayed awakening from anesthesia, ONSD measurement can guide further management [10].

For perioperative use, ONSD should be measured before patient positioning for surgery, as a baseline measurement.

8.4.1.3 Advantages

1. Noninvasive.
2. Can be used in patients with deranged coagulation profile.
3. Easy to master, quick, and reproducible technique and can be done in any patient position.
4. It does not involve extra cost as most of the operating rooms are equipped with point-of-care ultrasound machines.

8.4.1.4 Limitations

1. Acute changes in blood pressures (>10% of initial values) at the time of assessment can theoretically lead to blood pressure-induced changes in ONSD.
2. Cannot be performed in ophthalmic injuries such as ruptured globe.
3. Arguable predictive value in patients with glaucoma.

8.4.1.5 Procedure for Ocular Ultrasound

1. Probe selection.
   (a) A high resolution 7.5–10 MHz or higher linear array ultrasound transducer, held with a pencil grip.
2. Probe—eye interface preparation:
   (a) Cover eyelids with a sterile transparent dressing (Tegaderm) to prevent contamination or trauma during the scan procedure (Fig. 8.9a, b).
   (b) Apply adequate amount of water-based gel (ultrasound gel) onto the interface of tegaderm and ultrasound probe.
   (c) Apply very gentle pressure over the eye, while keeping your hand on the patient's face so as to avoid discomfort/trauma to the eye.
3. Ultrasound image:
   (a) Eye is scanned to assess normal anatomy and landmarks.
   (b) Following structures are visualized from anterior to posterior direction to gain a proper orientation, before proceeding with any measurements (Fig. 8.10) (Table 8.3) [11].
4. Target depth:
   (a) A point 3 mm posterior to the optic disc is considered the target point. Optic nerve is considered to be most distensible and hence representative of rise in ICP at this particular point (Fig. 8.11a, b).
   (b) Optic nerve is seen as anechoic (black) linear structure bounded by hyperechoic (bright) lines, i.e., optic nerve sheath at this level (behind the optic disc).
5. Scan protocol: Ultrasound examination is carried out at two axes perpendicular to each other.

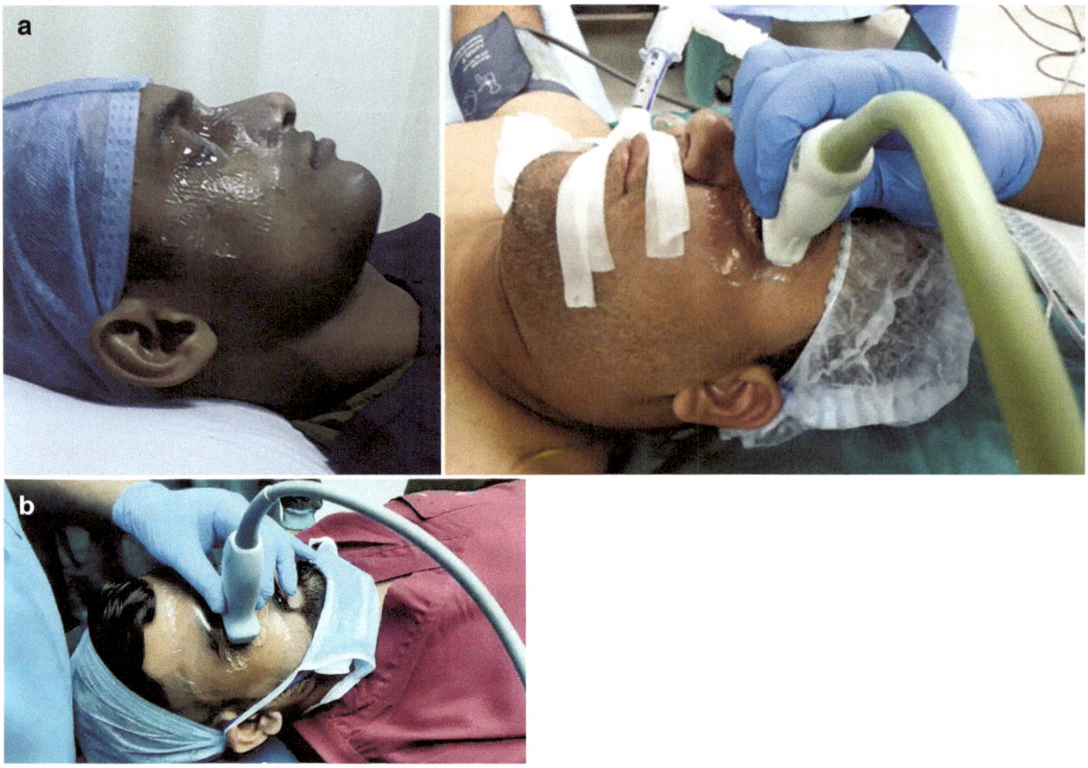

Fig. 8.9 (**a**) Preparation of eye *(tegaderm and jelly application)* and probe placement for Ocular Ultrasound. (**b**) Tegaderm application over eye and position of probe

Fig. 8.10 Ultrasound appearance of Ocular structures

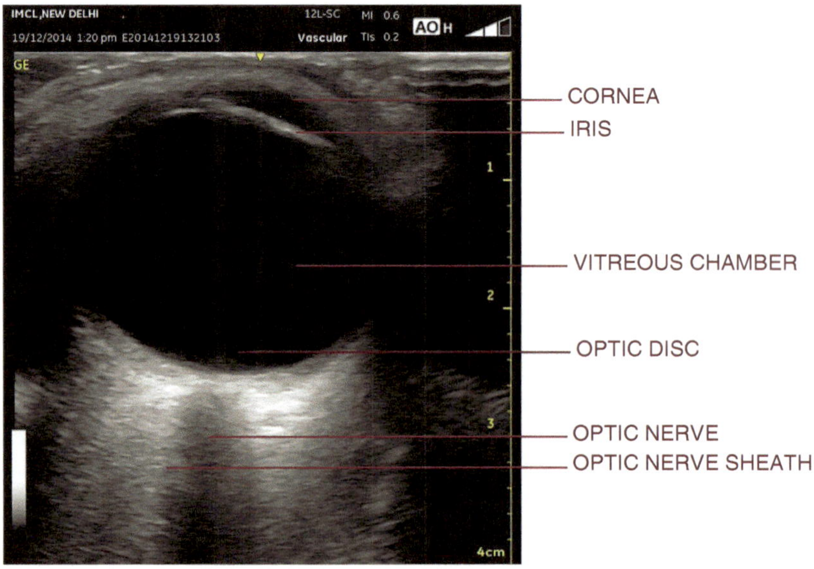

Table 8.3 Ultrasound correlation of Ocular structures

Structure	Echogenicity	Relative USG anatomy (normal eye)
Cornea	Hypoechoic	Thin hypoechoic layer parallel to the eyelid
Anterior chamber	Anechoic	Anechoic area between cornea, iris, and anterior reflection of lens capsule
Lens capsule	Hyperechoic	Curvilinear anterior and posterior lines enclosing anechoic lens
Iris and ciliary body	Hyperechoic	Linear structures extending from the peripheral globe towards lens
Posterior chamber	Anechoic	Hollow spherical structure behind lens capsule
Retina/choroid/sclera (covering layers of eyeball)	Hyperechoic	Spherical covering outlining the eyeball, cannot be differentiated from each other
Retro-orbital region (EOM/orbit)	Heterogeneously hyperechoic	Posterior to globe
Optic nerve with its covering sheath	Anechoic linear structure enclosed in hyperechoic sheath (optic nerve sheath)	Linear structure radiating away from the globe

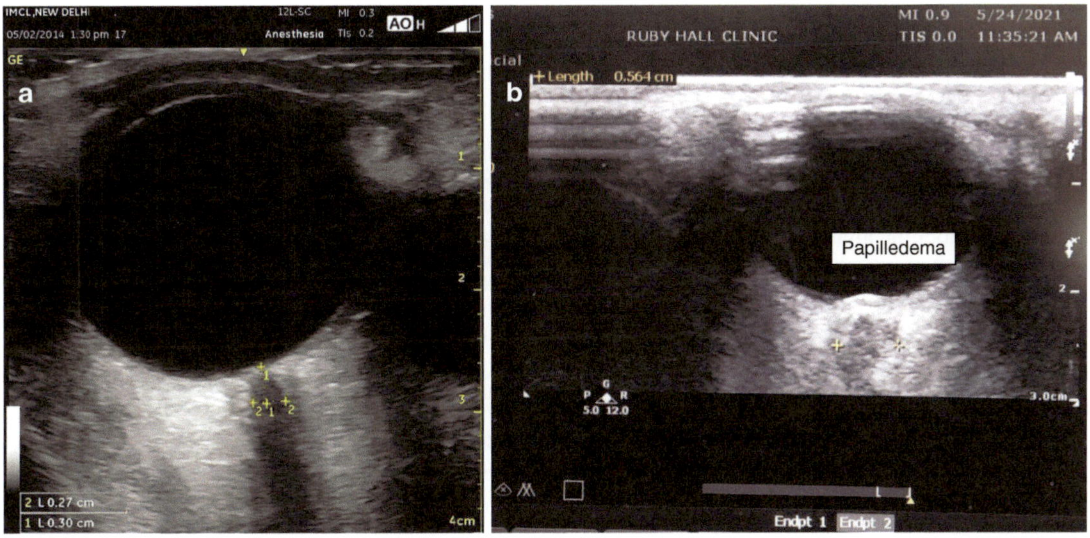

Fig. 8.11 (**a**) Measurement of Optic Nerve Sheath Diameter (0.27 cm in the above figure). (**b**) Papilledema bulging into retina with grossly dilated optic nerve sheath diameter

(c) Horizontal Scan: Probe is placed in a line joining both canthi, i.e., horizontal axis.
(d) Vertical Scan: Probe is placed in a plane perpendicular to first plane, i.e., vertical axis.
(e) Measurements are taken in both axes and a mean of ONSD in both transverse and vertical axes is taken as final reading, representative of ONSD.

8.4.1.6 Conclusion

1. Technique of ONSD measurement by ultrasound of the eye is an established screening tool for predicting raised ICP in trauma patients.
2. The cut-off values of ONSD for predicting a raised ICP vary from 0.48 to 0.59 cm in different studies.

3. A serial change in ONSD is more important than an absolute single value, though this has to be validated.

8.4.2 Consensual Light Reflex [12]

8.4.2.1 Introduction

Ultrasound examination of the eye can be used to assess consensual light reflex in patients who cannot open an ipsilateral eye for pupillary examination because of reasons like trauma, swollen eyelid, perifacial edema, etc.

Probe selection and preparation remain the same as for ONSD measurement.

Patients can be in a sitting or upright position for this procedure (Fig. 8.12).

8.4.2.2 Ultrasound Views

Iris can be visualized in either of the two ways:

1. Transverse/sagittal view:
   (a) Probe is placed transverse or para-sagittal over the eyeball, with ultrasound beam directed towards the back of the eye. Intraocular anatomy can be identified, as mentioned in the table. Iris can be seen as a linear structure extending from the peripheral globe towards the lens. It can be observed as a smiling face, with eyes representing iris and smiling lips representing lenses.

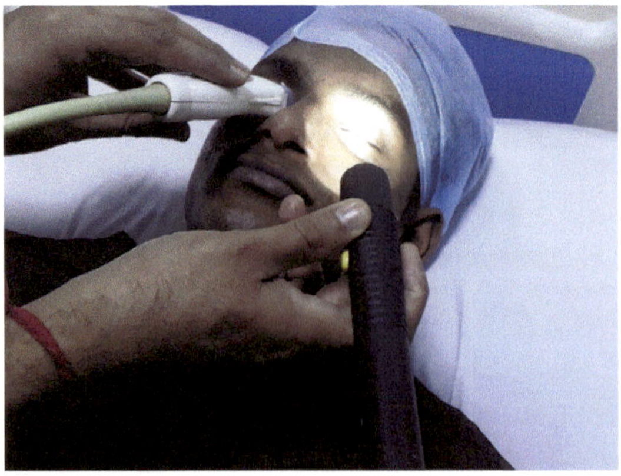

Fig. 8.12 Method to assess consensual light reflex *(probe placed over the eye to be examined and light shown over the opposite eye)*

2. Coronal view:
   (a) Patient is asked to look with his gaze down. Probe is placed over the lower part of the eyeball with ultrasound beam pointing cranially. Iris with pupil can be identified in coronal orientation.

8.4.2.3 Assessment of Consensual Light Reflex

(a) Light is directed to the opposite eye and consensual response in the form of pupillary constriction is observed with ultrasound in the eye to be examined. In both views (transverse and coronal), pupils will be seen to contract. Pupillary activity along with maximum and minimum pupillary diameters can be assessed (Fig. 8.13).

8.4.2.4 Central Retinal Artery Occlusion (CRAO) [13]

Ultrasound examination of the eye can help to diagnose Central Retinal Artery Occlusion in cases of sudden blurring or loss of vision, e.g., after major spine surgery, long-duration prone position ventilation in ARDS patients or intubated patients of COVID-19, etc.

It is observed as a hyperechoic spot (ditzel) in the center of the Optic nerve (Retro-bulbar Spot sign). This hyperechogenic spot represents thrombosis of the Central Retinal Artery. Retinal blood flow occlusion can be confirmed with the use of color Doppler, accuracy of which itself depends upon the angle of insonation of ultrasound beam.

A false positive assessment can be made in case of Optic Nerve Drusen, which is a calcific material deposit in the head of Optic nerve/retina and also presents clinically as blurring or loss of vision.

Ocular ultrasound provides high specificity but low sensitivity to confirm diagnosis of CRAO.

8.4.2.5 Vitreous Versus Retinal Detachment [14]

Ultrasound examination of the eye can help to diagnose and differentiate between retinal and vitreous detachment, in cases of emergency scenarios.

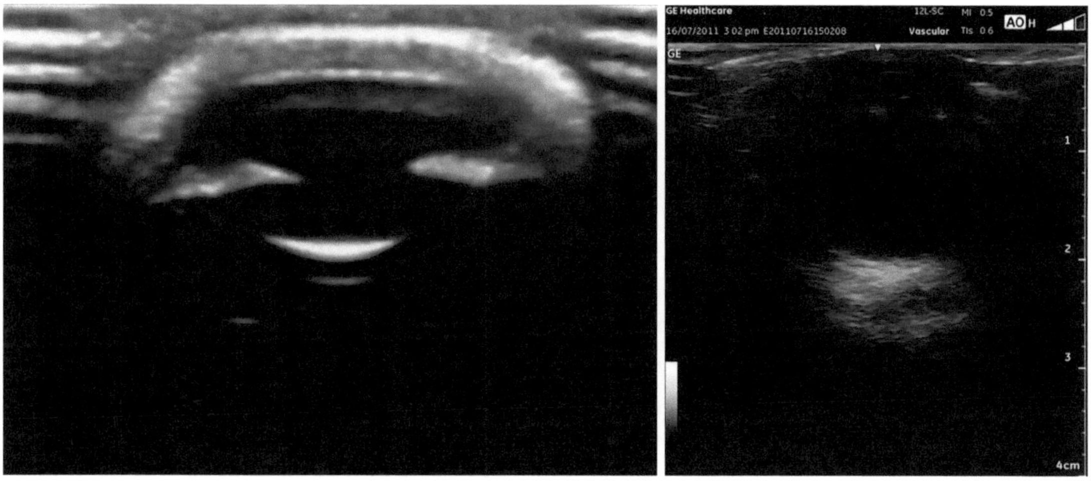

Fig. 8.13 Transverse and Coronal views of the iris (pupil)

Retinal detachment:

Appears as a bright, continuous, smooth and somewhat folded membrane within the vitreous, and freely moving on real-time imaging and is seen coming out of the optic nerve.

Vitreous detachment:

Posterior vitreous detachment is seen as a freely mobile hyperechoic membrane that swirls away from the optic disc with movement of eye.

The mobile membrane is seen to cross the midline, with the optic disc representing the midline, i.e., the line is seen crossing over the optic nerve and not attached to it.

Use of ocular ultrasound can also detect globe rupture and intraocular foreign body which is beyond the scope of this book.

8.5 Point-of-Care Obstetric Ultrasound

8.5.1 Introduction

Point-of-care ultrasound (POCUS) is used to provide an accurate assessment of gestational age, fetal number, presence or absence of cardiac activity, and placental location.

POCUS may also aid in the diagnosis of underlying obstetric pathologies, such as fetal demise, premature rupture of membranes (PROM), and antenatal hemorrhage from abnormal placentation, such as placenta previa or accreta. Additionally, POCUS can be used in the assessment of various other conditions that impact pregnant women, including abdominal pain and maternal trauma.

It is especially useful in health care centers located in remote locations where radiologists are not easily available. Complete obstetric ultrasound is the domain of radiologists.

8.5.2 Anatomical Correlation

The enlarging uterus will displace the normal position of surrounding structures and this can affect the ultrasound appearance of intra-abdominal pathology (Fig. 8.14).

8.5.3 Scope of a POCUS in Second- or Third-Trimester Ultrasound Examination

Obstetric POCUS can aid in assessing the following conditions:

1. Fetal lie and presentation.

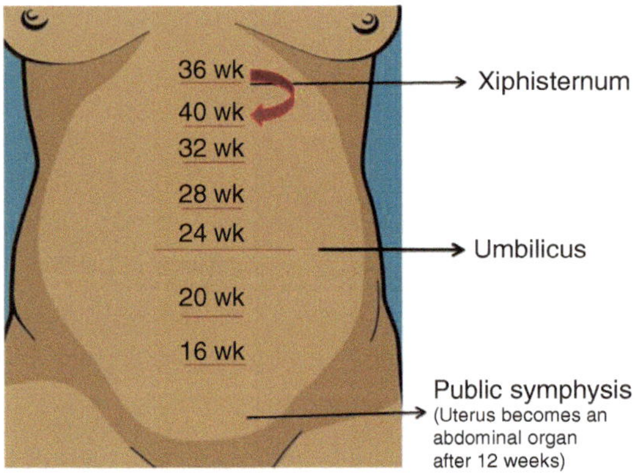

Fig. 8.14 Gravid uterus abdominal assessment on palpation

2. Fetal cardiac activity.
3. Fetal number (singleton, twin, triplet, or higher order multiple gestation).
4. Amniotic fluid volume.
5. Placental localization and assessment.
6. Fetal biometry.

8.5.4 Image Acquisition

Two techniques are generally used for examination

- Transabdominal Ultrasound examination.
- Transvaginal Ultrasound examination.

8.5.5 Scanning Procedure for Transabdominal Examination Technique (Figs. 8.15 and 8.16)

- Patient positioning for ultrasound examination.

  The patient should be supine with the lower abdomen exposed. A full bladder is preferred because it provides an acoustic window to visualize the uterus and adnexa. Patient's upper body and head are slightly inclined and supported by a soft pillow or cushion. In the latter part of pregnancy, a pillow may be placed under the patient's right side to provide left lateral tilt and relieve aortocaval compression.

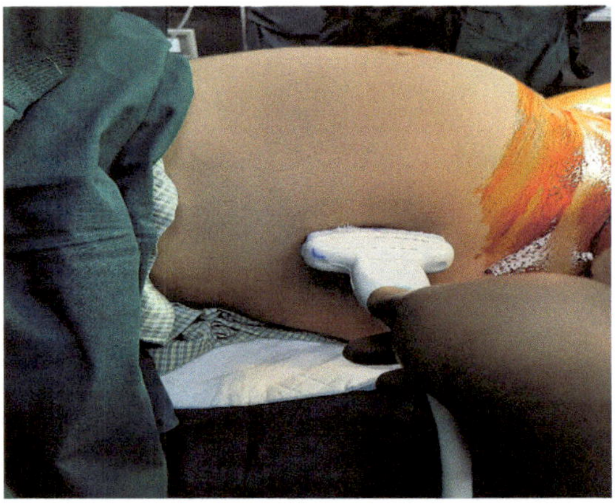

Fig. 8.15 Sagittal scan for obstetric POCUS

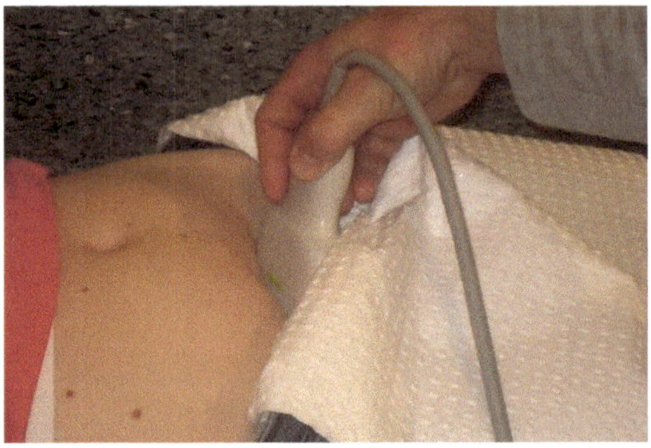

Fig. 8.16 Transverse scan for obstetric POCUS

- Probe selection:

  A low-frequency, curvilinear ultrasound probe (2–5 Hz) is preferred with a wide field of view and adequate penetration for pelvic imaging. An obstetric exam preset should be selected to perform some key measurements and calculations.
- Scan protocol:

  A transverse scan is performed in midline examining in a caudocranial direction. This is followed by a sagittal scan extending from either side and also in the craniocaudal direction.

  An optimal pressure should be maintained while performing this transabdominal ultrasound scan. An excessive probe pressure over a gravid uterus is not desirable.

For a transverse view of the uterus, the transducer is placed immediately above the pubic symphysis with the marker pointing to the patient's right side. A sagittal view is obtained in the same position by rotating the transducer 90 degrees clockwise with the transducer marker pointing cephalad.

- Ultrasound correlation of surrounding anatomy:

  In a transverse orientation, the bladder is seen in the near field with the uterus immediately posterior to it. Within the uterus, the myometrium surrounds the endometrium and is less echogenic by comparison.

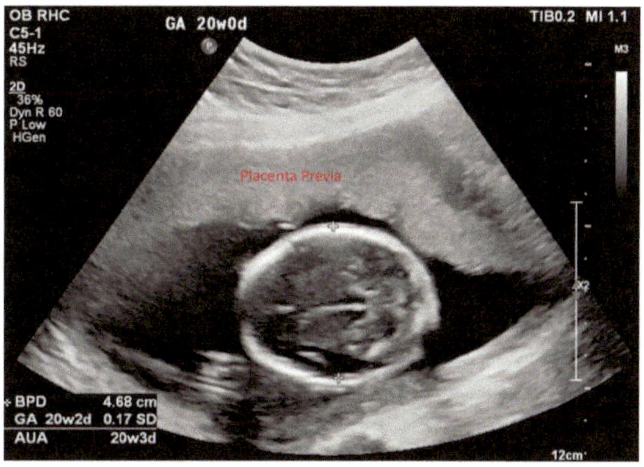

Fig. 8.18 Transverse scan suggestive of placenta adherent to the anterior uterine wall in the lower segment

8.5.6 Applications

- Fetal cardiac activity:

  Quick bedside obstetric ultrasound can detect fetal cardiac activity, fetal heart rate, and thereby fetal distress. This technique is also useful for decision-making in suspected patients of intrauterine fetal death (IUFD). Doppler ultrasound usage is desirable for picking up fetal heart rate.
- Placental localization, fetal lie, and fetal presentation:

  Point-of-care approach can help in anticipating difficult labor as with obstetric ultrasound we can also detect placental localization (placenta previa, placenta accreta, etc.) (Figs. 8.17 and 8.18) fetal lie (Fig. 8.19), fetal number, and fetal presentation with its presenting part (Fig. 8.20), e.g., transverse lie occurs when the fetal spine is positioned perpendicular to the maternal spine (Fig. 8.21). Antenatal detection of placenta previa decreases the fetal and maternal mortality [15].
- Multiple cords around fetus's neck:

  Color Doppler interrogation can detect number of cords around fetus's neck which can be very useful information to the attending pediatrician (Fig. 8.22).

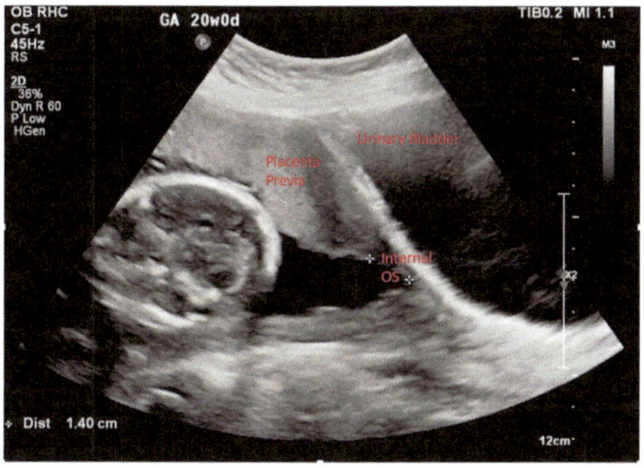

Fig. 8.17 Placenta Previa with anticipated difficult normal labor

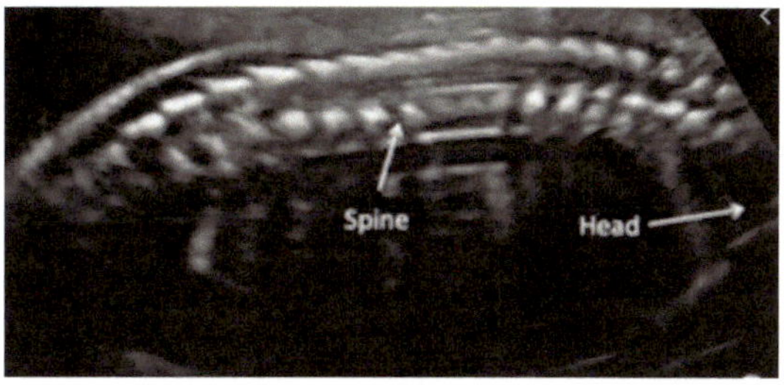

Fig. 8.19 Transverse scan with fetal spine perpendicular to maternal spine suggestive of transverse lie

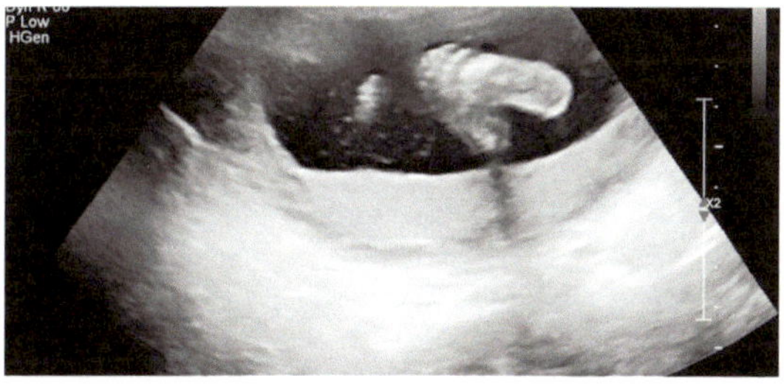

Fig. 8.20 Footling presentation

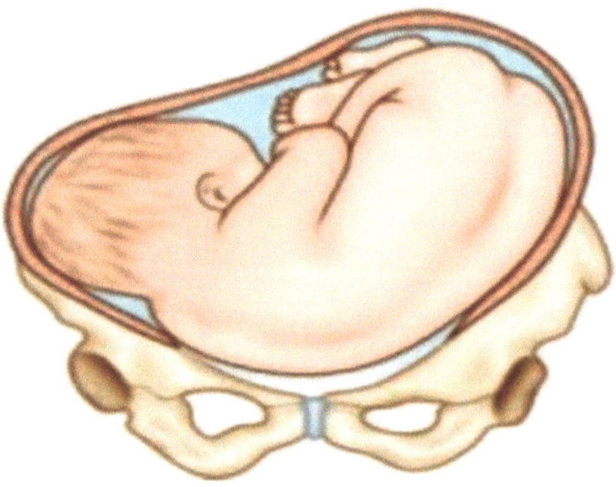

Fig. 8.21 Transverse lie

8.5.7 Limitations

Amniotic fluid volume assessment and fetal biometry including head circumference and femur length is beyond the scope of this chapter.

Questions

1. Which type of resolution is primarily determined by the width of the ultrasound beam?
   A. Axial
   B. Lateral

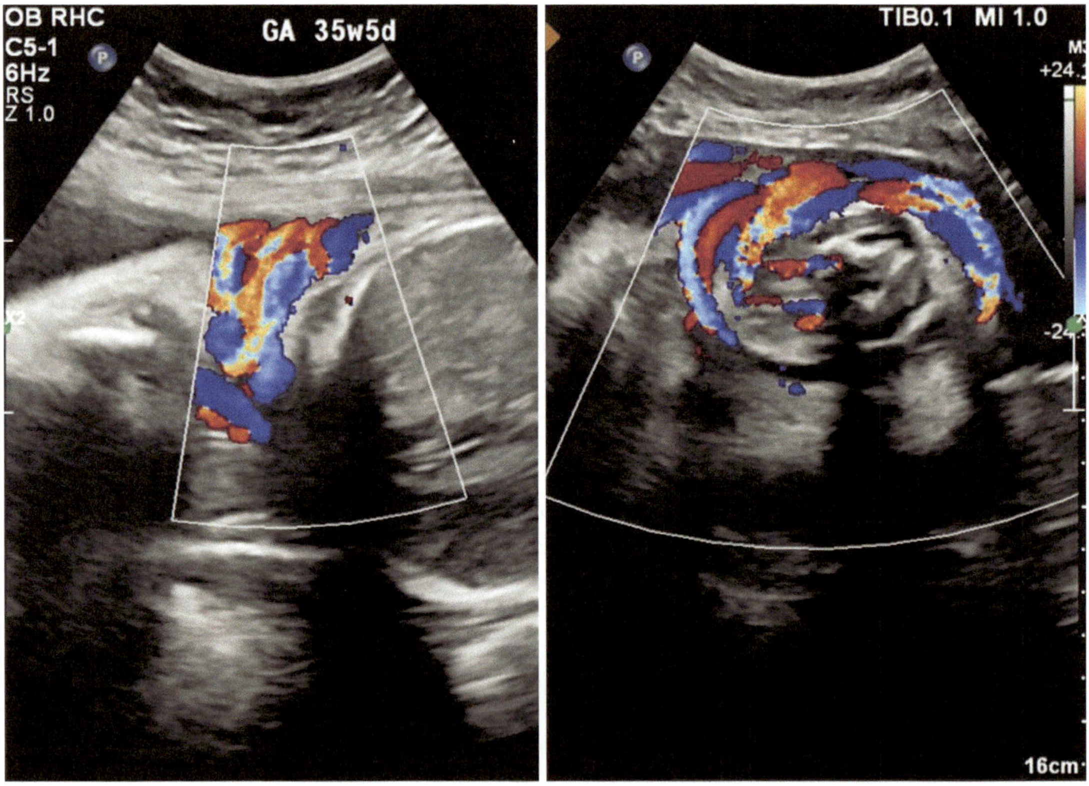

Fig. 8.22 Multiple cords around fetus's neck using color Doppler

C. Elevational
D. Temporal

2. Which transducer type is most commonly used for ocular ultrasound?
A. Curvilinear
B. Intracavitary
C. Linear
D. Phased array

3. How will you adjust the ultrasound settings to improve the quality of transverse scan of urinary bladder, as shown in Fig. 8.23?
A. Decrease depth
B. Increase depth
C. Increase gain
D. Decrease gain

4. Which of the following patient characteristics facilitates ultrasound imaging of the abdominopelvic cavity?
A. Asplenia
B. Subcutaneous emphysema
C. Urine-filled bladder
D. Gas-filled loops of bowel

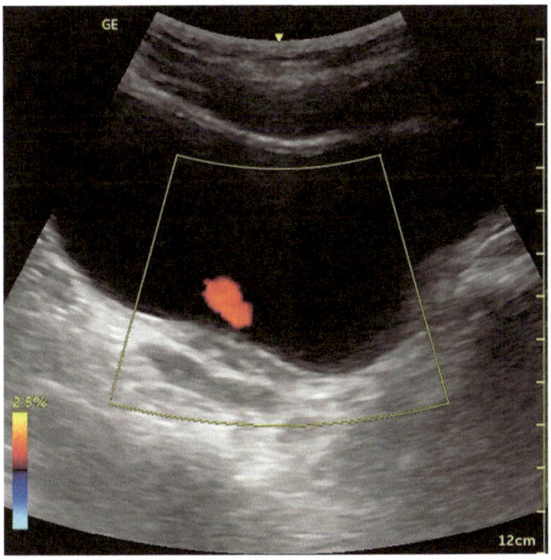

Fig. 8.23 Transverse scan of urinary bladder

5. When point-of-care ultrasound detects peritoneal free fluid in the pelvis, it is always a pathologic finding in both men and women.
A. True
B. False

6. Which of the following artifacts is usually seen posterior or deep to a fluid-filled bladder?
A. Acoustic shadowing
B. Edge artifact
C. Mirror artifact
D. Acoustic enhancement

7. Which ultrasound imaging mode is used to best visualize ureteral jets?
A. A. Two-dimensional grayscale
B. M-mode
C. Spectral Doppler
D. Power Doppler

8. Which of the following formulas is most often used to calculate bladder volume?
A. 0.25 × width × length × height
B. 0.35 × width × length × height
C. 0.50 × width × length × height
D. 0.75 × width × length × height

9. Which dimension best describes prostatic hypertrophy by ultrasound?
A. Transverse diameter > 5 cm
B. Longitudinal diameter > 5 cm
C. Transverse diameter > 2.5 cm
D. Longitudinal diameter > 2.5 cm

10. A 19-year-old man presents with acute unilateral eye pain and visual impairment after sustaining direct trauma to the eye. Which of the following complications of traumatic eye injury would NOT be detected by ocular ultrasound?
A. Globe rupture
B. Retinal detachment
C. Corneal abrasion
D. Hyphema
E. Extraocular motor dysfunction

11. Which of the following is the correct location to measure the optic nerve sheath diameter?
    A. At the optic disc where the optic nerve sheath engages the retina
    B. 1 mm posterior to where the optic nerve sheath engages the retina
    C. 3 mm posterior to where the optic nerve sheath engages the retina
    D. 5 mm posterior to where the optic nerve sheath engages the retina
12. Which of the following statements regarding cleaning and disinfection of ultrasound transducers is TRUE?
    A. If a disposable sterile probe cover is used over an endocavitary transducer during contact with mucous membranes, high-level disinfection is not necessary after disposal of the probe cover.
    B. Alcohol-based disinfecting wipes are recommended after scanning patients with Clostridium difficile infection.
    C. Ultrasound transducers should be autoclaved after use on patients with multidrug-resistant bacteria, especially Pseudomonas aeruginosa.
    D. Transducers that do not make contact with mucous membranes can be cleaned with nonabrasive soap, or low- or intermediate-level disinfectant wipes after each use.
13. Which vessels determine the correct location in visualizing the antrum of stomach when performing a gastric ultrasound examination?
    A. Superior mesenteric vessels
    B. Abdominal aorta
    C. Inferior vena cava
    D. All of the above

References

1. Van de Putte P, Perlas A. Ultrasound assessment of gastric content and volume. Br J Anaesth. 2014;113(1):12–22.
2. Perlas A, Chan VWS, Lupu CM, Mitsakakis N, Hanbidge A. Ultrasound assessment of gastric content and volume. Anesthesiology. 2009;111:82–9.
3. El-Boghdadly K, Wojcikiewicz T, Perlas A. Perioperative point-of-care gastric ultrasound. BJA Education. 2019;19(7):219e226.
4. Sharma G, Jacob R, Mahankali S, Ravindra MN. Preoperative assessment of gastric contents and volume using bedside ultrasound in adult patients: a prospective, observational, correlation study. Indian J Anaesth. 2018;62:753–8.
5. Perlas A, Van de Putte P, Van Houwe P, Chan VW. I-AIM framework for point-of-care gastric ultrasound. Br J Anaesth. 2016 Jan;116(1):7–11.
6. Matsumoto M, Tsutaoka T, Yabunaka K, Handa M, Yoshida M, Nakagami G, et al. Development and evaluation of automated ultrasonographic detection of bladder diameter for estimation of bladder urine volume. PLoS One. 2019;14(9):e0219916.
7. Dicuio M, Pomara G, Fabris FM, Ales V, Dahlstrand C, Morelli G. Measurements of urinary bladder volume: comparison of five ultrasound calculation methods in volunteers. Arch Ital Urol Androl. 2005;77(1):60–2.
8. Garagliano J, Madhok J. POCUS for visulalization and facilitation of urinary catheter placement. POCUS J. 2020;5(2):35.
9. Dubourg J, Javouhey E, Geeraerts T, Messerer M, Kassai B. Ultrasonography of optic nerve sheath diameter for detection of raised intracranial pressure: a systematic review and metaanalysis. Intensive Care Med. 2011;37:1059–68.
10. Lin J-J, Chen AE, Lin EE, Hsia S-H, Chiang M-C, Lin K-L. Point-of-care ultrasound of optic nerve sheath diameter to detect intracranial pressure in neurocritically ill children - a narrative review. Biomed J. 2020;43(3):231–9.
11. Lorente-Ramos RM, Armán JA, Muñoz-Hernández A, Gómez JMG, de la Torre SB. US of the eye made easy: a comprehensive how-to review with ophthalmoscopic correlation. Radiographics. 2012;32:E175–200.
12. Sargsyan AE, Hamilton DR, Melton SL, Amponsah D, Marshall NE, Dulchavsky SA. Ultrasonic evaluation of pupillary light reflex. Crit Ultrasound J. 2009;1:53–7.
13. Stoner-Duncan B, Morris SC. Early identification of central retinal artery occlusion using point-of-care ultrasound. Clin Pract Cases Emerg Med. 2019;3(1):13–5.
14. Gottlieb M, Holladay D, Peksa GD. Point-of-care ocular ultrasound for the diagnosis of retinal detachment: a systematic review and meta-analysis. Acad Emerg Med. 2019;26(8):931–9.
15. American College of Obstetricians and Gynecologists: ACOG committee opinion no. 560: medically indicated late-preterm and early-term deliveries. Obstet Gynecol. 2013;121(4):908–10.

9 POCUS: What does the Future Hold?

Rachel Hui Xuan Chia and Balakrishnan Ashokka

9.1 Introduction

The invention of the stethoscope revolutionized the practice of medicine in the 1800s. Fast forward two centuries later, the era of "Point-of-Care Ultrasound" (POCUS) arrived, heralding a great milestone in the practice of medicine. POCUS is well-established in the field of emergency medicine and trauma management. It is emerging as a valuable tool in a wide range of applications including procedural guidance for general and regional anesthesia, vascular access, decision-making in intensive care, perioperative care, goal-directed management, and therapeutics. Now, real-time ultrasound-guided assessment of inpatients in the wards is within reach for many clinicians. Medical schools are also including ultrasound interpretation skills in their curriculum. In the next decade, it would be unsurprising to see POCUS become the new standard of care. As advances in imaging technology develop further in parallel with the continued upgrading of ultrasound skills of clinicians, the future of POCUS could bring about enhancements in visualization and accuracy, while minimizing the cognitive load on the operator. The future of POCUS can be simply summarized in a few words: *"What is advanced today, may be basic tomorrow."*

R. H. X. Chia (✉) · B. Ashokka
Department of Anaesthesia, National University Health System, Singapore, Singapore
e-mail: rachel_hx_chia@nuhs.edu.sg

9.2 Artificial Intelligence

Imagine a world where the expertise of a doctor could be supported by the power of computer-assisted decision-making. The combined efforts of multiple experts in the field of computer science, medicine, robotics, and more have made this a reality. There is a plethora of reasons why traditional technologies in healthcare should embrace artificial intelligence (AI). In the field of imaging technology, AI has an extraordinary ability to not only make sense of images but also reveal to the clinician, potentially hidden patterns that would evade even the most highly trained human eye. In other words, AI is training the computer to see what the human eye cannot.

9.2.1 Deep Learning

The demand for greater accuracy and more objective imaging assessments have led to the incorporation of deep learning technology into the field of ultrasonography. Deep learning is a machine learning technique where artificial neural networks, inspired by the human brain, are able to make sense of data themselves. As one of the top ten breakthrough technologies of 2013 [1], deep learning has solidified its position as the leading machine learning tool in imaging analysis [2]. In 2020, the US Food and Drug Administration approved the first cardiac ultrasound automated

A. Chakraborty, B. Ashokka (eds.), *A Practical Guide to Point of Care Ultrasound (POCUS)*,
https://doi.org/10.1007/978-981-16-7687-1_9

software [3], which uses deep learning technology to guide the operator to acquire images of diagnostic quality. It accomplishes this via real-time prescriptive guidance of the user's hand motions and transducer positions to obtain the desired image [4]. Once this image is captured, the ejection fraction can be automatically calculated. With this novel technology, even novice operators with no formal training in ultrasound will be able to obtain high-quality cardiac images, allowing rapid assessment and decision-making.

Automated software has also been deployed in other ultrasound applications such as to identify and track endocardial structures to calculate indices of myocardial function in commercially available platforms (HeartModelA.I., Philips Healthcare) [5, 6]. In the field of regional anesthesia, identification of nerves can be considered one of the more challenging tasks for the novice provider and image recognition technology could potentially be incorporated into ultrasound-guided regional nerve blocks. A machine learning model has been employed in ultrasound images of the femoral nerve and brachial plexus [7, 8]. Besides nerve identification, AI-powered systems in ultrasound have also been deployed to increase the accuracy of spinal landmark identification for complex anatomical presentations in neuraxial anesthesia (uSINE™) [9]. Indeed, AI allows clinicians to look forward to exciting future applications in clinical use, as well as in regional anesthesia training.

Despite its unique capabilities in refining diagnostic accuracy and sensitivity in medical imaging, users of AI-powered systems need to be cognizant of certain potential perils. A study on screening mammograms showed that deep learning is no more sensitive than radiologists in detecting cancer, but was consistently less specific, i.e., higher false-positive rates [10]. The powerful ability of AI to detect minor changes in images may potentially be a double-edged sword, as increased sensitivity leads to overdiagnosis of subclinical diseases with minimal impact on morbidity and mortality. Undoubtedly, AI-powered systems have promising clinical applications with the potential to improve public health. However, more research into finetuning of its capabilities in detecting lesions is warranted to prevent overdiagnosis and wastage of resources and man-hours.

9.3 Handheld Ultrasound (HHU)

In the field of POCUS-enabled healthcare advancements, the demand for "pocket sized" devices is increasing [11]. The hallmark of HHU is its accessibility, making it readily available to virtually every patient in the hospital that is limited by the need for large bulky equipment and perpetually busy qualified ultrasound technologists. This complements and enhances any point-of-care ultrasound assessment. A variety of handheld devices with different characteristics are currently available in the market. Some products have single or multiple probes, while some have the ability to stream images onto a mobile device. A few devices have incorporated AI systems, aiding the novice operator to obtain high-quality images and estimate certain measurements of interest, such as ejection fraction in echocardiography [12].

Traditionally, the piezoelectric effect is the cornerstone of ultrasound, which is commonplace in the transducers of heavier cart-based ultrasound machines. Few disadvantages of piezoelectric technology include high cost of production and need for separate probes for the analysis of high and low frequencies [13]. The inherent limitations of piezoelectric technology have inspired the development of a novel *ultrasound-on-chip technology*. Known as Capacitive Micromachined Ultrasound Transducers (CMUT), piezoelectric crystals are replaced with a single silicon chip, which converts electrical currents into ultrasound waves [12]. The advantage of using an ultrasound chip is its lower cost of production and ability to analyze a wider range of frequencies without the use of multiple probes. In addition, images can be displayed on a mobile device, further enhancing portability (Butterfly iQ) [13].

Image quality in HHU has been an area of concern as some historical evidence suggests that they are slightly inferior to traditional standalone devices [12, 14–16]. HHUs classically utilize 2D and color Doppler imaging and lack the capability to visualize all abnormalities. Indeed, image quality in HHU may be inadequate in performing a comprehensive ultrasound examination; however, users need to understand that the use of POCUS is to function as an adjunct to physical examination in order to answer a focused clinical question. In a systematic review comparing handheld ultrasound with high-end ultrasound systems, the authors showed that there was a good overall correlation when the use of HHU is limited to a distinct focused clinical question [16]. This consensus is supported by several studies that have also found HHU to be a valuable tool in the various settings, displaying images of sufficient quality to detect ascites, hydronephrosis and even screening for abdominal aorta aneurysms and measuring aortic diameters [17–22].

In the field of obstetric anesthesia, the placement of epidural catheters for labor analgesia traditionally relies on the palpation of body surface landmarks. First pass success rates with palpation alone have been reported to be as low as 20% [23]. In the first study of its kind, Seligman et al. studied the accuracy of a HHU device (Accuro, Rivanna Medical, Charlottesville, VA) (Fig. 9.1) in estimating depth to epidural space compared to using the conventional method of Tuohy epidural needle depth (depth to loss of resistance to saline) [24]. The authors found that the HHU accurately estimated the epidural depth, with a mean difference of −0.61 cm [95% CI, −0.79 to −0.44] compared to needle depth, and furthermore showed a high first pass rate of 87% with HHU-guided identification of the lumbar interspace. In fact, the Accuro HHU has also shown that it is comparable to a console ultrasound machine in estimating epidural depth [25].

9.4 Contrast-Enhanced Ultrasound (CEUS)

The development of Contrast-Enhanced Ultrasound (CEUS) could be a major paradigm shift in the field of imaging. CEUS was first introduced in the 1960s, where the injection of agitated saline bubbles produced a detectable signal change on ultrasound [25]. Decades of research have culminated in the discovery of novel ultrasound contrast agents (UCA), which are microbubbles of perfluorocarbon, nitrogen gas, or sulfur hexafluoride stabilized in a phospholipid membrane [26]. The backscatter of ultrasound waves is enhanced when UCA microbubbles are injected into the vasculature, which provides information on microvascular blood flow and tissue perfusion. The analysis of microvasculature therefore confers a benefit when compared to Doppler ultrasound [27, 28].

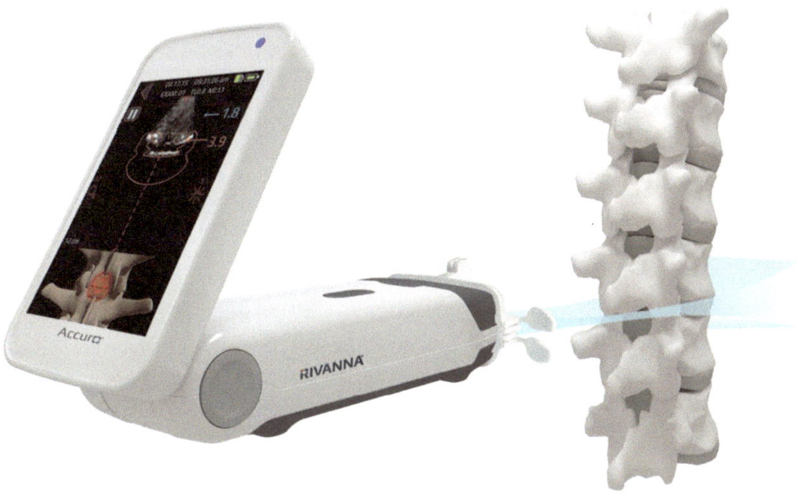

Fig. 9.1 The Accuro spinal navigation system. (Reproduced with permission, Accuro, Rivanna Medical, Charlottesville, VA)

With contrast agents no longer restricted to computed tomography (CT), magnetic resonance imaging (MRI), and angiography, the application of CEUS in various clinical settings could benefit patients significantly. Major advantages of CEUS include its low cost, radiation sparing effects, bedside accessibility, lack of need for sedation, and lack of nephrotoxicity. In addition, its lack of iodine content, which is present in other contrast media avoids the risk of thyroid function impairment [29]. Contrast agents are foreign materials and although it has a good safety profile, hypersensitivity reactions have been reported in about 0.002% of abdominal studies [30, 31]. The incidence of hypersensitivity in CEUS is lower than the use of iodine contrast in CT and comparable to the use of Gadolinium contrast in MRI [31]. The main contraindications for the use of CEUS include patients with known coronary artery disease, severe arrhythmias, right-to-left shunts, severe pulmonary hypertension, prosthetic valves, and patients with acute respiratory distress syndrome [32].

CEUS has been widely used in abdominal and cardiac imaging for decades throughout Asia and Europe. Yet, it was only in recent years, its use was approved by the US Food and Drug Administration for diagnostic liver imaging in adults and children [33]. The characterization of liver lesions has been one of the most well-established clinical applications of CEUS, with several published reports claiming its success [34–36] (Fig. 9.2). Various studies have shown that CEUS has an excellent accuracy in detecting liver lesions, with a reported 87–91% sensitivity [37]. Contrast-enhanced imaging of liver lesions were found to be related to phagocytosis of the UCA microbubbles [38]. CEUS is highly accurate in differentiating benign and malignant liver lesions as well, with a sensitivity of 96–97.2% and a negative predictive value (NPV) of 94.1–98.5% [39]. With such remarkable results in

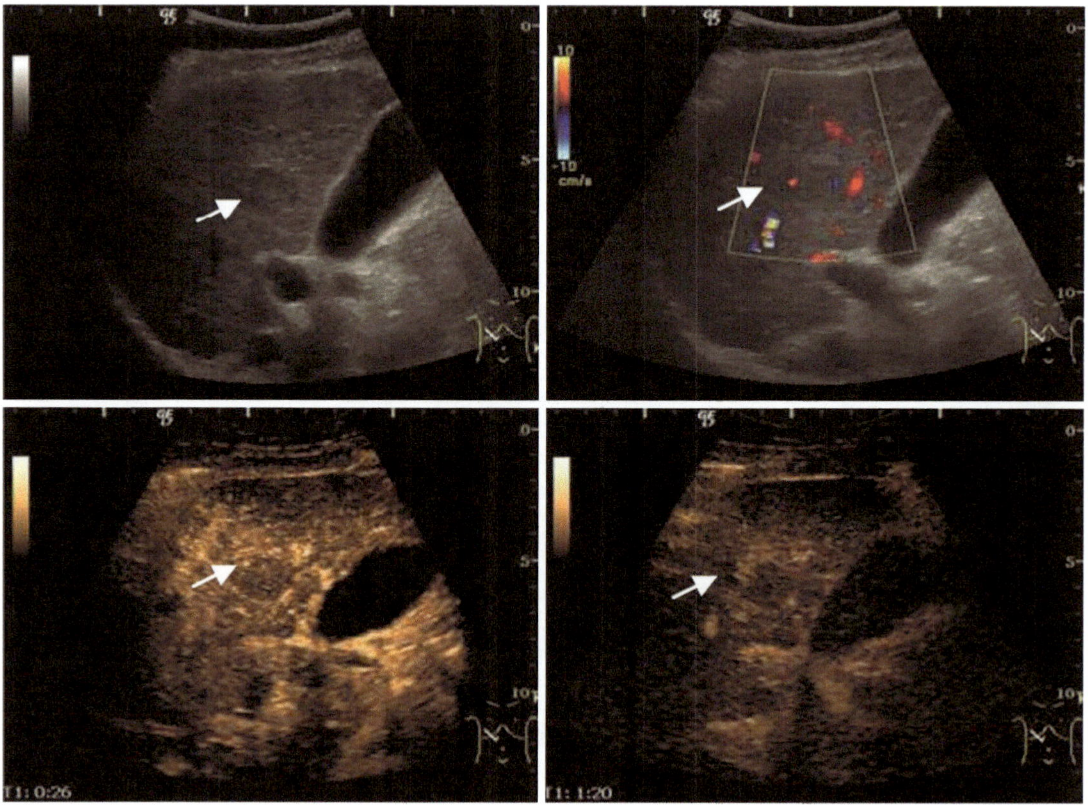

Fig. 9.2 "File:Ultrasonography of a dysplastic nodule.jpg" by R. Badea and Simona Ioanitescu, CC BY 3.0

liver imaging, CEUS has found its way into a wide variety of non-hepatic imaging applications, examples of which are the detection and differentiation of kidney lesions, clearer delineation of pancreatic cancer and the adjacent vessels, evaluation of aortic or other vascular abnormalities, and the evaluation solid organ injuries in blunt abdominal trauma [29]. A novel territory within the field of POCUS, CEUS has gained popularity in the trauma setting, where it was able to detect avascular laceration planes as well as pseudoaneurysms and active bleeding [40, 41]. The expansion of the use of CEUS in emergency medicine has recently garnered the interest of intensivists caring for critically ill COVID-19 patients. A case report by Yusuf et al. proved CEUS to be a useful tool in point-of-care lung ultrasound. With its well-known ability to distinguish perfused from avascular tissues, CEUS was able to identify microvascular lung infarcts classically seen in COVID-19 patients with immune-mediated thrombotic events. The authors also showed that the degree of lung infarction correlated with clinical status, providing relevant prognostic and diagnostic information to guide management [42].

CEUS is emerging as a promising imaging technique for POCUS applications and more research into its diagnostic accuracy, healthcare costs, and patient safety profile is warranted to prove its value in various clinical settings. These techniques when developed into critical care protocols can help in early diagnosis, timely initiation of definitive management, and more importantly minimize transfer of critical ill ventilated patients to radiology suites. Where dissemination of infective pathogens is a concern, the use of these techniques help to prevent the occurrences of super spreader events from patient transit within the hospital.

9.5 Tele-Ultrasound

Tele-medicine has been on the rise in the past few decades, but the recent COVID-19 pandemic has given it a major boost in popularity, as healthcare systems become overwhelmed throughout the world. Tele-medicine offers healthcare providers a unique opportunity to provide remote consults, and at the same time increase the opportunity for patients globally to receive proper assessments and diagnoses. As data transmission technology in healthcare grows in parallel with the miniaturization of ultrasound devices, this has spurred the development of the tele-ultrasound practice. Tele-ultrasound could potentially eliminate a major limitation of traditional ultrasound, as with the aid of a remote expert interpreter, the lack of image interpretation skills may no longer pose a problem [43].

The bulk of the tele-ultrasound application can be found in the field of obstetric and fetal medicine, majority of which relates to the confirmation of pregnancy, assessing for pregnancy-related complications, and monitoring fetal growth [44]. In recent years, the scope of tele-ultrasound has reached various clinical applications involving echocardiography to imaging of trauma patients as well as guided procedures [45, 46]. The assessment of trauma patients relies heavily on physical examination supplemented by the use of ultrasound for rapid diagnosis and decision-making. The Focused Assessment with Sonography for Trauma (FAST) scan is traditionally performed by emergency medicine physicians to rapidly diagnose life-threatening injuries requiring immediate management. Recently, systems have been developed to enable ultrasound-novice paramedics to perform prehospital ultrasound scans in trauma victims and obtain FAST images under the remote direction of emergency medicine physicians, allowing the medical team to obtain an early diagnosis and prepare for any emergency procedures [47].

In the most extreme example of a remote location, astronauts aboard the International Space Station (ISS) with limited ultrasound training were guided by remote experts in the Mission Control Center (MCC) to aid the diagnosis of several medical ailments commonly occurring in crew members [48]. Examples of which are musculoskeletal pain secondary to joint contusions or effusions, trauma injuries when crew members engage in heavy-duty tasks, and even ocular injuries. Eye foreign bodies are a common problem as small particles float freely in space. It was reported that an untrained astronaut had used ultrasound to perform an eye examination with remote guidance from the MCC, and was capable of visualizing the anatomical structures of the globe, iris, and pupil [49].

As telecommunication systems and data transmission technologies improve, tele-ultrasound could potentially be ubiquitous around the globe. The remote interpretation of ultrasound images requires software, hardware, and video-conferencing platforms which are costly and could be a major barrier in implementing tele-ultrasound in developing countries [50]. While video streaming might require higher Internet streaming capacities, short video clips and popular 1 min social media and networking platforms could help in rapid transmission of video content and timely interpretation by the experts. In low resource settings and remote hospitals, there has been some evidence of its clinical feasibility in emergency medicine however more rigorous research is needed to evaluate its diagnostic accuracy and effectiveness before tele-ultrasound can be fully utilized with confidence [51].

9.6 Conclusion

The introduction of POCUS has revolutionized the process of bringing diagnostic imaging possibilities and clinical interpretation is possible in a more time-sensitive manner. The advances in technology and data processing have helped in the development of pattern recognition software that enhance the accuracy of decision-making through large data points from machine learning. Applying these could enhance the safety of healthcare, minimizing errors and potentially reducing healthcare costs. Bulkier imaging equipment and long wait in obtaining specialist and expert opinions can now be supplemented with portable, hand help and modern technology. With the advent of enhanced connectivity help is now available rapidly. These advances in ultrasound technology and the application of POCUS are a welcome promise of the near future with scope for reduction in patient morbidity and mortality.

Self-Test MCQ (20 Questions)

1. Fluid appears _____ on the ultrasound screen
   A. White
   B. Black
   C. Grey
   D. Not seen
2. The linear probe has a range of frequency of
   A. 2–5 MHz
   B. 4–7 MHz
   C. 5–10 MHz
   D. 10–15 MHz
3. If the image on the monitor screen is too dark, you should
   A. Increase depth
   B. Use more ultrasound gel
   C. Decrease gain
   D. Increase gain
4. Which of the following is a piezoelectric material?
   A. Nickel
   B. Tourmaline
   C. Iron
   D. None of the above
5. Speed of ultrasound is the fastest when traveling through
   A. Bone
   B. Air
   C. Water
   D. Muscle
6. Properties of sound waves include
   A. Amplitude
   B. Frequency
   C. Wavelength
   D. All of the above
7. The main factor affecting attenuation is
   A. Scattering
   B. Divergence
   C. Absorption
   D. Reflection
8. Which of the following are not reported benefits of using artificial intelligence (AI) in ultrasonography?
   A. Improved survival rates
   B. Enhanced diagnostic accuracy
   C. Wide clinical applications
   D. Image capture assistance

9. Which of the following statements regarding artificial intelligence (AI) is FALSE?
   A. Deep learning technology is one of the machine learning techniques used in AI
   B. AI-powered systems may lower false-positive rates in cancer detection
   C. Untrained operators may obtain diagnostic quality imaging
   D. AI allows automated calculation of cardiac ejection fraction
10. Which of the following statements regarding handheld ultrasound is FALSE?
    A. Piezoelectric crystals have a lower cost of production compared to Capacitive Micromachined Ultrasound Transducers (CMUT)
    B. Devices may use single or multiple probes
    C. 2D imaging is classically used
    D. Epidural depth is one of the parameters that can be measured
11. Which of the following is not a benefit of handheld ultrasound compared to traditional cart-based ultrasound?
    A. Low cost
    B. Improved image quality
    C. Portable
    D. Reduced examination time
12. Current ultrasound contrast agents in the market consist of
    A. Hydrofluorocarbons
    B. Agarose gel
    C. Galactose and air
    D. Sulfur hexafluoride
13. The incidence of hypersensitivity reactions with the use of contrast-enhanced ultrasound (CEUS) is reported to be
    A. 2%
    B. 0.2%
    C. 0.002%
    D. 0.0002%
14. Which of the following is not a contraindication of contrast-enhanced ultrasound (CEUS)
    A. Coronary artery disease
    B. Acute respiratory distress syndrome
    C. Acute kidney injury
    D. Arrhythmias
15. Which of the following statements regarding contrast-enhanced ultrasound (CEUS) is FALSE?
    A. The US was the first country to approve the use of CEUS
    B. CEUS may be used in pediatric patients
    C. POCUS lung ultrasound may benefit from CEUS in detecting lung infarcts
    D. CEUS is highly accurate in differentiating benign and malignant lesions
16. The gold standard for diagnosis of hepatocellular carcinoma (HCC) is
    A. Computed tomography (CT) perfusion
    B. Liver biopsy
    C. Contrast-enhanced ultrasound (CEUS)
    D. Magnetic resonance imaging (MRI)
17. In contrast-enhanced ultrasound of the liver, microbubbles are taken up by
    A. Sinusoid cells
    B. Kupffer cells
    C. Stellate cells
    D. Hepatocytes
18. Which of the following regarding POCUS lung ultrasound is FALSE?
    A. B-lines are artifacts caused by acoustic impedance due to the underlying lung
    B. Loss of lung sliding is sensitive to pneumothorax
    C. In M-mode, the "barcode" sign suggests a pneumothorax
    D. "Lung point" is the most specific sign of pneumothorax
19. Which of the following regarding the FAST exam is true?
    A. It leads to few diagnostic peritoneal lavages
    B. FAST can be repeated for serial examinations
    C. It is safe for use in pregnant and pediatric patients
    D. All of the above
20. Regarding the FAST exam
    A. FAST is more sensitive in obese patients
    B. Solid organ injuries are easily identified
    C. Peritoneal free fluid will not be detected until more than 500 ml is present
    D. Diagnostic accuracy differs significantly between radiologists and non-radiologists

References

1. Wang G. A perspective on deep imaging. IEEE Access. 2016;4:8914–24.
2. Liu S, Wang Y, Yang X, Lei B, Liu L, Li SX, Ni D, Wang T. Deep learning in medical ultrasound analysis: a review. Engineering. 2019;5(2):261–75. https://doi.org/10.1016/j.eng.2018.11.020. ISSN 2095-8099
3. U.S. Food and Drug Administration. FDA authorizes marketing of first cardiac ultrasound software that uses artificial intelligence to guide user. 2020. https://www.fda.gov/news-events/press-announcements/fda-authorizes-marketing-first-cardiac-ultrasound-software-uses-artificial-intelligence-guide-user
4. Cheema BS, Walter J, Narang A, Thomas JD. Artificial intelligence-enabled POCUS in the COVID-19 ICU: a new spin on cardiac ultrasound. JACC Case Rep. 2021;3(2):258–63. https://doi.org/10.1016/j.jaccas.2020.12.013.
5. Volpato V, Mor-Avi V, Narang A, et al. Automated, machine learning-based, 3D echocardiographic quantification of left ventricular mass. Echocardiography. 2019;36(2):312–9. https://doi.org/10.1111/echo.14234.
6. Medvedofsky D, Mor-Avi V, Byku I, et al. Three-dimensional echocardiographic automated quantification of left heart chamber volumes using an adaptive analytics algorithm: feasibility and impact of image quality in nonselected patients. J Am Soc Echocardiogr. 2017;30(9):879–85. https://doi.org/10.1016/j.echo.2017.05.018.
7. Huang C, Zhou Y, Tan W, et al. Applying deep learning in recognizing the femoral nerve block region on ultrasound images. Ann Transl Med. 2019;7(18):453. https://doi.org/10.21037/atm.2019.08.61.
8. Smistad E, Johansen KF, Iversen DH, Reinertsen I. Highlighting nerves and blood vessels for ultrasound-guided axillary nerve block procedures using neural networks. J Med Imaging (Bellingham). 2018;5(4):044004. https://doi.org/10.1117/1.JMI.5.4.044004.
9. KKH collaborates with NUS to develop world-first AI-powered system to enhance accuracy of spinal anaesthesia. https://www.kkh.com.sg/news/research/kkh-collaborates-with-nus-to-develop-world-first-ai-powered-system-to-enhance-accuracy-of-spinal-anaesthesia
10. Becker AS, Marcon M, Ghafoor S, Wurnig MC, Frauenfelder T, Boss A. Deep learning in mammography: diagnostic accuracy of a multipurpose image analysis software in the detection of breast cancer. Investig Radiol. 2017;52:434–40.
11. Baran JM, Webster JG. Design of low-cost portable ultrasound systems. In Annual International Conference of the IEEE Engineering in Medicine and Biology Society, IEEE; 2009. pp. 792–795.
12. Baribeau Y, Sharkey A, Chaudhary O, Krumm S, Fatima H, Mahmood F, et al. Handheld point-of-care ultrasound probes: the new generation of POCUS. J Cardiothorac Vasc Anesth. 2020;34(11):3139–45. https://doi.org/10.1053/j.jvca.2020.07.004.
13. Malik AN, Rowland J, Haber BD, et al. The use of handheld ultrasound devices in emergency medicine. Curr Emerg Hosp Med Rep. 2021;9(3):73–81. https://doi.org/10.1007/s40138-021-00229-6.
14. Galusko V, Bodger O, Ionescu A. A systematic review of pocket-sized imaging devices: small and mighty? Echo Res Pract. 2018;5(4):113–38.
15. Zardi EM, Franceschetti E, Giorgi C, Palumbo A, Franceschi F. Accuracy and performance of a new handheld ultrasound machine with wireless system. Sci Rep. 2019;9(1):14599. https://doi.org/10.1038/s41598-019-51160-6.
16. European Society of Radiology (ESR). ESR statement on portable ultrasound devices. Insights Imaging. 2019;10(1):89. https://doi.org/10.1186/s13244-019-0775-x.
17. Barreiros AP, Cui XW, Ignee A, De Molo C, Pirri C, Dietrich CF. EchoScopy in scanning abdominal diseases: initial clinical experience. Z Gastroenterol. 2014;52:269–75.
18. Stock KF, Klein B, Steubl D, Lersch C, Heemann U, Wagenpfeil S, Eyer F, Clevert D-A. Comparison of a pocket-size ultrasound device with a premium ultrasound machine: diagnostic value and time required in bedside ultrasound examination. Abdom Imaging. 2015;40:2861–6.
19. Andrea S, Giovanna L, Pietro C, Luca F. Teaching echoscopy for the early diagnosis of ascites in cirrhosis: assessment of an objective structured clinical examination (OSCE). J Ultrasound. 2017;20:123–6.
20. Esposito R, Ilardi F, Schiano Lomoriello V, Sorrentino R, Sellitto V, Giugliano G, Esposito G, Trimarco B, Galderisi M. Identification of the main determinants of abdominal aorta size: a screening by pocket size imaging device. Cardiovasc Ultrasound. 2017;15:2.
21. Bonnafy T, Lacroix P, Desormais I, Labrunie A, Marin B, Leclerc A, Oueslati A, Rollé F, Vignon P, Aboyans V. Reliability of the measurement of the abdominal aortic diameter by novice operators using a pocket-sized ultrasound system. Arch Cardiovasc Dis. 2013;106:644–50.
22. Dijos M, Pucheux Y, Lafitte M, Réant P, Prevot A, Mignot A, Barandon L, Roques X, Roudaut R, Pilois X, et al. Fast track echo of abdominal aortic aneurysm using a real pocket-ultrasound device at bedside. Echocardiography (Mount Kisco, NY). 2012;29:285–90.
23. Grau T, Leipold RW, Conradi R, Martin E, Motsch J. Ultrasound imaging facilitates localization of the epidural space during combined spinal and epidural anesthesia. Reg Anesth Pain Med. 2001;26:64–7.
24. Seligman KM, Weiniger CF, Carvalho B. The accuracy of a handheld ultrasound device for neuraxial depth and landmark assessment: a prospective cohort trial. Anesth Analg. 2018;126(6):1995–8. https://doi.org/10.1213/ANE.0000000000002407.

25. Carvalho B, Seligman KM, Weiniger CF. The comparative accuracy of a handheld and console ultrasound device for neuraxial depth and landmark assessment. Int J Obstet Anesth. 2019;39:68–73. https://doi.org/10.1016/j.ijoa.2019.01.004. Epub 2019 Jan 11
26. Wilson SR, Greenbaum LD, Goldberg BB. Contrast-enhanced ultrasound: what is the evidence and what are the obstacles? AJR Am J Roentgenol. 2009;193(1):55–60. https://doi.org/10.2214/AJR.09.2553.
27. Greis C. Technology overview: SonoVue (Bracco, Milan). Eur Radiol. 2004;14(Suppl 8):P11–5.
28. Sontum PC. Physicochemical characteristics of Sonazoid, a new contrast agent for ultrasound imaging. Ultrasound Med Biol. 2008 May;34(5):824–33.
29. Chung YE, Kim KW. Contrast-enhanced ultrasonography: advance and current status in abdominal imaging. Ultrasonography. 2015;34(1):3–18. https://doi.org/10.14366/usg.14034.
30. Piscaglia F, Bolondi L. Italian Society for ultrasound in medicine and biology (SIUMB) study group on ultrasound contrast agents the safety of Sonovue in abdominal applications: retrospective analysis of 23188 investigations. Ultrasound Med Biol. 2006;32:1369–75.
31. Sidhu PS, Choi BI, Nielsen MB. The EFSUMB guidelines on the nonhepatic clinical applications of contrast enhanced ultrasound (CEUS): a new dawn for the escalating use of this ubiquitous technique. Ultraschall Med. 2012;33:5–7.
32. The European Agency for the Evaluation of Medicinal Products. Public statement on SONOVUE (Sulphur hexafluoride) new contraindication in patients with heart disease: restriction of use to non-cardiac imaging. London: The European Agency for the Evaluation of Medicinal Products; 2014.
33. Seitz K, Strobel D. A milestone: approval of CEUS for diagnostic liver imaging in adults and children in the USA. Ultraschall Med. 2016;37(3):229–32. English. https://doi.org/10.1055/s-0042-107411.
34. Wilson SR, Jang HJ, Kim TK, Burns PN. Diagnosis of focal liver masses on ultrasonography: comparison of unenhanced and contrast-enhanced scans. J Ultrasound Med. 2007;26(6):775–87; quiz 788-90
35. Leen E, Ceccotti P, Kalogeropoulou C, Angerson WJ, Moug SJ, Horgan PG. Prospective multicenter trial evaluating a novel method of characterizing focal liver lesions using contrast-enhanced sonography. AJR Am J Roentgenol. 2006;186(6):1551–9.
36. Ding H, Wang WP, Huang BJ. Imaging of focal liver lesions low-mechanical-index real-time ultrasonography with SonoVue. J Ultrasound Med. 2005;24(3):285–97.
37. Cabassa P, Bipat S, Longaretti L, Morone M, Maroldi R. Liver metastases: Sulphur hexafluoride-enhanced ultrasonography for lesion detection: a systematic review. Ultrasound Med Biol. 2010;36(10):1561–7.
38. Yanagisawa K, Moriyasu F, Miyahara T, Yuki M, Iijima H. Phagocytosis of ultrasound contrast agent microbubbles by Kupffer cells. Ultrasound Med Biol. 2007;33(2):318–25. https://doi.org/10.1016/j.ultrasmedbio.2006.08.008.
39. Sawatzki M, Meyenberger C, Brand S, Semela D. Contrast-enhanced ultrasound (CEUS) has excellent diagnostic accuracy in differentiating focal liver lesions: results from a Swiss tertiary gastroenterological centre. Swiss Med Wkly. 2019;149:w20087. https://doi.org/10.4414/smw.2019.20087.
40. Sidhu PS, Cantisani V, Dietrich CF, et al. The EFSUMB guidelines and recommendations for the clinical practice of contrast-enhanced ultrasound (CEUS) in non-hepatic applications: update 2017 (long version). Ultraschall Medi. 2018;39(02):e2–e44.
41. Catalano O, Aiani L, Barozzi L, Bokor D, et al. CEUS in abdominal trauma: multi-center study. Abdom Imaging. 2009;34(2):225–34.
42. Yusuf GT, Wong A, Rao D, et al. The use of contrast-enhanced ultrasound in COVID-19 lung imaging. J Ultrasound. 2020;25(2):319–23. https://doi.org/10.1007/s40477-020-00517-z.
43. Whitson MR, Mayo PH. Ultrasonography in the emergency department. Crit Care. 2016;20:227. Pmid:27523885
44. Ferreira AC, Mahony E, Oliani AH, Junior AE, da Silva CF. Teleultrasound: historical perspective and clinical application. Int J Telemed Appl. 2015;2015:306259. pmid:25810717
45. Sheehan FH, Ricci MA, Murtagh C, Clark H, Bolson EL. Expert visual guidance of ultrasound for telemedicine. J Telemed Telecare. 2010;16(2):77–82.
46. Law J, Macbeth PB. Ultrasound: from earth to space. McGill J Medi. 2011;13(2):59–65.
47. Pian L, Gillman LM, McBeth PB, et al. Potential use of remote telesonography as a transformational technology in underresourced and/or remote settings. Emerg Med Int. 2013;2013:986160.
48. Law J, Macbeth PB. Ultrasound: from earth to space. Mcgill J Med. 2011;13(2):59.
49. Chiao L, Sharipov S, Sargsyan AE, Melton S, Hamilton DR, McFarlin K, Dulchavsky SA. Ocular examination for trauma; clinical ultrasound aboard the International Space Station. J Trauma. 2005;58(5):885–9.
50. Crawford I, McBeth PB, Mitchelson M, Ferguson J, Tiruta C, Kirkpatrick AW. How to set up a low cost tele-ultrasound capable videoconferencing system with wide applicability. Crit Ultrasound J. 2012;4(1):13.
51. Marsh-Feiley G, Eadie L, Wilson P. Telesonography in emergency medicine: a systematic review. PLoS One. 2018;13(5):e0194840. https://doi.org/10.1371/journal.pone.0194840.

Answer Keys

Chapter 1

Answers: 1C, 2D, 3A, 4C, 5D, 6B, 7C, 8B, 9D, 10B

Chapter 2

Answers: 1E, 2B, 3E, 4E, 5D, 6E, 7E, 8E, 9A, 10D, 11E, 12A, 13B, 14A, 15E, 16B, 17C, 18D, 19C, 20D

Chapter 3

Answers: 1A, 2D, 3B, 4C, 5C, 6A, 7D, 8C, 9D, 10D, 11A, 12C, 13B, 14B, 15A, 16C, 17A, 18A, 19C, 20D

Chapter 4

Answers: 1C, 2A, 3B, 4C, 5C, 6C, 7A, 8C, 9C, 10D, 11C, 12D, 13B, 14A, 15D, 16B, 17A, 18F, 19D, 20A

Chapter 6

Answers: 1C, 2C, 3C, 4D, 5D, 6B, 7D, 8B, 9B, 10C, 11B, 12B, 13D, 14A, 15D, 16E, 17E, 18B, 19E, 20D

Chapter 7

Answers: 1D, 2C, 3A, 4B, 5A, 6C, 7B, 8C, 9D, 10B, 11C, 12B, 13A, 14D, 15B, 16A, 17D, 18D, 19A, 20B

Chapter 8

Answers: 1B. Lateral resolution is determined primarily by the width of the ultrasound beam. The focal zone, or narrowest portion of the ultrasound beam, is where the highest lateral resolution is obtained. Ideally, the target structure(s) should be positioned within the focal zone to maximize resolution.

2C. Linear transducers produce the highest resolution images of superficial structures (<6 cm) as they transmit high-frequency ultrasound waves in a parallel orientation. Linear transducers are used to image any superficial structures, including blood vessels, skin/soft tissues, joints, eyes, testicles, thyroid, lymph nodes, and nerves.

3B. Only the anterior portion of the bladder is visualized. Increasing the depth will allow visualization of the entire bladder, including the posterior wall.

4C. Fluid-filled structures serve as acoustic windows for sound waves to travel into the abdomino-pelvic cavity to generate ultrasound images. The blood-filled liver and spleen serve as acoustic windows in the right and left upper quadrants. Similarly, a urine-filled bladder is an

A. Chakraborty, B. Ashokka (eds.), *A Practical Guide to Point of Care Ultrasound (POCUS)*, https://doi.org/10.1007/978-981-16-7687-1

ideal acoustic window for the visualization of pelvic structures. Gas-filled loops of the bowel scatter sound waves and prevent visualization of deep structures in the abdomen and pelvis. Subcutaneous emphysema and asplenia also limit ultrasound imaging of the abdomino-pelvic cavity.

5B. A small amount of physiologic free fluid may be detected with point-of-care ultrasound in the pelvic cavity of women. However, in women with a positive pregnancy test and abdominal pain, the presence of abdomino-pelvic free fluid is an ectopic pregnancy until proven otherwise.

6D. Acoustic enhancement, or posterior acoustic enhancement, is an artifact that is seen deep in fluid-filled structures. Due to the low acoustic impedance of a fluid-filled body, such as the bladder, a disproportionately high number of echoes return to the transducer from tissues deep into the fluid-filled body, resulting in these tissues appearing hyperechoic, or brighter, than usual.

7D. Power Doppler is particularly well suited for low-flow states, such as ureteral jets. The ureteral jets appear as bright yellow-orange emissions streaming from the base of the bladder towards its center. Power Doppler does not display directional information, like color flow Doppler. None of the other imaging modalities listed is used for the detection of ureteral jets.

8D. Past research has demonstrated a close correlation between the estimated bladder volume using the formula above (bladder volume = 0.75 × width × length × height) compared to the actual catheterized volume (correlation factor = 0.983). It is noteworthy that bladder shape has a considerable impact on the accuracy of US estimation of bladder volume. Though applying the corresponding correction coefficient to volume calculations will improve the accuracy of the estimation, the correction factor 0.75 yields the closest approximation regardless of bladder shape.

9A. The prostate sits deep in the bladder and normally encircles the bladder neck. Normally, the prostate measures less than 5 cm in transverse diameter.

10C. The differential diagnosis for traumatic vision loss includes corneal abrasion, hyphema, traumatic iritis, lens dislocation, foreign body, retinal detachment, vitreous hemorrhage, traumatic optic neuropathy, acute maculopathy, and globe rupture. Ocular ultrasound serves as a useful tool in the setting of trauma to assess pupillary function, extraocular muscle function, lens position, and globe abnormalities, and to evaluate for evidence of increased intracranial pressure. All of the conditions listed above can be diagnosed by ocular ultrasound, except corneal abrasion.

11C. The subarachnoid space in the optic nerve sheath does not dilate uniformly. The most pronounced response to increased fluid in the subarachnoid space due to increased intracranial pressure occurs 3 mm posterior to the optic nerve—retina junction. The optic nerve sheath diameter should be measured in transverse and sagittal planes and compared to measurements obtained on the contralateral side. An optic nerve sheath diameter greater than 5 mm is considered abnormal in patients with clinical concern for elevated intracranial pressure.

12D. It is true that transducers that have only been in contact with intact skin can be cleaned with a nonabrasive soap or with low- or intermediate-level disinfectant wipes. Statements A through C are false. Use of disposable sterile transducer covers followed by cleaning with a nonabrasive soap and high-level disinfection is recommended for endocavitary transducers that have been in contact with mucous membranes. Transducers exposed to patients with Clostridium difficile infection should be cleaned with a hypochlorite-based or hydrogen peroxide-based solution to kill the bacterial spores. Ultrasound transducers should never be autoclaved or subjected to high heat, electricity, or pressure because the piezoelectric elements can be damaged.

13D. The transducer is placed in the parasagittal plane of the epigastric region to obtain general qualitative observations of the gastric antrum and body, the stomach cavity, and the stomach contents. It is scanned curving from right to left. The antrum is generally seen in the parasagittal plane immediately to the right of the midline. Reference points to be considered are the left anterior lobe or caudal lobe of the liver, the pancreas head, and the superior mesenteric vessels with the vena cava inferior or abdominal aorta.

Chapter 9

Answers: 1B, 2C, 3D, 4B, 5A, 6D, 7C, 8A, 9B, 10A, 11B, 12D, 13C, 14C, 15A, 16B, 17B, 18A, 19D, 20C